Praise for *Mastering Simulation, Second E...*

"Mastering Simulation *by Janice Palaganas, Beth Ulrich, and Beth Mancini, is a veritable treasure trove of useful ideas, practical insights, and underpinning conceptual frameworks that will help discerning simulation educators improve their practice, programs, and performance. Drawn from a who's who of US clinical simulation experts, the second edition's content is comprehensive, inclusive, and clearly presented. A welcome and definitive contribution to the scholarly practice of simulation in healthcare."*

–Ian Curran, BSc, MBBS (London), AKC, FRCA (UK), Pg Dip Med Ed (Distinction), FFPMRCA (UK), FAcadMEd (UK), FSSH (USA), FRCP Edinburgh, FAOrthoA (Australia), FRCP (London), FAMS (Singapore)
Vice Dean of Education, Duke–NUS Medical School
Co-Director, SingHealth, Duke–NUS, Academic Medical Education Institute

"An inspired vision of how we holistically transform our profession across the continuum of health to imagine how we fully embrace a world of technology, virtual presence, digital health, avatars, and adaptive learning—reshaping the economy, our lives, and our humanity. A brilliant work of art and science that creates a compelling case for a leap of faith into a new reality."

–Cole Edmonson, DNP, RN, NEA-BC, FACHE, FAONL, FNAP, FAAN
Chief Experience and Clinical Officer, AMN Healthcare

"These renowned editors have thought of everything! From novice to expert simulationists, there is something for everyone. This book takes the reader through the various stages of simulation design and application, with considerations for both academic and clinical environments. The chapters on research, operations, and career building round out an already exceptional book. If you are involved in simulation, you must have this book on your shelf."

–Nicole Harder, PhD, RN, CHSE, CCSNE
Assistant Professor, College of Nursing
Mindermar Professor in Human Simulation, Rady Faculty of Health Sciences
Winnipeg, Manitoba, Canada
Editor-in-Chief, *Clinical Simulation in Nursing*

"I have watched the evolution of simulation since my initial exposure as a CPR instructor in the 1980s. The science of simulation has advanced significantly since that time, as demonstrated by the content of this invaluable text. Whether you are new to simulation or an expert, you will find this text to be a must-have resource."

–Kenneth W. Dion, PhD, MSN, MBA, RN, FAAN
Assistant Dean for Business Innovation
Johns Hopkins School of Nursing

Mastering Simulation

Second Edition

A Handbook for Success

Janice C. Palaganas, PhD, RN, NP, ANEF, FAAN, FSSH

Beth Tamplet Ulrich, EdD, RN, FACHE, FAONL, FAAN

Mary E. (Beth) Mancini, PhD, RN, NE-BC, FAHA, FSSH, ANEF, FAAN

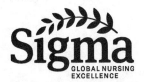

Sigma
GLOBAL NURSING
EXCELLENCE

Sigma Theta Tau International Honor Society of Nursing (Sigma) is a nonprofit organization whose mission is developing nurse leaders anywhere to improve healthcare everywhere. Founded in 1922, Sigma has more than 135,000 active members in over 100 countries and territories. Members include practicing nurses, instructors, researchers, policymakers, entrepreneurs, and others. Sigma's more than 540 chapters are located at more than 700 institutions of higher education throughout Armenia, Australia, Botswana, Brazil, Canada, Colombia, England, Eswatini, Ghana, Hong Kong, Ireland, Israel, Jamaica, Japan, Jordan, Kenya, Lebanon, Malawi, Mexico, the Netherlands, Nigeria, Pakistan, Philippines, Portugal, Puerto Rico, Scotland, Singapore, South Africa, South Korea, Sweden, Taiwan, Tanzania, Thailand, the United States, and Wales. Learn more at www.sigmanursing.org.

Sigma Theta Tau International
550 West North Street
Indianapolis, IN, USA 46202

To order additional books, buy in bulk, or order for corporate use, contact Sigma Marketplace at 888.654.4968 (US and Canada) or +1.317.634.8171 (outside US and Canada).

To request a review copy for course adoption, email solutions@sigmamarketplace.org or call 888.654.4968 (US and Canada) or +1.317.634.8171 (outside US and Canada).

To request author information, or for speaker or other media requests, contact Sigma Marketing at 888.634.7575 (US and Canada) or +1.317.634.8171 (outside US and Canada).

ISBN:	9781948057332
EPUB ISBN:	9781948057349
PDF ISBN:	9781948057356
MOBI ISBN:	9781948057363

Library of Congress Cataloging-in-Publication Data

LCCN: 2020023406

First Printing, 2020

Publisher: Dustin Sullivan
Acquisitions Editor: Emily Hatch
Development Editor: Kate Shoup
Cover Designer: Michael Tanamachi
Interior Design/Page Layout: Rebecca Batchelor
Indexer: Joy Dean Lee

Managing Editor: Carla Hall
Publications Specialist: Todd Lothery
Project Editor: Todd Lothery
Copy Editors: Erin Geile, Todd Lothery
Proofreaders: Jane Palmer, Gill Editorial Services

Ancillary Materials, Free Downloads, and Additional Book Materials

Find more information about ancillary materials, free downloads, and any additional book-related materials, go to https://www.sigmanursing.org/MasteringSimulation2.

You can also access these additional materials through the QR codes placed alongside the web link or URL. A QR Code is a two-dimensional barcode that contains information about an item. It can be scanned on a smartphone with a camera, sometimes requiring a mobile app.

Dedications

To my students, who teach me how to take theory to practice, challenge me to think outside the box, teach me how to be a better educator, and make me a better person through our learning together.

To our readers, I hope that you'll take what you need from this book and apply it in ways that move patient safety forward.

To my daughter Jianna, my son Jayden, and my brother Gerr, who challenge and inspire my thinking and being every day.

–Janice C. Palaganas, PhD, RN, NP, ANEF, FAAN, FSSH

To my colleagues who see no boundaries to the contributions that the nursing profession can make, who lead us into bold new worlds, and who day after day serve as vocal patient advocates—and, when necessary, as the last line of defense to ensure that patients receive safe, high-quality care.

To my daughter Blythe, who inspires me in so many ways; my grandson Henry, through whose eyes I see new wonder in the world every day; and my husband Walter, who supports even my craziest ideas and projects.

–Beth Tamplet Ulrich, EdD, RN, FACHE, FAONL, FAAN

To David, Laura, Jake, Carla, and Michael: love you forever; love you for always.

–Mary E. (Beth) Mancini, PhD, RN, NE-BC, FAHA, FSSH, ANEF, FAAN

Acknowledgments

It takes a lot of people with many different sets of knowledge and skills to create a book such as this one. Thanks first and foremost to our wonderful contributors. They are experts and leaders in the use of simulation in healthcare education and practice, and we very much appreciate their willingness to share their knowledge and expertise. Thanks to Carla Hall, Managing Editor extraordinaire, and the fantastic Sigma staff, who inspire, plan, nag (when needed), organize, encourage, create, facilitate, and so much more—all to turn an idea into a book that benefits nurses and ultimately their patients.

About the Authors

Janice C. Palaganas, PhD, RN, NP, ANEF, FAAN, FSSH

Janice C. Palaganas is the Director of Educational Innovation and Development for the Center for Medical Simulation in Boston, Massachusetts, Department of Anesthesia and Critical Pain Management, Harvard Medical School. She is also Associate Professor in Interprofessional Studies and Associate Director of the PhD Health Profession Programs at the Massachusetts General Hospital (MGH) Institute of Health Professions. Palaganas received her bachelor of science in nursing and two master's degrees—adult nurse practitioner and geriatric nurse practitioner—from the University of Pennsylvania. She earned her PhD in nursing from Loma Linda University, where she explored healthcare simulation as a platform for interprofessional education.

Palaganas has developed a passion for teamwork from her background as an emergency nurse, trauma nurse practitioner, director of emergency and critical care services, and faculty for schools of medicine, nursing, allied health, management, a physician assistant program, and emergency medicine. As a behavioral scientist and former clinical nurse and hospital administrator, Palaganas focuses on using healthcare simulation as a platform for interprofessional education (IPE). She has served as a committee member for the publication of the National Academy of Medicine (formerly the Institute of Medicine) report on measuring the impact of IPE on practice. Palaganas's primary role is to develop health profession educators in an IPE setting. She previously led the Center for Medical Simulation instructor course, which teaches simulation to educators all over the world. She developed the Center for Medical Simulation Interprofessional Virtual Campus as the principal investigator of a board grant awarded by the Josiah Macy Jr. Foundation. She is currently the chair of the Credentialing Commission for the Society for Simulation in Healthcare (SSH), overseeing the Accreditation, Certification, and Fellows Academy.

Palaganas has shaped the field of simulation, leading the development of the SSH's accreditation and certification programs; served as Editor-in-Chief for the SSH's first textbook, *Defining Excellence in Simulation Programs*; authored seminal articles; and coauthored field-changing research, including the National League for Nursing (NLN) study for high-stakes assessment using simulation. As the Associate Director of PhD Programs for Health Professions Education at MGH Institute of Health Professions, she has led the development and the launch of the first PhD Program in Simulation and in IPE. She has been invited as a keynote speaker for numerous national and international conferences.

Beth Tamplet Ulrich, EdD, RN, FACHE, FAONL, FAAN

Beth Tamplet Ulrich is a nationally recognized thought leader known for her research in nursing work environments and the experiences of new graduate nurses as they transition from nursing school into the workforce. Ulrich is also recognized for her leadership in developing the roles of nephrology nurses and improving the care of nephrology patients. Ulrich has extensive experience as a healthcare executive, educator, and researcher. She currently serves as Professor at the Cizik School of Nursing at the University of Texas Health Science Center in Houston, where she teaches in the doctoral program, and as Editor-in-Chief of the *Nephrology Nursing Journal*, the official journal of the American Nephrology Nurses' Association (ANNA). Ulrich previously served as the Vice President of Hospital Services for CAE Healthcare; has extensive senior executive experience in CNO, COO, and Senior Vice President positions in both hospitals and large healthcare systems; and has held graduate and undergraduate faculty positions. She has been a co-investigator on a series of national nursing workforce and work environment studies and on four studies of critical care nurse work environments conducted for the American Association of Critical-Care Nurses, and the primary investigator on two ANNA national studies on nephrology patient and nurse safety.

Ulrich received her bachelor's degree from the Medical University of South Carolina, her master's degree from the University of Texas Health Science Center at Houston, and her doctorate from the University of Houston in a collaborative program with Baylor College of Medicine. She is a Past President of the American Nephrology Nurses' Association, a Fellow in the American College of Healthcare Executives, a Fellow in the American Organization for Nursing Leadership, and a Fellow in the American Academy of Nursing. She was recognized as the Outstanding Nursing Alumnus of the Medical University of South Carolina in 1989 and as a distinguished alumnus of the University of Texas Health Science Center at Houston School of Nursing in 2002, and she received the Outstanding Contribution to the American Nephrology Nurses' Association award in 2008. In 2018, she received the Marguerite Rodgers Kinney Award for a Distinguished Career from the American Association of Critical-Care Nurses. She has numerous publications and presentations to her credit on topics including nephrology nursing, nurses' work environments, and how new graduate nurses transition into professional nurses. Both the first and the second editions of her landmark book *Mastering Precepting* received *American Journal of Nursing* Book of the Year Award recognitions in two different categories. In 2014, Ulrich and Beth Mancini collaborated to publish the first edition of *Mastering Simulation: A Handbook for Success*, which was also honored with an *AJN* Book of the Year award.

Mary Elizabeth (Beth) Mancini, PhD, RN, NE-BC, FAHA, FSSH, ANEF, FAAN

Mary (Beth) Mancini is Professor and Senior Associate Dean for Education Innovation at The University of Texas at Arlington College of Nursing and Health Innovation, where she holds the Baylor Professorship for Healthcare Research. Before moving to an academic role in 2004, Mancini was Senior Vice President for Nursing Administration and Chief Nursing Officer at Parkland Health & Hospital System in Dallas, Texas, a position she held for 18 years.

Mancini received an ADN from Rhode Island Junior College, a BSN from Rhode Island College, a master's in nursing administration from the University of Rhode Island, and a PhD in public and urban affairs from The University of Texas at Arlington. She completed a Johnson & Johnson Wharton Nurse Executive Fellowship at the Wharton School of Business of the University of Pennsylvania and a National Association of Public Hospitals Management Fellowship program through the Robert F. Wagner Graduate School of Public Service at New York University.

Mancini is internationally recognized for her groundbreaking work in simulation and in high-quality, high-volume, accelerated online education. Her work in this area resulted in UTA's College of Nursing becoming the country's largest college of nursing in a public university and led to the College of Nursing receiving the Texas Higher Education Coordinating Board's prestigious Star Award in 2012. In recognition for her many contributions to the fields, Mancini was inducted as a Fellow in the American Academy of Nursing, the National League for Nursing's Academy of Nurse Educators, the American Heart Association, and the Society for Simulation in Healthcare. In 2013, she was recognized with a Regent's Outstanding Teaching Award from the University of Texas system and was appointed a visiting scholar in innovation and simulation at the University of Pennsylvania School of Nursing. In 2014, she was reappointed as a visiting scholar in simulation and curriculum.

Mancini is an active volunteer with numerous professional organizations. She currently serves as a member of the National Academies of Science Global Task Force on Innovations in Health Professions Education and a member of the American Heart Association's Educational Science and Program committee, as well as its Get With The Guidelines–Resuscitation work group. She is also co-chair of the Basic Life Support Task Force for the International Liaison Committee on Resuscitation. She has served as President of the Society for Simulation in Healthcare and is a member of the Royal College of Physicians and Surgeons of Canada's Simulation Task Force and the World Health Organization's Initiative on Training, Simulation, and Patient Safety.

Mancini's research interests include innovations in education, interprofessional collaborative practice, and the development of high-performing healthcare teams through the use of simulation. She has received more than $6.5 million in competitive grants, has more than 100 publications to her credit, and is a sought-after speaker at local, national, and international conferences on topics such as simulation in health professions education; innovations in online education; development of high-volume, high-quality educational programs; patient safety; outcomes related to basic and advanced life support education; and work redesign.

Contributing Authors

Pamela Andreatta, EdD, PhD, MFA, MA, FSSH, is a Professor of Surgical Education at the Uniformed Services University. She is a passionate educator and researcher and an expert human-performance specialist dedicated to supporting the acquisition and implementation of abilities in critical and complex health services environments. She is a proficient analyst specializing in outcomes-based research and evidence-based evaluation leading to high-impact quality of care and safety initiatives in medicine, surgery, nursing, and the health professions. Andreatta has deep expertise in assessment, evaluation, theoretical and empirical systems of practice, professional development, and instructional design that incorporates optimal technologies and simulation-supported methods for achieving performance mastery in all disciplines. She is an experienced and globally recognized leader in medical, surgical, nursing, and health profession education, including administrative and executive leadership roles.

Eric B. Bauman, PhD, RN, FSSH, an award-winning educational designer and author, is a proven innovation leader who promotes the integration and evaluation of emerging technology for health professions education. He is founder and managing member of Clinical Playground LLC, a consulting service focusing on the nexus of academic and industry collaboration with demonstrated success and extensive experience leveraging simulation, mobile technology, game-based learning, and virtual environments to support paradigm shifts in the educational processes. Bauman received his PhD from University of Wisconsin–Madison School of Education, where he studied with renowned scholars at the forefront of the game-based learning movement. Bauman is a sought-after collaborator and speaker. He has authored and coauthored numerous academic articles, books, and chapters on simulation and game-based teaching and learning. Bauman is a Society for Simulation in Healthcare Fellow (FSSN) and a member of Sigma Theta Tau International Honor Society of Nursing (Sigma) and of the International Nursing Association for Clinical Simulation and Nursing.

Deborah Becker, PhD, RN, ACNP, BC, CHSE, FAAN, is a Practice Professor of Nursing at the University of Pennsylvania. Becker served as Director of the Helene Fuld Pavilion for Innovative Learning and Simulation from 2013 to 2018. There, she oversaw the integration of simulation into both undergraduate and graduate curricula in collaboration with course and program faculty. Becker has taught simulation for more than 25 years in hospital and academic settings and consults nationally and internationally on the meaningful use of simulation for teaching and evaluation. Recently she has focused on developing interprofessional education and collaborative programs using simulated scenarios as the vehicle to test approaches to tackling global problems.

Stephanie D. Boyd, PhD, is a Research Associate in the Division of Emergency Medicine and the Center for Simulation and Research at Cincinnati Children's Hospital, where she has worked for the past three years. Since arriving at Cincinnati Children's, her primary focus has been on the development of effective outcomes measures in simulation education. Previously, she was a Research Associate at the Center for Evaluation and Program Improvement at Vanderbilt University, where she contributed to the development and evaluation of communication trainings using standardized patients in novel scenarios.

Teresa Britt, MSN, RN, CHSE, is the Director of Education at the Center for Healthcare Improvement and Patient Simulation (CHIPS) at the University of Tennessee Health Science Center. In her current role, she serves as a simulation mentor to faculty from six different colleges and assists community clinical partners with their simulation courses. She was one of the founding board members for the Tennessee Simulation Alliance and is currently President of that organization. In 2016, Britt was selected by the National League for Nursing as a Simulation Leader and continues to work on projects with this group. She served as team leader at the Interprofessional Education Collaborative Institute and is one of the founding members of the Mid-South Interprofessional Health Education Collaborative. She serves actively on committees for the International Nursing Association for Clinical Simulation and Learning, the Association of Standardized Patient Educators, and the Society for Simulation in Healthcare. Britt's interests are in faculty development, patient safety, and simulation for replacement of traditional clinical training.

Sandra Caballero, MSN, RN, CHSE, is the Director of Simulation at the F. Marie Hall SimLife Center at the Texas Tech University Health Sciences Center (TTUHSC), Assistant Professor at the TTUHSC School of Nursing, and a site coordinator for the TTUHSC School of Nursing's accelerated program. Caballero has obtained her certification in simulation education and contributes in online as well as on-site modules relating to all aspects of simulation pedagogy. She also serves as a debriefing coach for the National League for Nursing. Caballero has presented at local, state, and international conferences. She is a sim leader alumni of the National League for Nursing. Caballero received both her bachelor's and master's degrees from the TTUHSC School of Nursing.

Carol Noe Cheney, MS, CCC-SLP, began her career in 1995 as an acute medical speech-language pathologist for Banner Health, a large nonprofit healthcare system. In 2005, she assumed the position of Operations Director of the Simulation Education and Training Center (SimET) at Banner Good Samaritan Medical Center in Phoenix, Arizona, while it was still in the conceptual and development stage. Cheney led the planning, design, and development of a 55,000-square-foot simulation medical center at Banner Mesa. In 2011, Cheney became the Senior Director of Clinical Education and Simulation for Banner Health, responsible for simulation education and nursing, physician, and multidisciplinary clinical education, including electronic medical record training. Cheney is now the Vice President of staffing and staff recruiting for Banner Health.

Jane Crofut, RN, MAOM, is a Healthcare Planning and Medical Education Specialist at GSBS Consulting. With more than 25 years of experience in healthcare and medical education, Crofut is a respected developer and leader of simulation lab designs that support rapidly evolving, experiential learning pedagogies. Crofut's expertise in business analytics, curriculum delivery requirements, and quality patient care give her a unique perspective that enables her to combine operational optimization with future-forward, flexible space design. It's a perspective gained through a varied career that began as a trauma flight nurse and spans advocacy for patient safety and outcomes, roles in academia and healthcare administration, and architectural planning. In the past 15 years, Crofut has helped more than 40 institutions implement innovative health and educational programs with visioning, business planning, funding, space design, specialty equipment selection, curriculum development, program implementation, and faculty education.

Sharon I. Decker, PhD, RN, FSSH, ANEF, FAAN, is the Associate Dean for Simulation at Texas Tech University Health Sciences Center (TTUHSC), Professor at the TTUHSC School of Nursing, Executive Director for the TTUHSC simulation program, a TTUHSC Grover E. Murray Professor, and the Covenant Health System Endowed Chair in Simulation and Nursing Education. Decker has been the recipient of the Texas Tech Chancellor's Council Distinguished Teaching Award and several TTUHSC President's Awards for Academic Achievement. She is a Fellow in the Academy of Nursing Education and American Academy of Nursing and an inaugural member of the Society for Simulation in Healthcare Academy. Decker's scholarship relates to using the pedagogy of simulation to promote clinical reasoning and reflective thinking. She has presented at conferences and provided consultation on a national and international basis, and she has received numerous grants to support her research. Decker received her bachelor's degree from Baylor University, her master's degree from the University of Texas at Arlington, and her doctorate from Texas Woman's University.

Chad A. Epps, MD, FSSH, is the Executive Director of the Center for Healthcare Improvement and Patient Simulation (CHIPS). CHIPS is a 45,000-square-foot, stand-alone simulation building at the University of Tennessee Health Science Center, where he is also a Professor in the departments of anesthesiology and interprofessional education. Epps trained in anesthesiology and completed a fellowship in healthcare simulation at the Mount Sinai Medical Center in New York City. As a fellow, faculty, and director of simulation, he has been active in simulation education, research, assessment, and center management for the past 15 years. He is a Past President of the Society for Simulation in Healthcare and a past chair of the Council on Accreditation of Healthcare Simulation Programs. Epps has published in the areas of simulation-enhanced interprofessional education and co-edited the textbook *Defining Excellence in Simulation Programs*.

Crystel L. Farina, MSN, RN, CNE, CHSE, is the Director of Simulation and Experiential Learning at the George Washington University School of Nursing (GWSON), where she leads simulation experiences for graduate and undergraduate nursing students. Farina studies and creates new simulation and debriefing models that serve as substitutes for traditional clinical experiences to better prepare nurses for today's increasingly complex healthcare environment. Before joining GWSON, Farina was the Director of Simulation for Health Professions at Chesapeake College in Wye Mills, Maryland. There, she launched the Chesapeake Institute for Medical Simulation (CIMS) in the Health Professions and Athletic Center. The CIMS provides simulation-learning activities for nursing, EMS, surgical technology, and radiologic technology professionals. She leveraged CIMS to increase revenue by developing professional development programs with Compass Regional Hospice, hosting the Mid-Atlantic Regional Human Patient Simulator Network with CAE Healthcare, and collaborating with the Maryland Film Office to film *Investigative Discoveries*. Farina has presented at international and regional meetings on debriefing, failure to rescue, and core concepts in simulation. Farina serves on the faculty of the Maryland Clinical Simulation Resource Consortium (MCSRC) and is a member of the MCSRC Steering Committee. She is also the Chief Financial Officer of SIMPL Simulation LLC.

Gary Geis, MD, is a Professor in the Department of Pediatrics at the University of Cincinnati College of Medicine, Division of Emergency Medicine, Cincinnati Children's Hospital Medical Center. He is the Medical Director of the Center for Simulation and Research at Cincinnati Children's Hospital Medical

Center. He has led the development of an internationally recognized simulation center and is a leader in the area of in situ simulation for systems integration.

Teresa N. Gore, PhD, DNP, FNP-BC, NP-C, CHSE-A, FAAN, is an Associate Professor and Assistant Dean of Experiential Learning and Simulation at the University of South Florida College of Nursing in Tampa, Florida. She is a Past President of the International Nursing Association for Clinical Simulation and Learning (INACSL). Major themes of Gore's work are the dissemination of the INACSL "Standards of Best Practice: Simulation" and how to operationalize the standards. These have been demonstrated by her involvement in the establishment of the INACSL and its development of the first standards of best practice, which were incorporated into the National Council of State Boards of Nursing (NCSBN) National Simulation Study. Gore has combined her expertise in clinical skills and simulation to advance the science of nursing by authoring multiple book chapters and journal articles. She is one of 35 Certified Healthcare Simulation Educators-Advanced (CHSE-A) worldwide. A recognized simulation expert, she has been invited to speak throughout North America, Europe, and China. Her unique knowledge base has enabled her to teach educators how to operationalize high-fidelity simulation templates using INACSL standards for baccalaureate and advanced practice nursing students.

Katie Anne Haerling, PhD, RN, is an Associate Professor at the University of Washington Tacoma in the Nursing and Healthcare Leadership Program. She earned her PhD in nursing from Washington State University in Spokane, Washington. Her current research includes the use of simulation to examine the effects of incivility on emotional status, team behavior, and performance, and a cost-utility analysis comparing virtual and mannequin-based simulation activities. Haerling's mission is to help identify the most effective and efficient ways to prepare the next generation of healthcare professionals and to contribute to the evidence base supporting better healthcare education. She believes improving healthcare providers' education will support improved healthcare and a healthier nation and world. Her clinical expertise includes maternal-child and medical-surgical nursing.

Valerie M. Howard, EdD, MSN, RN, CNE, FAAN, is the Associate Dean for Academic Affairs at Duke University School of Nursing. She has more than 21 years of experience in higher education, with the past 14 years dedicated to researching, developing, implementing, and evaluating innovative teaching methods as well as leadership and team-building experiences across the curriculum. Before joining the faculty at Duke, Howard served as Dean of the School of Nursing and Health Sciences and Assistant Dean for External Affairs at Robert Morris University (RMU). Howard created the Society for Simulation in Healthcare-accredited RMU Regional Research and Innovation in Simulation Education (RISE) Center and served as its founding director. She was President of the International Nursing Association of Clinical Simulation and Learning (INACSL) from 2011 to 2013 and received the INACSL Excellence Award in Research in 2010. Howard worked with a team to develop the inaugural Elsevier Simulation Learning System, a curricular support system to assist with the implementation of simulation experiences that is now used at more than 400 schools of nursing. She also developed the STRIVE Model to guide educators in designing and planning simulation programs at their institutions. She created the RMU Leadership in Simulation Instruction and Management Certificate Program to prepare faculty to implement simulation in their curricula. Howard earned her EdD in higher education administration and MSN (nursing education) from the University of Pittsburgh and her BSN from Indiana University of Pennsylvania.

Pamela R. Jeffries, PhD, RN, FAAN, ANEF, FSSH, Professor and Dean of George Washington University School of Nursing, is internationally known for her research and work in nursing education and simulation. Throughout the academic community, she is well-regarded for her scholarly contributions to the development of innovative teaching strategies, experiential learning techniques, new pedagogies, and the delivery of content using technology. Jeffries's accomplishments have been recognized through prestigious teaching and research awards and honors from a number of national and international organizations, including NLN, AACN, Sigma Theta Tau International, and the INACSL.

Karen Josey, MEd, BSN, RN, CHSE, is the Simulation Senior Director for Banner Health. She has more than 41 years in nursing, with a background in leadership, simulation, ICU, medical imaging, and training center operations. Josey has worked in simulation since 2007, when Banner opened its first simulation center. Her scope includes leadership and operations of four simulation centers that cover six states. Josey has been integral in standardizing simulation throughout the Banner system as well as achieving accreditations through the American College of Surgeons and the Society for Simulation in Healthcare in all five standards. Josey is passionate about delivering realistic innovative products, from complex critical care mega-simulations for 500-plus learners, to in-situ simulations, to collaborating in the development of OB and trauma 360 virtual reality simulation videos for just-in-time education anywhere. She has been a Certified Healthcare Simulation Educator (CHSE) since 2012 and participated in the initial CHSE pilot. Josey has numerous publications, including work on in-situ mock codes at a system level that produced positive patient outcomes.

Benjamin T. Kerrey, MD, MS, is an Associate Professor in the emergency medicine division at Cincinnati Children's Hospital. He became a faculty member there 10 years ago, after completing his pediatric residency and pediatric emergency medicine fellowship. Kerrey is the Research Director for the Center for Simulation and Research and co-leads the Medical Resuscitation Committee, overseeing peer review, quality assurance, and research activities for the shock trauma suite in the hospital's pediatric emergency department. His major academic focus is improving critical care delivery in high-acuity, low-frequency environments, with a focus on systems integration, in-situ simulation, and video-based data collection.

Steve Kopp, AIA, ACHA, is an Associate Vice President and Senior Designer at CannonDesign, an innovative architecture-engineering firm that specializes in healthcare, education, and research. As an interior architect with 20 years of experience in healthcare and medical education, Kopp believes that evidence-based design can be integrated with beautiful interior architecture to create functional and cost-effective solutions for institutional clients. He has completed large healthcare building projects for Kaiser Permanente and Texas Children's Hospital, as well as medical simulation projects for Houston Methodist and the Cizik School of Nursing at UTHealth. Kopp is a registered architect in California and Texas.

Thomas E. LeMaster, MSN, MEd, RN, CHSE, FSSH, is responsible for the operation of the simulation program at the University of Florida Center for Experiential Learning and Simulations. This includes the development, implementation, and evaluation of simulation educational program policies and procedures. He is also responsible for administrative tasks related to the simulation program. He assists teams to determine gaps in skills, care delivery, and critical thinking. With the assistance of content experts, LeMaster conducts formative evaluations, assesses clinical competencies, and coordinates and directs in-situ simulations in the hospital setting, including multidisciplinary team training. Previously, LeMaster served as Manager of Simulation at St. Jude Children's Research Hospital, National Manager of SIMCARE Operations at Chamberlain College of Nursing, and Director of Operations for the Cincinnati Children's Hospital simulation program. This work included operations manual development, facilitation of education, and scenario development. In addition, LeMaster developed, implemented, and directed healthcare simulation education, and focused on teamwork, communication, and patient safety. He has participated and played a key role in operationalizing research activities including several federal AHRQ grants. LeMaster is a registered nurse with experience in pediatric and adult care.

Joseph O. Lopreiato, MD, MPH, CHSE-A, was commissioned as an ensign in the United States Navy Medical Corps in 1977 and received his MD degree from Georgetown University in 1981 under the Health Professions Scholarship Program. He completed his pediatric internship and residency at the National Naval Medical Center in Bethesda, Maryland, in 1984. He was then assigned as staff pediatrician and general medical officer at several locations before being assigned to the Uniformed Services University (USU) of the Health Sciences in Bethesda, Maryland. There, he became an Assistant Professor of pediatrics and clerkship coordinator. He completed a fellowship in faculty development at Michigan State University. He then completed a two-year fellowship in academic general pediatrics and earned a master's of public health at the University of Texas. In 1999, Lopreiato was named Program Director of the National Capital Consortium pediatric residency program. In 2003, he became the medical director of the Val G. Hemming Simulation Center at USU—a 30,000-square-foot facility that uses standardized patients, human patient simulators, task trainers, and virtual reality simulations to train 170 medical students, 45 advanced practice nurses, and several residency and fellowship programs in the Washington, DC, area. In 2009, he completed a 31-year career in the United States Navy Medical Corps and became a civilian employee of the Department of Defense, directing programs at the simulation center. He is currently the Associate Dean for Simulation Education and Professor of Pediatrics, Medicine and Nursing at USU.

Jody R. Lori, PhD, CNM, FACNM, FAAN, is Professor and Associate Dean for Global Affairs at the University of Michigan School of Nursing, where she also serves as Director of the PAHO/WHO Collaborating Center for Nursing and Midwifery. A Fellow in the American College of Nurse Midwives and the American Academy of Nursing, Lori's work uses community-based participatory research to develop and test new models of care to address the high rates of maternal and newborn mortality in sub-Saharan Africa. Her research has examined the impact of maternity waiting homes as a system-based intervention to increase access to quality intrapartum and postpartum care for women and newborns in Liberia and Zambia living far from a health facility. Lori conducted the first trial of group antenatal care in sub-Saharan Africa and is currently conducting a cluster randomized controlled trial in Ghana to test the efficacy of group antenatal care.

Jennifer L. Manos, MBA, MSN, RN, is the Executive Director for the Society for Simulation in Healthcare (SSH). Prior to her employment with SSH, she was a critical care nurse and simulation education specialist at Cincinnati Children's Hospital Medical Center (CCHMC). She received her bachelor of science in nursing, master of science in nursing, and master of business administration degrees from Indiana Wesleyan University. Manos has been involved in nonprofit management for 10 years. She has directly managed the development and implementation of the SSH accreditation program, the International Meeting on Simulation in Healthcare, the Asia Pacific Meeting on Simulation in Healthcare, the Regional SimOps conference, SSH general operations, and financial oversight for the organization. Manos was a pediatric critical care and trauma resuscitation nurse for 10 years and an education specialist with the Center for Simulation and Research at CCHMC for seven years. She developed and implemented various programs at CCHMC, including the Pediatric Emergency Management Simulation course, the Cardiac Intensive Care and Pediatric Intensive Care Serious Safety Event Reduction courses, an institution-wide simulation mock code program, and simulation curriculum for testing new spaces and healthcare teams.

David Marzano, MD, has a strong background in the field of medical education. He serves as an educator for medical students at all levels of learning and for residents as the OBGYN Residency Program Director at Michigan Medicine. His area of research interest includes the use of simulation for educational purposes and the development of interprofessional team training to improve patient safety. As a member of the American College of Obstetrics and Gynecology Simulation Working Group, he has been active in developing simulated-based curricula for the care of pregnant patients. He has also developed curricula addressing multidisciplinary care of pregnant patients as well as training modules for gynecologic surgical procedures.

Juli C. Maxworthy, DNP, MSN, MBA, RN, CNL, CPHQ, CPPS, CHSE, FNAP, FSSH, has been a nurse for more than 30 years. She began her career working in an open heart and trauma unit. After her last clinical position as VP of Quality and Risk at a district hospital, she moved into academia full time and is currently a tenured Associate Professor at the University of San Francisco (USF). Her roles at USF have included teaching in the doctor of nursing practice (DNP)/executive leadership DNP program and the healthcare simulation program, working as Director of the Healthcare Simulation Program, and serving as chair of the Healthcare Leadership and Innovations Department. For more than a decade, Maxworthy has been involved in healthcare simulation. She served as the Secretary on the International Board of Directors for the Society for Simulation in Healthcare (SSH) from 2017 to 2019 and is currently a Director at Large. She has led the revision of accreditation standards; is an accreditation program reviewer; is an Editor of the leading healthcare simulation textbook, *Defining Excellence in Simulation Programs*; and has written multiple articles, chapters, and textbooks on a variety of subjects. In 2017, she was inducted into the inaugural class of the SSH Fellows Academy. Maxworthy also served as Vice President on the International Board of Directors of Sigma Theta Tau International. In 2008, she founded a successful consulting firm called WithMax Consulting Inc. to provide healthcare consulting and medical writing services for the clinical development of experimental drugs.

Chris McClanahan, DNP, RN, CHSE, is the Director of Simulation and Interprofessional Education at St. David's School of Nursing, Texas State University. McClanahan is a highly motivated, focused, outcomes-oriented educator with experience operating and managing multiple interprofessional simulation centers within large universities in Central and West Texas. A dynamic and aggressive path has led McClanahan to progressive leadership development, equitable systems management, and successful educator and management roles. McClanahan received his BSN and MSN from Lubbock Christian University in 2009 and 2010, respectively, and his DNP from Texas Tech University in 2014. McClanahan's doctoral research took a deep dive into the operational and management practices of clinical simulation centers in the US. He received his Certified Healthcare Simulation Educator (CHSE) certification in 2017. McClanahan holds membership in numerous professional organizations, has served as a reviewer for the Society for Simulation in Healthcare's annual conference poster and podium presentations, and has served as chair of the Directors of SIM Centers SIG.

Gerald R. Moses, PhD, FSSH, is the Director of Medical Simulation Training at the Anne Arundel Medical Center. He has more than 20 years of pioneering experience in advanced telesurgical and simulation training. He has demonstrated expertise in developing, directing, and leading simulation training of healthcare providers in academic medical centers and government facilities. Moses is a proven developer of medical simulation training and certification, helping to establish the technology as a viable education tool at more than 400 centers. He is skilled at coordinating and directing medical simulation training for medical residents, students, and healthcare providers in academic, medical, and research environments.

Mary D. Patterson, MD, MEd, FSSH, is a pediatric emergency medicine physician. She is the Associate Dean of Experiential Learning and the Lou Oberndorf Professor of Healthcare Technology at the University of Florida, where she directs the Center for Experiential Learning and Simulation. Previously, she served as Associate Vice Chair of Medical Education and Executive Director of Simulation at the Children's National Medical Center and as Medical Director of the Cincinnati Children's Center for Simulation and Research. She is a Past President of the Society for Simulation in Healthcare. She currently serves on the board of directors for the International Pediatric Simulation Society. Patterson completed a master's in education at the University of Cincinnati and a patient safety fellowship at Virginia Commonwealth University. Her primary research interests relate to the use of medical simulation to improve patient safety, team performance, and human factors work related to patient safety. She is a federally funded investigator in these areas.

Shelly J. Reed, PhD, DNP, APRN, CNE, is an Associate Teaching Professor at Brigham Young University. She teaches in the area of maternal, child, and global health. She is the coordinator of an obstetric and pediatric simulation course. Reed began researching aspects of simulation debriefing in 2007. Both her DNP thesis and her PhD dissertation investigated this topic. Reed developed a tool called the Debriefing Experience Scale that evaluates the participant's debriefing experience and has shared this tool with researchers in the US and internationally. Recently, she developed a second debriefing evaluation tool that evaluates learning and engagement behaviors during debriefing. Clinically, Reed works as a nurse practitioner in OB emergency services. She has experience as a nurse practitioner and registered nurse in obstetrics, pain management, and pediatrics. Reed teaches obstetric and neonatal resuscitation courses internationally with LDS Charities.

Pamela W. Slaven-Lee, DNP, RN, FNP-BC, CHSE, is an Associate Clinical Professor and the Senior Associate Dean for Academic Affairs at the George Washington University School of Nursing. Slaven-Lee is an accomplished nurse educator and higher education administrator. A Sigma Theta Tau International Experienced Nurse Faculty Leadership Academy Scholar, Slaven-Lee has extensive expertise in clinical education and simulation in nurse practitioner education. Her research on the families of US military service members and service to the National Committee for Quality Assurance (NCQA) Clinical Practice Committee directly influence evidence-based practice standards that affect healthcare quality measures and population health. She a founding board member of the Wreaths Across America military service organization.

Andrew E. Spain, MA, EMT-P, is the Director of Certification for the Society for Simulation in Healthcare. He has been a paramedic for 25 years—first in the Denver, Colorado, area, and later in the state of Missouri—doing both ground and air ambulance work. This evolved into directing an EMS education program for five years before moving to SSH. He has an MA in political science and is currently working on his dissertation for a PhD in education (with an emphasis in educational leadership and policy analysis) at the University of Missouri.

Linda Tinker, MSN, RN, is Director of Simulation for Banner Health. She has nearly 38 years of nursing experience, with a background focused primarily on leadership, education, and emergency nursing. Banner Health covers six states, has more than 50,000 employees, and runs four simulation centers, all accredited by the Society for Simulation in Healthcare and the American College of Surgeons. Tinker has spent the last 10 years of her career with the Banner Simulation System. She was part of the initial CHSE pilot. Her responsibilities include operations and leadership for two of the four centers, the design of a 55,000-square-foot virtual hospital, and the redesign and rebuilding of a 10,000-square-foot virtual-simulation hospital unit on site at one of Banner's university medical centers.

Cynthia Walston, FAIA, is a Principal with CannonDesign. A nationally recognized leader in laboratory and medical education design, Walston has designed more than 2.6 million square feet of academic and science facilities. She is a founding member of the American College of Healthcare Architects and speaks regularly at national conferences about laboratory design and equipment planning. In 2013, Walston achieved the highest level of her profession, FAIA, due in large part to her accomplishments in lab design.

Table of Contents

Foreword

By Suzan Kardong-Edgren, PhD, RN, ANEF, CHSE, FSSH, FAAN

I am writing this foreword as the extended fallout from the COVID-19 pandemic continues to affect education and healthcare in nations around the world, in ways we are all still trying to understand. Thank goodness simulation educators have been honing their craft for the past 20 years and were ready to step into the breach and take up the slack at an unprecedented time in modern history.

No one expected a "black swan" event that would force so many health professions students out of their clinical practice environments. The same is true for many of their clinical educators, who may have been aware of simulation but never practiced it. Countless educators are suddenly being thrust into the simulation arena with little or no preparation. Many are literally one step ahead of their students. Thus, the timing for a second edition of *Mastering Simulation: A Handbook for Success* couldn't be better!

This book is a one-stop shop for both novice and experienced simulation educators to gain or refresh foundational simulation knowledge. This text is edited by three of our most experienced educators and leaders in healthcare and simulation: Janice Palaganas, Beth Ulrich, and Beth Mancini. The editors have assembled some of the best simulationists in the field to provide updated chapters that seamlessly take the reader through simulation history, basic theory and practice, various uses of simulation, increased professionalization of the discipline through certification, and careers in simulation. They end with a glimpse into the future of simulation—a future that experienced simulationists knew would eventually come but maybe not in this way. It is a future made all the brighter because simulation was well positioned to provide an alternative to traditional educational methods in this unprecedented time.

–Suzan Kardong-Edgren, PhD, RN, ANEF, CHSE, FSSH, FAAN
Nurse Scientist, Texas Health Harris Methodist Hospital Ft. Worth and Frisco, Texas
Senior Fellow, Center for Medical Simulation, Boston, Massachusetts

Foreword

By David Marshall, JD, DNP, RN, FAAN, FAONL

My earliest introduction to caring for others was when I was an 11-year-old Boy Scout earning my very first merit badge—the first aid badge. I remember the first time I pinched a bandage between my fingers and carefully rolled it around an ankle. I learned to splint a fracture, apply pressure to stop bleeding, and use lifesaving resuscitation techniques.

Even after 35 years as a licensed professional, I trace my desire to become a nurse to this first spark of knowledge that I could help alleviate someone's pain and suffering—maybe even save a life—with those basic skills I practiced on my fellow Scouts using supplies our leader wrangled from a local hospital. This feeling has sustained my nursing career at the bedside and as an executive.

Another important lesson of that first merit badge is the crucial role simulation plays in acquiring skills. Instead of practicing on my fellow Scouts, though, I work at an institution that has a state-of-the-art center with computer-controlled virtual patients that can breathe, bleed, and blink. We can practice high-fidelity simulations—everything from delivering a baby to performing an emergency intubation. Well beyond the basics I approached in boyhood, we re-create realistic scenarios for every imaginable aspect of acute care, ambulatory care, critical care, procedures, and surgeries.

Rapid innovations and advances in technology make this an incredible time to work in patient care. At the same time, our patients are increasingly sophisticated. Even the simplest online search turns up in-depth information about patient outcomes and safety. Nurses have never been asked to do more, and the expectations placed on them have never been higher. Simulation is our best training tool, allowing an interdisciplinary team to practice as a cohesive unit. It's also a powerful tool for achieving what every caregiver ultimately wants most: better outcomes for our patients.

This compassionate drive to be the best we can be for our patients fuels the culture of learning in nursing. We are never done training. We are never done acquiring and honing our skills. Day after day, I see nurses balance efficiency, effectiveness, and technical proficiency with personal caring to meet the diverse needs of their patients. Every day that nurses report to their unit, round on a patient, or scrub in for surgery, they encounter something new. The only prescription for handling the unexpected is again borrowed from my Boy Scout past: Be prepared.

Janice Palaganas, Beth Ulrich, and Beth Mancini recruited the finest interprofessional simulation experts to contribute to this volume. It serves as a practical guide for practitioners and students alike to translate the potential of simulation as a training tool into a powerful instrument that improves the outcomes of patients at their own institutions.

–David Marshall, JD, DNP, RN, FAAN, FAONL
Senior Vice President & Chief Nursing Executive
Cedars-Sinai, Los Angeles, California

Introduction

"Simulation is the key to patient safety and medical quality."
–John Nance, *author of*
Why Hospitals Should Fly

One of the biggest challenges we face in healthcare is how to educate and train healthcare professionals without endangering patients—especially when we are teaching the management of high-stakes situations such as codes, trauma care, chest pain, or anaphylactic shock, in which any delay in treatment threatens the outcome. Often, new healthcare practitioners enter their profession without ever having seen—much less gotten experience with—many high-risk/low-volume patient conditions.

The use of simulation is growing exponentially in academic and service settings. Simulation can enable students, new graduates, and experienced clinicians to develop clinical competence and confidence in caring for patients in a learning environment that is cognitively and emotionally realistic and safe for the learner—and does not compromise patient safety or outcomes. Simulation can be applied to many clinical situations—far more than a learner can be exposed to in a live clinical environment. Simulation activities need not be bound by one profession, time, or place. Simulation can be expanded to include the systems dynamics of care, interprofessional teamwork, and considerations for hospital technology and equipment at any point in the healthcare continuum.

In a clinical setting, simulation can be used to onboard new graduates and experienced staff. Simulation also offers the ability to objectively assess the performance of healthcare professionals based on a well-defined standard of practice. Many organizations carefully assess the competency and performance of new staff, but—other than perhaps yearly skills fairs—do little to ensure that existing staff continue to meet standards of practice and follow evidence-based and best practice processes and protocols. Renewing nursing or medical licenses generally requires only paying a fee and completing continuing education programs—*not* demonstrating continued competence. Simulation can be developed for continued development of staff and educators. Although we know much more about healthcare education today than we did 20 years ago, much has yet to be discovered. Research is changing healthcare practice on an almost daily basis. To assume that all professionals who renew their licenses are competent in the knowledge and skills needed to practice in the current environment is naive at best and dangerous at worst—something Florence Nightingale knew and was passionate about more than 100 years ago. It often surprises people to learn that Nightingale opposed the registration of nurses. The reason was that she thought you could not know whether a nurse was competent based on just the fact that the nurse had finished nursing school or passed a written examination. In an 1888 letter to the probationer nurses at St. Thomas Hospital, Nightingale wrote:

> She [the nurse] may have gone to a first rate course—plenty of examinations. And we may find nothing inside. It may be the difference between a nurse nursing and a nurse reading a book on nursing. Unless it bear fruit, it is all gilding and veneering; the reality is not there, growing, growing every year. Every nurse must grow. No nurse can stand still, she must go forward, or she will go backward, every year. And how can a certificate or public register show this?

Simulation can be used to improve an organization's ability to ensure that all its clinicians maintain competence. Knowing is not doing. Simulation can demonstrate the successful application of knowledge.

There is also growing evidence that simulation is effective in developing, assessing, and improving the performance of healthcare teams. Much as the aviation industry first used flight simulators to teach the "hard" skills of piloting airplanes, such as takeoffs, landings, and handling mechanical emergencies, healthcare began using simulators to teach the "hard" skills of caring for patients—diagnosing and using medications and other interventions in response to a patient's physiological changes. A series of high-fatality plane crashes caused the aviation industry to look beyond the hard-skill training solutions to improve how their people worked together and communicated with each other. This led to the development of what is now called crew resource management (CRM). CRM redefined roles and expectations; created a culture of transparency; encouraged people to learn from errors; and pushed for the development of training, processes, and standards to enable leaders to quickly create highly functional teams from a group of crew members who very often have never worked together. All these practices have been integrated into the aviation industry's simulation experiences. As a result, air travel is safer than ever. Like the aviation industry, the healthcare industry has come to understand that how healthcare professionals work together can have a major impact on patient safety and improving patient outcomes. Just as aviation uses simulation to teach CRM to its professionals, healthcare can use simulation to develop highly functional teams.

Simulation can contribute to risk management and quality improvement activities. It can be used to identify latent threats to patient and clinician safety, allow clinicians to test "what if" scenarios (e.g., what if we used another drug? Or, what if we did intervention B before intervention A?), and perform trial runs of new techniques, equipment, and patient-care areas.

Who Should Read This Book?

The primary audience for this book is healthcare professionals in both academic and service settings who are currently using or anticipate using simulation, including schools of nursing and medicine, EMT training programs, the military, and hospitals and healthcare systems. The availability of education for simulation professionals and others involved peripherally with simulation has not kept up with the rapid growth of simulation use in academic and service settings. Many simulation professionals are receiving their education on simulation through on-the-job, just-in-time training.

This book is designed as a professional resource and as a support text for simulation courses. It is also a book for healthcare leaders who want to learn more about what simulation can offer their organizations, who are looking for ways to standardize how healthcare is delivered, and who understand that ensuring that competency is maintained is equally or more important than determining competency when healthcare professionals enter their professions.

This book is a handbook for individuals working in or preparing to work in simulation and for academic and service organizations that are using or are planning to use simulation. The book is both evidence-based and pragmatic. It is written in a style that can be easily read by busy healthcare professionals and provides strategies that can be immediately integrated into practice.

Second Edition

Since the first edition of this book was published, healthcare simulation has taken the stage as the most innovative educational methodology due to its many advantages. Many academic and hospital organizations, researchers, and credentialing bodies have encouraged and promoted its use, holding simulation as a gold standard of healthcare education. Since we wrote the first edition of this book, there has been increasing and renewed interest in developing the field of healthcare simulation. This edition continues to draw on foundational thoughts and findings while integrating current evidence in healthcare, education, behavioral science, neuroscience, and related fields as we seek to provide a balance of theory, evidence, and practical approaches.

In this edition, all chapters have been updated with the most current information. We have also added a new chapter, Chapter 7, on the use of simulation along a continuous learning system. This chapter suggests ways in which we can expand our current activities to bridge gaps in education and practice and facilitate the longitudinal sustainment and improvement of knowledge. We hope that in future editions of this book, we will be able to include new evidence that you, our readers, develop as you apply what you read here to your practice.

Book Content

Whether you are looking for a primer on simulation or information to improve your existing knowledge and expertise in the simulation specialty, *Mastering Simulation* has content for you.

- The book begins with an overview of the foundations of simulation in Chapter 1, familiarizing the reader with simulation terminology, philosophic foundations, and educational principles and describing the range of simulator typology that is currently available.

- Chapter 2 discusses competence and confidence, the relationships between them, and how simulation can be used to develop both in clinical performance.

- Chapter 3 describes the necessity and means of creating effective simulation environments that encourage participants to suspend disbelief and fully engage in the simulation as if they were caring for a live patient.

- Developing and planning scenarios, including detailed scripts for simulations and simulation environments, are discussed in Chapter 4.

- Chapter 5 offers information on the debriefing component of the simulation experience—including how to guide simulation participants through reflecting on their experiences.

- In Chapter 6, strategies and techniques to evaluate simulation effectiveness are described.

- In Chapter 7, the use of simulation along a continuous learning system is discussed.

- Simulations with specific learner populations are discussed in Chapter 8.

- The importance of interprofessional education and practice is increasingly being recognized. Chapter 9 is dedicated to understanding how simulation can be used to develop and enhance high-functioning teamwork.

- Using simulation in academic environments is the topic of Chapter 10.

- A discussion on how to use simulation to improve outcomes in hospitals and healthcare systems is found in Chapter 11.

- Chapter 12 addresses using simulation for risk management and quality improvement, including identifying latent threats and improving processes.

- Chapter 13 provides information on designing and implementing simulation-based research.

- Chapter 14 is a resource for individuals who want to enter or expand their careers in the field of simulation, as well as for simulation programs, providing descriptions of simulation roles and positions.

- Credentialing of individuals and simulation programs is described in Chapter 15.

- Chapter 16 offers the information you need to develop and build a simulation center—from the initial planning and assessment process to space and design recommendations.

- The final chapter of the book, Chapter 17, looks to the future and describes the issues, challenges, and opportunities that are evolving around the use of simulation in healthcare.

Final Thoughts

We wrote this book with two goals in mind: to provide a comprehensive resource for simulation professionals and to raise awareness of the depth of knowledge and expertise required to use simulation strategies efficiently and effectively in healthcare. Although there are identified best practices related to the implementation of simulation methodologies, there is no single best way to integrate simulation into health profession education or healthcare practice. Simulation has many techniques, many places to be used, and many ways in which the impact can be measured.

Every week, we hear of new ways that simulation is improving patient care and enhancing patient safety. At this point in the life cycle of simulation, we need to stay nimble and innovative, being careful not to become too rigid or tied to any one method or way to do things. We also need to actively look outside the domain of healthcare for guidance; the lessons learned by aviation, military science, and others who use simulation successfully are applicable to healthcare.

The use of simulation in healthcare is limited only by our creativity and imagination.

-Janice C. Palaganas, PhD, RN, NP, ANEF, FAAN, FSSH
jpalaganas@harvardmedsim.org

-Beth Tamplet Ulrich, EdD, RN, FACHE, FAONL, FAAN
BethTUlrich@gmail.com

-Mary E. (Beth) Mancini, PhD, RN, NE-BC, FAHA, FSSH, ANEF, FAAN
mancini@uta.edu

"No industry in which human lives depend on the skilled performance of responsible operators has waited for unequivocal proof of the benefits of simulation before embracing it."

–David M. Gaba, MD

Foundations of Simulation

1

Sharon I. Decker, PhD, RN, FSSH, ANEF, FAAN
Sandra Caballero, MSN, RN, CHSE
Chris McClanahan, DNP, RN, CHSE

Introduction to Simulation

Today's dynamic and complex healthcare environment requires healthcare providers to demonstrate evidence-based clinical judgment while providing safe, reliable, and effective care as a collaborative member of a healthcare team (Frankel, Haraden, Federico, & Lenoci-Edwards, 2017; Institute of Medicine [IOM], 2004a, 2011). National leaders, organizations, and accreditation agencies have challenged nurse educators to transform the current educational process to a learner-centered, active pedagogy.

In 2004, the IOM—renamed the National Academy of Medicine (NAM) in 2015—provided recommendations for evidence-based revisions in the clinical education of healthcare professionals. Multiple IOM/NAM reports (IOM, 2001, 2003, 2004a, 2011, 2015) have stressed the need for research in order to:

- Understand how to apply adult learning principles to clinical education

- Obtain empirical evidence to support the integration of new technologies, including simulation, into curricula

- Explore the outcomes achieved by different types of teaching technologies

- Understand the process of translating knowledge to clinical practice

- Perfect the science of team-based care

Simulation combined with other technologies facilitates the development of skills, competencies, and clinical judgment needed to provide safe, quality patient care (Benner, Sutphen, Leonard, & Day, 2010; Gaba, 2004; IOM, 2004a, 2004b, 2011). For example, the IOM (2004b) report *Keeping Patients Safe* states that simulation is the most useful approach for developing skills related

OBJECTIVES

- Describe the history of simulation and influential factors in its use.

- Identify the philosophical framework for simulation.

- Discuss adult learning principles that pertain to simulation-based activities.

- Recognize the legal and ethical issues common to simulation-based activities.

- Review published standards and guidelines for simulation-based activities.

- Understand the code of ethics for simulationists.

to unpredictable situations and crises. Similarly, Benner et al. (2010) support the development of clinical reasoning and interprofessional communication through new technologies such as simulation. Additionally, learning in a simulated environment is transferable to the clinical setting but enables educators to monitor learner progress without risk to patients (IOM, 2011). Simulation is a complement to—rather than a substitute for—actual patient care. It promotes a learner's ability to integrate theory into a patient-care situation in a safe and controlled environment (International Nursing Association for Clinical Simulation and Learning [INACSL] Standards Committee, 2016b).

Definition of Simulation

The definition of simulation has evolved over time:

- In 2004, Gaba described simulation as "a 'technique,' not a technology, to replace or amplify real experiences with guided experiences, often immersive in nature, that evoke or replicate substantial aspects of the real world in a fully interactive fashion" (p. i2).

- Jeffries (2005) described simulation as an educational process in which learning experiences are simulated to imitate the working environment. The learner is required to integrate skills (both technical and nontechnical) into a patient-care scenario and thus demonstrate clinical judgment. Jeffries and Rogers (2012) more recently described the simulation experience as "an environment that is experiential, interactive, collaborative, and learner centered" (p. 41).

- The INACSL Standards Committee (2016a), citing the work of Gaba (2004), defines simulation as "an educational strategy in

which a particular set of conditions are created or replicated to resemble authentic situations that are possible in real life. Simulation can incorporate one or more modalities to promote, improve, or validate a participant's performance" (p. S44).

- The Society for Simulation in Healthcare (SSH), in its *Healthcare Simulation Dictionary,* defines simulation as "a technique that creates a situation or environment to allow persons to experience a representation of a real event for the purpose of practice, learning, evaluation, testing, or to gain understanding of systems or human actions" (Lioce et al., 2020, p. 44).

Comparing these definitions reveals similarities—specifically, that simulation is a pedagogy that uses multiple tools (such as simulators, partial trainers, and standardized patients) to promote and assess learning.

Simulation Definitions: Resources

SSH Definitions: https://www.ssih.org/Dictionary

INACSL Definitions: https://www.nursingsimulation.org/article/S1876-1399(16)30133-5/fulltext

NLN Definitions: http://sirc.nln.org/mod/glossary/view.php?id=183

History of Simulation

The history of simulation has been well-documented (Aebersold, 2016; Gaba, 2004; Jones, Passos-Neto, & Braghiroli, 2015). Simulation has been used in the aviation, military, and medical fields. One common goal has driven its adoption in all these areas: increased safety. In the healthcare industry, there is increasing evidence of a link between simulation and patient safety. As a result, simulation continues to be a method of medical training to enhance vital skills for healthcare providers, including critical behaviors, communication, and teamwork (Aebersold, 2016).

Mannequins have been used since the early 16th century (Aebersold, 2016; Gaba, 2004; Jones et al., 2015). In 1911, the Chase Hospital Doll, more commonly called Mrs. Chase, became the first commercially available training mannequin. Mrs. Chase was used primarily for nursing education (Aebersold, 2016). In the 1960s, a Norwegian toymaker named Åsmund S. Lærdal further advanced clinical simulation with the development of the Resusci Anne mannequin. Resusci Anne was the first realistic and effective mouth-to-mouth resuscitation training aid (Cooper & Taqueti, 2004).

The next leap forward came from the University of Southern California in the late 1960s, with the development of SimOne, a computer-controlled, electronic mannequin capable of simulating vital signs, palpable pulses, inspiratory chest rise, eye blinking, and more (Bradley, 2006; Cooper & Taqueti, 2004). In 1968, Dr. Michael Gordon introduced Harvey, an anatomy-specific cardiopulmonary simulator that simulated 27 different cardiac pathologies (Rodgers, 2007). The Next Generation Harvey, used today, includes a total of 50 conditions and 10 standardized patient scenarios used in advanced patient assessment (Michael S. Gordon Center for Simulation and Innovation in Medical Education, n.d.).

In the late 1970s, the National Aeronautics and Space Administration developed a team training method called cockpit resource management with the goal of correcting communication deficiencies to decrease airline disasters. This method was later expanded to include the entire flight crew, error management, human factors, teamwork, and reporting systems for safety concerns and incidents. It was renamed crew resource management (CRM; Aebersold, 2016). Dr. David Gaba later applied CRM in the healthcare setting—developing a simulation-based program to help anesthesiologists manage crises (Aebersold, 2016). In the 1980s, the medical industry began using high-fidelity simulators for anesthesia training (Aebersold, 2016).

High-fidelity human patient simulators can simulate many functions of the human body, its physiological variables, and its responses to pharmacological and other care interventions. However, high-fidelity human patient simulators are not the only means of simulated learning used today. Standardized patients are also being utilized. A standardized patient is an actor who portrays the role of a real patient. In addition, the increased use of ultrasound technology in both the diagnostic and procedural arenas has led to the development of ultrasound-able human patient simulators that can reproduce multiple pathologies or simulate human anatomy. With the increased availability and affordability of technology, the use of augmented and virtual reality is becoming more common in the healthcare education industry. In the future, virtual simulations could be able to teach skills that nurses have historically learned by using task trainers. These new innovative technologies are expected to improve quality of care by increasing patient safety (Aebersold, 2018).

Influential Factors in the Use of Simulation

Clinical simulation is dynamic and ever-changing—constantly morphing as new technologies are developed, clinical knowledge increases, and new evidence-based practices are implemented. New patient safety requirements and the need for innovative modalities to educate clinicians drive clinical simulation forward. As noted by Benner et al. (2010), "New nurses [healthcare providers] need to be prepared to practice safely, accurately, and compassionately, in varied settings, where knowledge and innovation increase at an astonishing rate" (p. i).

Standards and Guidelines for Simulation-Based Activities

As the use of simulation has increased, standards and guidelines have been developed for simulation-based activities. Recognizing that simulation-based activities accelerate the learning process, providing learners and professionals with opportunities to develop skills competency, the World Health Organization published a recommendation related to the use of simulation methods in 2013: "Health professionals' education and training institutions should use simulation methods (high fidelity methods in settings with appropriate resources and lower fidelity methods in resource limited settings) in the education of health professionals" (p. 6).

The National Council of State Boards of Nursing (NCSBN) conducted a landmark national, longitudinal, multisite simulation study that concluded that simulation-based activities can be substituted for up to 50% of clinical experiences without impact on the learners' knowledge acquisition and clinical performance when specific guidelines are followed. These guidelines stress that:

> Simulation is a pedagogy that may be integrated across the prelicensure curriculum, provided that faculty are adequately trained, committed and in sufficient numbers; when there is a dedicated simulation lab which has appropriate resources; when the vignettes are realistically and

appropriately designed; and when debriefing is based on a theoretical model. (Hayden, Smiley, Alexander, Kardong-Edgren, & Jeffries, 2014, p. 5)

INACSL and the Association of Standardized Patient Educators (ASPE) have published standards of best practice for simulation. The INACSL standards emphasize that simulation-based activities should be based on the following (2016b):

- Expected outcomes of the experience

- Learner's knowledge and skills level

- Simulation modality being used

- Feedback and/or debrief method used

- Outcome assessment selected

The ASPE standards apply to activities that integrate standardized patients (Lewis et al., 2017). A standardized patient (SP) is "an individual who is trained to portray a real patient in order to simulate a set of symptoms or problems used for healthcare education, evaluation, and research" (Lioce et al., 2020, p. 49). The ASPE standards note that when trained appropriately, SPs can provide learner feedback and complete assessment instruments (Lewis et al., 2017; Lewis, Strachan, & Smith, 2012).

Patient Safety and Quality

Healthcare professionals need to become more astute and to critically analyze situations while providing evidence-based care. "Healthcare organizations have an absolute responsibility to deliver safe, reliable, and effective care to patients" (Frankel et al., 2017, p. 6) while also ensuring the engagement of patients and their families.

In the early 2000s, evidence-based research suggested that lack of communication and collaboration within interprofessional healthcare teams had a negative effect on the delivery of safe, quality care (IOM, 2003; Leonard, Graham, & Bonacum, 2004). The landmark IOM reports *To Err Is Human* (2000) and *Crossing the Quality Chasm* (2001) called for improvement in healthcare quality and safety by using strategies that prepared clinicians to:

- Work in interprofessional teams
- Use informatics
- Maintain an improved understanding of disease processes
- Provide leadership
- Provide safe, timely, efficient, and effective patient-centered care

Core Competencies for Interprofessional Collaborative Practice, a document initially published by the Interprofessional Education Collaborative (IPEC) in 2011 and updated in 2016, identified four domains of interprofessional competencies (IPEC, 2011, 2016):

- Values/ethics
- Roles/responsibilities
- Communication practices
- Teamwork and team-based practice

Providing realistic, interactive, simulation-based experiences that integrate the core competencies for interprofessional collaborative practice addresses the identified gaps in communication and collaboration between healthcare teams (D'Alimonte, McLaney, & Di Prospero, 2019). For example, research has demonstrated that using simulation to teach teamwork skills has improved team dynamics, communication, and patient care

(Black, 2018; Iverson et al., 2018; Parsons et al., 2018).

Technology

Changes in technology, safety issues, learner attitudes, and accreditation requirements have forced changes in educational strategies and delivery. Simulation as a pedagogy includes the use of a variety of technologies, from low-fidelity task trainers to mid-fidelity ultrasound-compatible mannequins to augmented reality. The pioneering development of virtual reality computer-based environments, haptic devices, and augmented reality provides realistic experiences in a risk-free environment with immediate feedback for the learner (Jenson & Forsyth, 2012).

With simulation, learners engage in reproducible clinical environments, interacting with virtual patients and interprofessional teams (Jenson & Forsyth, 2012). New integrated three-dimensional (3D) technologies, virtual reality, and augmented reality immerse the learner in realistic and clinically accurate anatomy models and environments. These change how concepts, skills, and clinical reasoning are developed. For example, ultrasound-compatible partial trainers and mannequins offer realistic representations of anatomical structures, facilitating proficiency in advanced skills such as central line insertion. The continued combination of low-fidelity task trainers and SPs creates hybrid scenarios, marrying true human interaction with skills acquisition and task performance. Advances in simulator technology augment opportunities for interprofessional learning experiences, improving patient safety and patient outcomes.

Transformation in Education

A decade ago, Benner and colleagues, noting the profound changes in nursing practice, called for a radical transformation in nursing education (Benner et al., 2010). The need for transformation in education has become even more critical with the shortage of experienced nurses and physicians. In addition, the growing lack of clinical placement availability has created many dilemmas in ensuring the competencies needed for graduating nurses (Jeffries, 2012; National League for Nursing [NLN], 2015).

The US Bureau of Labor Statistics (2019) has projected that RN jobs will increase 12% between 2018 and 2028—faster than the average for all occupations—due to growth and the need for replacements as older nurses phase into retirement. The Association of American Medical Colleges (2019) predicts a shortage of up to 112,000 physicians by 2032, largely due to a growing aging population. This critical shortage of qualified nurses and physicians amplifies the need to produce qualified, competent, and safe clinicians. At the same time, an increase in medical errors has revealed the need for additional patient safety education.

Regardless of the reasons for nursing shortages, developing innovative means of educating new nurses is paramount to combating the shortages. For almost two decades, the NLN has promoted simulation as an innovative strategy for transforming the education of nurses. Emphasis toward engaging students and preparing them for the increasing complexity of patient care by creating a realistic learning environment is key. This would address the growing lack of clinical placement availability (NLN, 2015).

Healthcare education has embraced the importance of simulation and the multiple simulation modalities. In its early days, simulation was seen as an "add-on" activity in nursing curricula—done to help relieve the shortage of clinical space. Today, nursing schools realize the importance of integrating simulation—including computerized mannequins, role-play, SPs, virtual and augmented reality, and virtual human and animal anatomy—throughout the entire curriculum. Simulation now assists nursing students not only in gaining skills competency but also in developing clinical reasoning abilities that lead to increased patient safety (Aebersold, 2018). Creating a realistic learning environment in simulation that engages students can help prepare them for the increasing complexity of patient care.

Studies on the effect of using high-fidelity simulation in undergraduate nursing curricula have found simulation to be effective in creating safer patient environments and care. Studies have validated that simulation can be used to effectively teach skill-based behaviors (including handwashing and medication safety) as well as communication and the acquisition and transfer of knowledge (Doolen et al., 2016). A review by Cant and Cooper (2017) revealed that students were able to reconcile theory with practice while using simulation. The most significant research to date was a two-part study conducted by the NCSBN. This study demonstrated that up to 50% of clinical hours can be effectively replaced by simulation (Hayden et al., 2014).

With the increased shortage of clinical sites and some of the restrictions students have in the clinical setting, simulation has become a well-accepted form of learning for students. However, simulation requires a thoughtful approach to ensure the success of both educators and learners. Simulation must be integrated into the curriculum and performed correctly. The goals and objectives in a simulated environment are different from those in the clinical setting. Educators must receive appropriate training to design, facilitate, and debrief after simulation-based experiences to meet these goals and objectives.

Kolb's Experiential Learning Theory and Reflective Learning

Simulation-based experiences use several educational learning theories and conceptual models. One popular learning theory is Kolb's (1984) experiential learning theory. This theory defines *learning* as "the process whereby knowledge is created through the transformation of experience. Knowledge results from the combination of grasping and transforming experience" (Kolb, 1984, p. 41). Grasping is achieved through concrete experiences and abstract conceptualization, while transforming experience is guided by the assimilation of reflective observations. More and more, health profession educators are adopting Kolb's experiential learning theory, which points them in the direction of using simulation (with debriefing) as a method in their teaching.

According to Kolb (1984), reflection is an essential component of experiential learning. It promotes insight leading to the discovery of new knowledge that can be applied in the future. *Reflection* can be defined as an active process of self-monitoring initiated by a state of puzzlement or uncertainty occurring during or after an experience (Kolb, 1984; Schön, 1983). Reflective learning can be facilitated in the debriefing stage of a simulation experience. Indeed, self-reflection is at the core of effective debriefing. Learning becomes meaningful when reflective debriefing is done. This in turn strengthens the ability of learners to handle the complexities they will face in the actual clinical setting (Hunter, 2016). For more information on debriefing and reflective practice, see Chapter 5.

The most common question with simulation used to be, "Does it work?" Now, the more common question is, "Under what conditions is simulation most effective?" (Walsh et al., 2018). For example, at the novice level, learners can use task trainers and role-play to develop basic technical and non-technical skills. After competencies in these skills are attained, educators should use scaffolding to shift the focus of the learners from producing replicable and predictable outcomes to developing the clinical reasoning required for competency by integrating unexpected issues into simulation-based scenarios. Educators can then provide students with opportunities to exercise and implement flexible clinical judgment and ethical comportment, and gain additional expertise in actual patient care situations (Benner et al., 2010).

Simulation Typology

Simulation typology varies in complexity and fidelity. *Fidelity* is defined as the "physical, psychological, and environmental elements" (Lioce et al., 2020, p. 18):

- **Low-fidelity mannequins** are static tools that may or may not provide isolated specific feedback to the learner. Low-fidelity mannequins include partial and full-body tasks trainers such as airway-management trainers. They are used mainly to develop and assess technical skills (Lioce et al., 2020).

- **Mid-fidelity mannequins/simulators** provide learners with isolated specific feedback. An example of a mid-fidelity trainer is a simulator used to generate heart and lung sounds without chest movement (Lioce et al., 2020).

- **High-fidelity simulators** provide realistic responses that can be modifiable to react to the situation and to learner input. High-fidelity simulators mimic human body functions at a very high level and provide realistic responses such as heart and lung sounds, chest movement, and palpable pulses. They are integrated into patient scenarios that require learners to demonstrate skill attainment while engaged in situations requiring clinical judgment (Jeffries & Rogers, 2012; Lioce et al., 2020).

The spectrum of simulation typologies is shown in Table 1.1. The appropriate use of the spectrum requires strategic planning. The type of simulation used must address identified learning needs and be suited to the expertise of the practitioner (Issenberg, McGaghie, Petrusa, Lee Gordon, & Scalese, 2005; Lioce et al., 2020).

Table 1.1   Simulation Typologies/Modalities

Simulation Typology/ Modality	Other Names/ Abbreviations	Definition
Task trainer	Part-task trainer Partial task trainer	Anatomical model or mannequin used to obtain competency in a specific skill or procedure
Peer-to-peer		Collaboration between peers used to learn and/or master specific skills
Computer-based training	Computer-based simulation Constructed simulation Screen-based simulation	Computer applications (software or web-based) to teach, provide feedback, and assess knowledge and clinical judgment
Gaming	Serious gaming Tabletop exercise	A simulation or program (board or computer-assisted game) that enables learners to interact, solve problems, and make decisions
Virtual reality	Virtual environment Virtual world Immersive virtual reality	An artificial projected environment that provides spatial dimensions and sensory stimuli through special glasses and sensors to promote authenticity
Augmented reality	Mixed reality Mixed reality human	The overlay of computer-generated information or images within the real-world environment
Haptic systems		A computer-generated environment that provides tactile and visual sensations as procedures are conducted
Standardized patient/ participant	SP Role player Simulated person	A volunteer or paid individual who portrays a patient in a case scenario in a realistic and consistent manner
Gynecological/ genitourinary teaching associate	GTA, MUTA, GUTA	A paid individual who teaches gender-specific physical examinations using his or her own body for demonstration
Objective Structured Clinical Examination	OSCE	Structured assessment of clinical or professional competence and skill with objectivity as a focus
Advanced patient simulators	High-fidelity simulator Manikin-based Mannequin-based	Computerized full-body mannequins that provide realistic physiologic responses

Source: Lioce et al., 2020

Simulation can be used to support lifelong learning at all levels—from novice learners to expert practitioners. In addition to assisting the practitioner in developing and maintaining competency in technical skills, simulation can help learners develop nontechnical skills such as communication and clinical reasoning, acquire new knowledge, and understand conceptual relationships (Cato, 2012; Gaba, 2004; INACSL, 2016b).

The IOM has recognized simulation as an effective strategy for healthcare learners and professionals to enhance their technical skills (IOM, 2001, 2011) and to acquire knowledge on an ongoing basis (IOM, 2004b). More advanced simulation technologies such as augmented and virtual reality are seen as ways to address the vexing problem of limited availability of clinical sites (Pappano, 2018).

The next sections discuss simulation typologies in more detail.

Task Trainers

Task trainers represent a specific body part or body system. They are used to acquire and assess technical skills. Task trainers facilitate the mastery of complex skills by subdividing the skills into segments—for example, the steps involved in inserting an intravenous catheter. Task trainers vary in complexity from static models to trainers that provide realistic heart, lung, and bowel sounds (Issenberg et al., 2005; Lioce et al., 2020).

Computer-Based Programs

Computer-based programs provide a computerized system or discovery learning in which the learner can interact with a situation and receive feedback on performed actions. These programs are relatively inexpensive and allow learners to work independently or in groups. Navigation options allow practitioners to tailor the learning to each learner's needs. The competencies of practitioners can be validated through case scenarios that require the integration of procedural and critical-thinking skills. Various levels of monitoring are integrated into the software to provide educators with written documentation of the learner's performance, including multiple choice test results and performance summaries (Issenberg et al., 2005; Lioce et al., 2020).

Virtual Reality

Virtual reality, developed as an offshoot of video-game technology, integrates interactive computer simulation with psychomotor and cognitive learning to immerse the learner in a simulated experience. Virtual reality provides cues through sensory stimulation (hearing, touch, and sight) to evoke feelings of reality. The practitioner engaged in virtual reality is required to integrate knowledge of anatomy and physiology while performing and validating clinical competency in specific procedures, such as intravenous catheter insertion, airway management, amniocentesis, endoscopy, and bronchoscopy (Kardong-Edgren, Farra, Alinier, & Young, 2019; Lioce et al., 2020).

Augmented Reality

A variant of virtual reality, augmented reality superimposes computer-generated or synthetic images (such as avatars) or data within the natural environment through devices such as glasses, goggles, or even a tablet. Where virtual reality re-creates the entire simulated environment, augmented reality projects 3D images into a real environment, so all human senses are engaged (Kardong-Edgren et al., 2019; Lioce et al., 2020).

Haptic Systems

Haptic (touch) systems integrate a feeling of resistance when the learner uses them, creating the illusion of direct contact with the patient's organs. Haptic systems are used primarily within surgical training programs and aid learners in laparoscopic and endoscopic procedures (Lioce et al., 2020).

Standardized Patients

An SP program integrates realistic case studies into role-play. Individuals (paid or volunteer) are taught to portray a "patient" in a realistic and consistent manner. The learner interacting with an SP is expected to demonstrate appropriate communication skills, behaviors, and attitudes while conducting interviews, performing physical examinations, and developing a plan of care (Lewis et al., 2017; Lioce et al., 2020). SPs have been successfully integrated into formative and summative assessments in both graduate and undergraduate nursing programs and provide a tool to validate the learner's knowledge, skills, and clinical judgment (Rutherford-Hemming, Alfes, & Breymier, 2019). SPs have been a component of the competency assessment component of the US Medical Licensing Examination (USMLE) since 2004. The clinical skills component of the USMLE requires the examinee to communicate effectively with an SP while developing a rapport, obtaining a health history, completing a focused assessment, and documenting the results (USMLE, 2012). SPs enhance learning by providing both verbal and nonverbal communication within an appropriate scenario. However, Holtschneider (2017) notes that there are some limitations in critical-care scenarios. For example, SPs cannot provide the realism needed to simulate an intravenous site, Foley catheter insertion, or tracheostomy suctioning. Wearable technology has been added to address this issue and enhance realism. The most common type is a chest piece known as a tracheostomy teaching device that interacts with the SP without the learner's knowledge. The SP receives a buzz, prompting the patient to respond when being suctioned too deep. Other wearable devices include intravenous sleeves and wearable genitalia. Diversity is another feature being developed for wearable technology.

Advanced Patient Simulators

Advanced patient simulators (also sometimes called human patient simulators) are full-body mannequins of various levels of complexity that can be programmed to respond in real time to pharmacological and other treatment modalities. Advanced patient simulators have palpable pulses, audible blood pressures, and chest movements with respirations; simulate various heart, lung, and bowel sounds; and provide verbal cues to the learner. Recent advances in patient simulator technology have increased the fidelity of these mannequins with the addition of augmented reality, muscle motion, eye tracking, skin pigmentation, and even hair. Such features—supplemented with monitors programmed to provide electrocardiogram waveforms, cardiac output, and pulse oximeter readings—add realism to clinical teaching scenarios. Additionally, the technology allows for objective measurement of the knowledge, technical skill level, and critical-thinking abilities of the learner (Lioce et al., 2020).

Simulated Learning Experience Requirements

Simulated learning experiences should:

- Be designed to replicate a realistic situation
- Have objectives that are learner-dependent and state the expected outcome of the experience
- Be based on current evidence and practice guidelines
- Be a complement to (not a substitute for) actual patient care to promote an individual's ability to develop competencies and clinical judgment
- Be conducted in a controlled, nonthreatening environment without risks to patients
- Be developed and conducted by trained simulationists
- Include a debriefing conversation focused on the learning objectives

Philosophical/Theoretical Foundation of Simulation

"Of the many cues that influence behavior, at any point in time, none is more common than the actions of others."

–Albert Bandura

The substructure for the pedagogy of simulation is grounded in the works of multiple philosophers such as Socrates (Johnson, 2012) and Dewey (1910, 1916, 1933). Various theoretical frameworks can be used in tangent to assist educators in supporting learning through simulation. For example, mastery of learning (Bloom, 1971, 1974), experiential learning (Kolb, 1984), reflective thinking (Schön, 1983, 1987), cognitive load (Sweller, 1988), social cognitive theory (Bandura, 1977, 2001), deliberate practice (Ericsson, 2004), and others. These theorists emphasize the synergistic relationship between the learning environment, the learner, the educator/facilitator, and a period of reflection to the development and transfer of new knowledge. The INACSL Standards of Best Practice and the NCSBN Guidelines highlight the importance

of formulating a simulation-based activity on a theoretical and/or conceptual framework (Alexander et al., 2015; INACSL, 2016b).

The Socratic methodology or questioning fosters critical thinking by posing questions to the learner (Johnson, 2012). The NCSBN Guidelines stress the importance of integrating Socratic questioning in debriefing, specifically recommending the use of "a standardized method of debriefing observed simulation using a Socratic methodology" (Hayden et al., 2014, p. 8). It is also recommended that the Socratic method be researched prior to use since health profession educators may have a flawed concept of the method (e.g., digging by using the learner's answer as a question is not Socratic method).

Dewey (1910) defined learning as "not learning things, but the meanings of things" (p. 176). According to Dewey (1933), the development of meaning or insight requires interaction, reflection, and time for personal discovery. Dewey (1933) described reflection as an active, emotional interaction that helps learners construct new knowledge based on past experiences and indicated that it is the responsibility of educators to facilitate this process.

Posed by Bloom (1971, 1974), mastery learning is an approach to competency-based learning based on the belief that most learners—regardless of their learning styles and rates—achieve the expected competency if provided time and appropriate learning conditions, which include giving the learner corrective feedback and opportunities to address identified learning gaps. If the learner does not demonstrate the predetermined level of mastery (competency) during a summative assessment, supplemental instruction is provided using alternative learning approaches and additional opportunities for practice (Bloom, 1971). The principles of mastery have been used successfully in teaching skills such as thoracentesis, nasogastric tube insertion, central line dressing changes, and basic life support (Braun et al., 2015; Cason et al., 2015; Dahlen, Finch, & Lambton, 2019) and have demonstrated translational outcomes—outcomes at the patient level (McGaghie, Issenberg, Barsuk, & Wayne, 2014).

Bandura (1977, 2001) discussed the relationship between an individual's behavior and attitudes and the environment to skills acquisition. According to Bandura, the environment includes the physical setting and interactions with others. Bandura's social learning (cognitive) theory (1977, 2001) proposes that behavior is learned through observation and imitation and is influenced by the observed consequences of the behavior. For example, if one observes positive outcomes from a behavior, one is more likely to emulate that behavior. Bandura stressed that optimal learning requires the individual to be proactive and goal-directed and to self-regulate. The self-regulated learner has an intrinsic motivation for learning, participates actively, sets personal learning goals, and engages in reflection. Additionally, the self-regulated learner uses learning outcomes to construct new knowledge. The process of engagement and self-regulation improves as the learner's self-confidence grows. According to Bandura (1977), the educator functions primarily as a role model or facilitator and is responsible for creating an environment conducive to learning.

According to Kolb (1984), the cycle of experiential learning represents the mandatory components for learning and requires a synergistic relationship between the learner and the environment. The cycle includes:

- **The integration of concrete experience:** Real-life experiences

- **Reflective observation:** Reflection or internalization of the experience

- **Abstract conceptualization:** Looking for patterns and meaning

- **Active experimentation:** Assimilation of thoughts in an effort to develop new understanding

Kolb (1984) stressed that learning occurs best in environments that replicate real-life situations that require the learner to seek patterns and meaning to promote insight. Kolb (1984) challenged educators to use various and multiple active strategies to support different learning styles. On a related note, the INACSL standard for simulation design (2016b) discusses the importance of using the appropriate fidelity to create the required perception of realism. This standard addresses the importance of physical, conceptual, and psychological considerations in simulation-based activities to "create the required perception of realism that will allow participants to engage in a relevant manner" (p. s7).

Schön (1987) proposed the use of a "reflective practicum" (p. 18)—an active learning experience based on a realistic event and completed in a realistic environment. Schön (1983) identified two specific types of reflection—reflection-in-action and reflection-on-action:

- *Reflection-in-action (self-monitoring)* occurs when one is engaged in an experience (thinking about an action while doing it). Schön (1987) describes reflection-in-action as the artistry displayed when a practitioner integrates knowledge from past experiences into new situations.

- *Reflection-on-action* (cognitive postmortem) is a conscious review after the experience. The goal of reflection-on-action is to "think back on what we have done" and uncover new understandings with the goal of applying this knowledge to future practice (Schön, 1987, p. 26).

When transferred and applied, reflection-in-action and reflection-on-action become knowing-in-action or knowing-in-practice (Schön, 1987). Knowing-in-action (constructions) is the knowing how or the spontaneous, skillful execution of tasks and/or procedures; it requires anticipation and "on the spot" adjustments. When we recognize knowing-in-action, the action can be converted to knowledge-in-action and yields to further thinking. When embedded into a profession, knowing-in-action can be referred to as knowing-in-practice (Schön, 1987).

According to Schön (1987), educators function as coaches to facilitate active learning and promote learning transfer. A simulation-based activity fulfills the requirements of a "reflective practicum" as discussed by Schön. Using the principles of a reflective practicum, educators can plan the learning experience to encourage reflection-in-action through the use of the Socratic method. The simulation-based environment allows learners to take risks and discover consequences while implementing patient care in a safe environment. Educators can facilitate reflection-on-action during debriefing, which can then be transferred to the patient care setting and be demonstrated as knowing-in-action or knowing-in-practice.

Deliberate practice, posed by Ericsson (2004), is a technique used to develop competence and confidence in clinical skills through purposeful, time-intensive, continued practice. The deliberate practice model (Ericsson, 2004, 2006) emphasizes the importance of time and intentional practice with immediate feedback to improve skill performance. Active learning experience requires problem solving. When engaged in deliberate practice, learners must be self-motivated. The goal of deliberate practice is for the learner to progress to an expert level of performance through constant improvement (Ericsson, 2004). Research has demonstrated that deliberate practice improves cognition, retention, and skills and promotes learning transfer (McGaghie et al., 2014).

Sweller (1988) posed the theory of cognitive load. It emphasizes the importance of effective sequencing. Cognitive load theory states that working memory has a limited capacity to process new information and that learning is impaired when this capacity is overloaded. However, when time is allowed, new knowledge and skills can be acquired, as they can be organized and placed in long-term memory. Therefore, with cognitive theory, an integrated sequencing approach that builds upon previously acquired knowledge and skills should be applied (Fraser, Ayres, & Sweller, 2015; Naismith & Cavalcanti, 2015; Reedy, 2015).

These theories emphasize the synergistic relationship between the learning environment, the learner, the educator/facilitator, and a period of reflection for the development and transfer of new knowledge. The INACSL Standards of Best Practice and the NCSBN Guidelines highlight the importance of formulating a simulation-based activity on a theoretical and/or conceptual framework (Alexander et al., 2015; INACSL, 2016b).

The pedagogy of simulation is grounded in the works of theorists who highlight the dynamic relationships of the learner, the educator, and the environment. Benner, Hooper-Kyriakidis, and Stannard (1999) emphasized this dynamic relationship and discussed the importance of time for reflection when they incorporated the Dreyfus model of skills acquisition into the learning process. The Dreyfus model states that the learner progresses through five levels of learning when acquiring and developing proficiency (Dreyfus & Dreyfus, 1980):

1. Novice

2. Advanced beginner

3. Competent

4. Proficient

5. Expert

However, they stress that experience is not obtained through the mere passage of time but should include the refinement of preconceived ideas through actual clinical practice. According to Dreyfus and Dreyfus (1980), experience facilitates progression through the stages.

Benner et al. (1999) define experiential learning as "clinical learning that is accomplished by being open to having one's expectations refined, challenged, or disconfirmed by the unfolding situation" (p. 568). As stressed by Benner (2000), nursing is a complex practice requiring continuous clinical knowledge development through experiential learning. Therefore, according to Benner and colleagues (1999), nurses who are learning to make good clinical judgments must become engaged in an ongoing process of experiential learning and reflection.

According to Knowles (1984) and Knowles, Holton, and Swanson (2011), adult learning principles that educators need to address when designing a learning experience include:

- Adults are internally motivated.

- Adults have past life experiences and expect these to be appreciated.

- Adults are goal directed.

- Adults expect to see relevancy of the learning.

- Adults want to be respected.

See Table 1.2 for details.

The ultimate goal for learning is the transfer of knowledge, skills, attitudes, and behaviors. Although limited research is available to demonstrate how and if simulation-based learning is transferred to the patient care setting, there are multiple ideas that can be integrated into healthcare. Table 1.3 presents some educational variables that affect the transfer of knowledge and strategies that educators can incorporate into simulated activities to promote this learning transfer.

Table 1.2   Incorporating Adult Learning Principles Into Simulated Experiences

Principle	Strategy
Adults are internally motivated.	Challenge the learner appropriately. For example, scenarios should become progressively more challenging throughout the curriculum.
	Lead the learner to inquiry through Socratic questioning. Ask questions that require deep thinking—questions that begin with why, what if, and what were you thinking when . . . ?
	Allow time for thought and actively listen to learners.
	Provide appropriate, regular, constructive feedback.
	Acknowledge goal attainment.
Adults have past life experiences and expect these to be appreciated.	Acknowledge life experiences and help learners connect these to the learning.
	Facilitate reflective thought using the Socratic method.
Adults are goal directed.	Link experiences to specific goals and expected outcomes.
	Base learning on realistic experiences (case scenarios).
Adults expect to see relevancy of the learning.	Allow learners to assist in designing learning experiences.
	Promote active learning and engagement by using multiple learning strategies.
Adults want to be respected.	Create a respectful, supportive environment.
	Establish an environment of trust to allow learners to express ideas.
	Allow learners to participate in self and peer feedback (peer debriefing).
	Foster active listening.
	Establish ground rules for the learning experience.

Table 1.3   Strategies to Promote Learning Transfer

Learner, Experience, and Environment Variables	Strategies to Promote Learning Transfer
Characteristics of the learner • Intrinsic motivation • Intellectual/cognitive ability • Self-efficacy • Openness or readiness to learn (There is a direct correlation between the listed learner characteristics and the demonstrated ability to transfer learning.)	Allow the learner to have input into the training. Validate usefulness of learning to current healthcare environment. Incorporate strategies that promote self-efficacy. Use Socratic questioning.
Specific stated behavioral objective and expected outcomes (Specific behavior objectives assist learners in directing effort and developing strategies for learning transfer.)	Establish learning objectives and expected outcomes for the experience that are attainable yet challenging. Integrating ground rules helps maintain the integrity of the experience.

continues

Table 1.3 Strategies to Promote Learning Transfer (cont.)	
Learner, Experience, and Environment Variables	**Strategies to Promote Learning Transfer**
Multiple active-learning instructional methodologies (Integrating multiple active-learning instructional methodologies improves the ability to transfer learning.)	Incorporate active learning activities, such as group work or case scenarios. Use various simulation modalities. Segment learning into manageable chunks. Model and demonstrate the desired knowledge, skill, attitude, and behavior changes.
Perceived value and relevance of the experience (The objectives are relevant to the learners, and the activities are structured to facilitate meeting that objective throughout the experience.)	Assist the learner in identifying the relevance of the learning. Assist the learner in transferring the knowledge, skills, and attitude developed through simulation-based learning activities to patient-care situations during debrief by asking "What would you . . . ?" questions. Assist the learner in developing action steps to take to implement the learned knowledge, skills, and behaviors.
Degree of practice and feedback (Focused practice and the integration of appropriate, regular feedback promotes learning transfer.)	Include deliberate practice into the experience. Provide positive yet corrective feedback. Incorporate periodic one-on-one coaching. Incorporate peer coaching and feedback.
Opportunity to apply learning (Develop active application methods and skills to identify opportunities for practice before, during, or after the learning session.)	Integrate a mixture of skills and knowledge into simulation-based activities. Provide opportunities for learners to apply new knowledge and skills to a situation as soon as possible after the learning.
Supportive work environment and commitment of the organization (Individuals who work in an environment that acknowledges new knowledge and skills demonstrate greater learning transfer.)	Recognize learning and provide incentives for it. (These could be financial or job-related, such as clinical ladder recognition.) Allow individuals to provide in-service education to colleagues to highlight new learning. Assist learners in recognizing their importance to the work setting.

In summary, the goal of experiential learning is for the learner to gain new ideas, knowledge, skills, and insight from experience. Under the principles of experiential learning, a simulated experience should be participant-centered, driven by appropriate objectives based on the learner's knowledge, and require active participation and engagement in reflection (INACSL, 2016b). As stressed by the NCSBN, simulation is a pedagogy that requires faculty to be adequately trained, that an appropriate learning environment and resources be provided, that realistic vignettes be used, and that debriefing based on a theoretical model occurs (Alexander et al., 2015).

Legal and Ethical Issues

Healthcare providers face many challenges:

- They must constantly keep up with new advances in technology.
- They must care for patients who have complex diseases.
- They must make split-second critical decisions with incomplete or inaccurate information.

These challenges are often the result of lack of communication and teamwork (IOM, 2011). A 2011 IOM report states that although progress had been noted on these challenges, the emphasis of interprofessional collaboration and communication to meet the complex needs of the population must continue. Nurses must continue to develop skills and competencies both in leadership and innovation, which requires collaboration with other healthcare professionals (IOM, 2015).

Communication and teamwork are addressed in many of The Joint Commission's 2020 National Patient Safety Goals (TJC, 2020). Improving the accuracy of patient identification is Goal 1 of all programs. In addition, the 2020 National Patient Safety Goals for hospital programs, ambulatory care programs, and office-based surgical programs all include improving the safety of using medications, reducing the risk of healthcare-associated infections, and the universal protocol for preventing wrong site, wrong procedure, and wrong person surgery.

An unforgettable IOM report published in 2000 called *To Err Is Human* stated that at least 44,000 people—and perhaps as many as 98,000—die in hospitals each year because of preventable mistakes by healthcare providers. That report revealed just how unsafe our healthcare system was. As noted by the report:

> The Quality of Health Care in America Committee of the Institute of Medicine (IOM) concluded that it is not acceptable for patients to be harmed by the healthcare system that is supposed to offer healing and comfort—a system that promises "First, do no harm."
> (IOM, 2000, p. 2)

This problem prompted healthcare regulatory and standards organizations to investigate its causes as well as what needed to be done to solve it. One answer was to change how healthcare professionals were trained. The times of didactic lectures to teach healthcare professionals how to deal with crises or rare situations are long gone. Active learning is needed to promote patient safety. Simulation introduces interesting and ethical education without the use of real patients, and with every bit of safety. Simulation has also improved risk management among healthcare providers (Sarfati et al., 2018).

The American Nurses Association (ANA) Code of Ethics for Nurses (2015) guides nurses in pursuing ethical behavior and decision-making. Nurses must respect human dignity and are held accountable and responsible for nursing judgment and actions. Above all, they are responsible for providing the most compassionate and competent care to meet all the health needs and concerns of their patients (ANA, 2015). The Code of Ethics for Nurses also stresses that nurse educators are directly responsible for ensuring that nursing students have achieved basic competencies prior to entry into practice (ANA, 2015).

This raises an important question: Is it ethical and legal to place healthcare providers into the clinical setting if they lack the training and experience to handle uncertainty and contingencies of practice for which they can prepare but never wholly predict? "Perhaps simulation's greatest value lies in providing access to the realities of a profession while providing protection from the consequences of error" (Strevens, Grimes, & Phillips, 2016, p. xvi). The simulated clinical setting allows learners to practice skills and experience different healthcare scenarios as many times as needed to achieve a level of comfort and competence to safely perform care in an actual clinical setting.

Benner et al. (2010) state that an adequate and credible process for assessing a nurse's skills and competencies is needed to prevent incidents that can lead to patient harm. The NLN (2019) defines *competence* as "the application of knowledge and interpersonal, decision-making and psychomotor skills in the performance of a task or implementation of a role" (p. 1) and stresses the importance of using reliable and valid instruments to assess these competencies. The Quality and Safety Education for Nurses (QSEN) project identifies patient-centered care, teamwork and collaboration, evidence-based practice, quality improvement, safety, and informatics as quality and safety competencies (QSEN Institute, 2012).

Simulation training helps identify ethical issues that can arise for healthcare providers (Carlson, 2011). These include the following:

- **Beneficence** is the moral obligation to respond in manners of benefit to others (Beauchamp & Childress, 2016). Pinar and Peksoy (2016) stress that beneficence is a moral obligation based in patient advocacy. Educators are challenged to ensure all providers have access to simulation-based

activities to develop the competence needed to provide safe, reliable, and effective care as a collaborative member of a healthcare team (Pinar & Peksoy, 2016).

- **Nonmaleficence** means doing no harm to others, whether it be emotional, physical, or financial (Beauchamp & Childress, 2016). Educators should provide simulation-based activities providing learners opportunities to engage in challenging realistic experiences prior to experience in actual patient care settings (Pinar & Peksoy, 2016).

- **Autonomy** means respecting the right of individuals to make their own decisions. Pertaining to health, this means ensuring that patients are given and understand all the information necessary to make the best possible decision (Beauchamp & Childress, 2016). Simulation-based activities could be designed to require learners to seek approval from the "patient" and protect the patient's freedom to choose and act voluntarily (Pinar & Peksoy, 2016).

- **Justice** is offering equal, fair, and proper treatment to patients (Beauchamp & Childress, 2016). Pinar and Peksoy (2016) state that individuals have a right to the equal and fair distribution of resources. Therefore, the principle of justice should be highlighted when proposals are submitted and in developing policy. A question to consider: Is it the simulation community's obligation to investigate innovative methods to provide sustainability and services?

Just as nurses are confronted with ethical dilemmas, simulationists face ethical challenges of their own. Research has indicated that educators and learners enjoy using simulation and develop increased confidence and ethical comportment. However, very little is known about simulation's role in transferring clinical judgment and ethical values to the patient care setting (Pinar & Peksoy, 2016). The *Healthcare Simulationist Code of Ethics* from SSH has begun to address this challenge (Park & Murphy, 2018). This code of ethics promotes and strengthens the ethical culture of individuals and organizations engaging in simulation. It recommends that all educational activities using simulation as a learning strategy be upheld to the highest ethical standards. The six values included in the *Healthcare Simulationist Code of Ethics* are as follows (Park & Murphy, 2018):

- Integrity
- Transparency
- Mutual respect
- Professionalism
- Accountability
- Results orientation

Conclusion

Clinical judgment and mastery of skills (technical and nontechnical) are necessary to provide safe, competent patient care. Educators are challenged to use evidence-based teaching strategies to promote the learner's clinical judgment. An experiential learning strategy, simulation provides a unique tool to promote clinical judgment. Simulation-based learning is consistent with experiential learning theory in that it requires interactivity, builds on prior knowledge, implements an ethical culture, and ensures knowledge transfer to provide safe, reliable, and effective care as a collaborative member of a healthcare team.

References

Aebersold, M. (2016). The history of simulation and its impact on the future. *AACN Advanced Critical Care, 27*(1), 56-61. doi:10.4037/aacnacc2016436

Aebersold, M. (2018). Simulation-based learning: No longer a novelty in undergraduate education. *Online Journal of Issues in Nursing, 23*(2). doi:10.3912/OJIN.Vol23No02PPT39

Alexander, M., Durham, C. F., Hooper, J. I., Jeffries, P. R., Goldman, N., Kardong-Edgren, S., ... Tillman, C. L. (2015). NCSBN simulation guidelines for prelicensure nursing programs. *Journal of Nursing Regulation, 6*(3), 39-42. doi:10.1016/S2155-8256(15)30783-3

American Nurses Association. (2015). *Code of ethics for nurses with interpretive statements*. Silver Spring, MD: Author.

Association of American Medical Colleges. (2019). 2019 update: The complexities of physician supply and demand: Projections from 2017 to 2032. Retrieved from https://www.aamc.org/data-reports/workforce/data/2019-update-complexities-physician-supply-and-demand-projections-2017-2032

Bandura, A. (1977). Self-efficacy: Toward a unifying theory of behavioral change. *Psychological Review, 84*(2), 191-215. doi:10.1037/0033-295X.84.2.191

Bandura, A. (2001). Social cognitive theory: An agentive perspective. *Annual Review of Psychology, 52*, 1-26. doi:10.1146/annurev.psych.52.1.1

Beauchamp, T. L., & Childress, J. F. (2016). *Principles of biomedical ethics* (7th ed.). New York, NY: Oxford University Press.

Benner, P. (2000). The wisdom of our practice. *American Journal of Nursing, 100*(10), 99-101.

Benner, P., Hooper-Kyriakidis, P., & Stannard, D. (1999). *Clinical wisdom and interventions in critical care: A thinking-in-action approach*. Philadelphia, PA: W. B. Saunders Company.

Benner, P., Sutphen, M., Leonard, V., & Day, L. (2010). *Educating nurses: A call for radical transformation*. San Francisco, CA: Jossey-Bass.

Black, S. E. (2018). Obstetric emergencies: Enhancing the multidisciplinary team through simulation. *British Journal of Midwifery, 26*(2), 96-102.

Bloom, B. S. (1971). Mastery learning. In J. H. Block (Ed.), *Mastery learning: Theory and practice* (pp. 47–63). New York, NY: Holt, Rinehart and Winston.

Bloom, B. S. (1974). Time and learning. *American Psychologist, 29*(9), 682–688.

Bradley, P. (2006). The history of simulation in medical education and possible future directions. *Medical Education, 40*(3), 254-262.

Braun, L., Sawyer, T., Smith, K., Hsu, A., Behrens, M., Chan, D., ... Lopreiato, J. (2015). Retention of pediatric resuscitation performance after a simulation-based mastery learning session: A multicenter randomized trial. *Pediatric Critical Care Medicine, 16*(2), 131-138. doi:10.1097/PCC.0000000000000315

Cant, R. P., & Cooper, S. J. (2017). Use of simulation-based learning in undergraduate nurse education: An umbrella systematic review. *Nurse Education Today, 49*, 63-71. doi:10.1016/j.nedt.2016.11.015

Carlson, E. (2011). Ethical consideration surrounding simulation-based competency training. *Journal of Illinois Nursing, 109*(3), 11-14.

Cason, M. L., Gilbert, G. E., Schmoll, H. H., Dolinar, S. M., Anderson, J., Nickles, B. M., ... Schaefer III, J. J. (2015). Cooperative learning using simulation to achieve mastery of nasogastric tube insertion. *Journal of Nursing Education, 54*(3 Suppl.), S47-51. doi:10.3928/01484834-20150218-09

Cato, M. L. (2012). Using simulation in nursing education. In P. R. Jeffries (Ed.), *Simulation in nursing education from conceptualization to evaluation* (pp. 1-12). New York, NY: National League for Nursing.

Cooper, J., & Taqueti, V. (2004). A brief history of the development of mannequin simulators for clinical education and training. *Quality and Safety in Health Care, 13*(Suppl. 1), i11-i18. doi:10.1136/qshc.2004.009886

Dahlen, B., Finch, M., & Lambton, J. (2019). Simulation-based mastery learning for central venous line dressing changes. *Clinical Simulation in Nursing, 27*, 35-38. doi:10.1016/j.ecns.2018.10.010

D'Alimonte, L., McLaney, E., & Di Prospero, L. (2019). Best practices on team communication: Interprofessional practice in oncology. *Current Opinion in Supportive and Palliative Care, 13*(1), 69-74. doi:10.1097/SPC.0000000000000412

Dewey, J. (1910). *How we think*. Boston, MA: D. C. Heath & Co..

Dewey, J. (1916). *Democracy in education*. Radford. VA: Wilder Publications LLC.

Dewey, J. (1933). *How we think: A restatement of the relation of reflective thinking to the educative process*. Boston, MA: D. C. Heath & Co.

Doolen, J., Mariani, B., Atz, T., Horsley, T. L., O'Rourke, J., McAfee, K., & Cross. C. L. (2016). High-fidelity simulation in undergraduate nursing education: A review of simulation reviews. *Clinical Simulation in Nursing, 12*(7), 290-302. doi:10.1016/j.ecns.2016.01.009

Dreyfus, S. E., & Dreyfus, H. L. (1980). *A five-stage model of the mental activities involved in directed skill acquisition*. Berkeley, CA: University of California. Retrieved from https://apps.dtic.mil/dtic/tr/fulltext/u2/a084551.pdf

Ericsson, K. A. (2004). Deliberate practice and the acquisition and maintenance of expert performance in medicine and related domains. *Academic Medicine, 79*(10, Suppl.), S70-S81.

Ericsson, K. A. (2006). The influence of experience and deliberate practice on the development of superior expert performance. In K. A. Ericsson, N. Charness, R. R. Hoffman, & P. J. Feltovich (Eds.), *The Cambridge handbook of expertise and expert performance* (pp. 683-703). New York, NY: Cambridge University Press.

Frankel, A., Haraden, C., Federico, F., & Lenoci-Edwards, J. (2017). *A framework for safe, reliable, and effective care*. [White Paper.] Cambridge, MA: Institute for Healthcare Improvement and Safe & Reliable Healthcare.

Fraser, K. L., Ayres, P., & Sweller, J. (2015). Cognitive load theory for the design of medical simulations. *Simulation in Healthcare, 10*(5), 295-307. doi:10.1097/SIH.0000000000000097

Gaba, D. M. (2004). The future vision of simulation in health care. *Quality and Safety in Health Care, 13*(Suppl. 1), i2-i10. doi:10.1136/qshc.2004.009878

Hayden, J. K., Smiley, R. A., Alexander, M., Kardong-Edgren, S., & Jeffries, P. R. (2014). The NCSBN national simulation study: A longitudinal, randomized controlled study replacing clinical hours with simulation in prelicensure nursing education. *Journal of Nursing Regulation, 5*(2), S1–S64. Retrieved from https://www.ncsbn.org/JNR_Simulation_Supplement.pdf

Holtschneider, M. E. (2017). Expanding the fidelity of standardized patients in simulation by incorporating wearable technology. *Journal for Nurses in Professional Development, 33*(6), 320-321. doi:10.1097/NND.0000000000000391

Hunter, L. A. (2016). Debriefing and feedback in the current healthcare environment. *The Journal of Perinatal & Neonatal Nursing, 30*(3), 174-178. doi:10.1097/JPN.0000000000000173

Institute of Medicine. (2000). *To err is human: Building a safer health system*. Washington, DC: The National Academies Press. Retrieved from https://www.nap.edu/catalog/9728/to-err-is-human-building-a-safer-health-system

Institute of Medicine. (2001). *Crossing the quality chasm: A new health system for the 21st century*. Washington, DC: The National Academies Press. Retrieved from https://www.nap.edu/catalog/10027/crossing-the-quality-chasm-a-new-health-system-for-the

Institute of Medicine. (2003). *Health professions education: A bridge to quality*. Washington, DC: The National Academies Press. Retrieved from http://www.nationalacademies.org/hmd/Reports/2003/health-professions-education-a-bridge-to-quality.aspx

Institute of Medicine. (2004a). *Academic health centers: Leading change in the 21st century*. Washington, DC: The National Academies Press. Retrieved from https://www.nap.edu/catalog/10734/academic-health-centers-leading-change-in-the-21st-century

Institute of Medicine. (2004b). *Keeping patients safe: Transforming the work environment of nurses.* Washington, DC: The National Academies Press. Retrieved from http://www.nationalacademies.org/hmd/Reports/2003/Keeping-Patients-Safe-Transforming-the-Work-Environment-of-Nurses.aspx

Institute of Medicine. (2011). *The future of nursing: Leading change, advancing health.* Washington, DC: The National Academies Press. Retrieved from http://www.nationalacademies.org/hmd/Reports/2010/The-Future-of-Nursing-Leading-Change-Advancing-Health.aspx

Institute of Medicine. (2015). *Assessing progress on the Institute of Medicine report the future of nursing.* Washington, DC: The National Academies Press. Retrieved from http://www.nationalacademies.org/hmd/Reports/2015/Assessing-Progress-on-the-IOM-Report-The-Future-of-Nursing.aspx

International Nursing Association for Clinical Simulation and Learning Standards Committee. (2016a). INACSL standards of best practice: Simulation: Simulation glossary. *Clinical Simulation in Nursing, 12*(S), S39–S47. http://dx.doi.org/10.1016/j.ecns.2016.09.012. Retrieved from https://www.nursingsimulation.org/article/S1876-1399(16)30133-5/pdf

International Nursing Association for Clinical Simulation and Learning Standards Committee. (2016b). INASCL standards of best practice: Simulation participation evaluation. *Clinical Simulation in Nursing, 12,* S26–S29. doi:10.1016/j.ecns.2016.09.009. Retrieved from https://www.inacsl.org/INACSL/document-server/?cfp=INACSL/assets/File/public/standards/SOBPEnglishCombo.pdf

Interprofessional Education Collaborative. (2016). Core competencies for interprofessional collaborative practice: 2016 update. Retrieved from https://hsc.unm.edu/ipe/resources/ipec-2016-core-competencies.pdf

Interprofessional Education Collaborative Expert Panel. (2011). *Core competencies for interprofessional collaborative practice.* Retrieved from https://www.aacom.org/docs/default-source/insideome/ccrpt05-10-11.pdf?sfvrsn=77937f97_2

Issenberg, S. B., McGaghie, W. C., Petrusa, E. R., Lee Gordon, D., & Scalese, R. J. (2005). Features and uses of high-fidelity medical simulations that lead to effective learning: A BEME systematic review. *Medical Teacher, 27*(1), 10–28.

Iverson, L., Bredenkamp, N., Carrico, C., Connelly, S., Hawkins, K., Monaghan, M. S., & Malesker, M. (2018). Development and assessment of an interprofessional education simulation to promote collaborative learning and practice. *Journal of Nursing Education, 57*(7), 426–429. doi:10.3928/01484834-20180618-08

Jeffries, P. R. (2005). A framework for designing, implementing, and evaluating simulations used as teaching strategies in nursing. *Nursing Education Perspectives, 26*(2), 96–103.

Jeffries, P. R. (Ed.) (2012). *Simulation in nursing education, from conceptualization to evaluation* (2nd ed.). New York, NY: National League for Nursing.

Jeffries, P. R., & Rogers, K. J. (2012). Theoretical framework for simulation design. In P. R. Jeffries (Ed.), *Simulation in nursing education from conceptualization to evaluation* (pp. 25–41). New York, NY: National League for Nursing.

Jenson, C. E., & Forsyth, D. M. (2012). Virtual reality simulation: Using three-dimensional technology to teach nursing students. *Computers, Informatics, Nursing, 30*(6), 312–318. doi:10.1097/NXN.0b013e31824af6ae

Johnson, P. (2012). *Socrates: A man for our times.* New York, NY: Penguin Books.

The Joint Commission. (2020). *National patient safety goals.* Retrieved from http://www.Jointcommission.org/standards/national-patient-safety-goals/

Jones, F., Passos-Neto, C. E., & Braghiroli, O. F. M. (2015). Simulation in medical education: Brief history and methodology. *Principles and Practice of Clinical Research, 1*(2), 56–63.

Kardong-Edgren, S., Farra, S. L., Alinier, G., & Young, H. M. (2019). A call to unify definitions of virtual reality. *Clinical Simulation in Nursing, 31,* 28–34.

Knowles, M. S. (1984). *Andragogy in action: Applying modern principles of adult learning.* San Francisco, CA: Jossey-Bass.

Knowles, M. S., Holton, E. F., & Swanson, R. A. (2011). *The adult learner: The definitive classic in adult education and human resource development* (7th ed.). Oxford, UK: Butterworth-Heinemann.

Kolb, D. A. (1984). *Experiential learning: Experience as the source of learning and development.* Englewood Cliffs, NJ: Prentice-Hall.

Leonard, M., Graham, S., & Bonacum, D. (2004). The human factor: The critical importance of effective teamwork and communication in providing safe care. *Quality & Safety in Health Care, 13*(Suppl. 1), i85–i90.

Lewis K. L., Bohnert C. A., Gammon, W. L., Hölzer, H., Lyman, L., Smith, C., … Gliva-McConvey, G. (2017). The Association of Standardized Patient Educators (ASPE) standards of best practice (SOBP). *Advances in Simulation, 2,* 10. doi:10.1186/s41077-017-0043-4. Retrieved from https://advancesinsimulation.biomedcentral.com/articles/10.1186/s41077-017-0043-4

Lewis, R., Strachan, A., & Smith, M. M. (2012). Is high fidelity simulation the most effective method for the development of non-technical skills in nursing? A review of the current evidence. *The Open Nursing Journal, 6,* 82–89. doi:10.2174/1874434601206010082

Lioce, L. (Ed.), Lopreiato, J. (Founding Ed.), Downing, D., Chang, T. P., Robertson, J. M., Anderson, M., … the Terminology and Concepts Working Group. (2020). *Healthcare simulation dictionary* (2nd ed.). Rockville, MD: Agency for Healthcare Research and Quality. AHRQ Publication No. 20-0019. doi: https://doi.org/10.23970/simulationv2

McGaghie, W. C., Issenberg, S. B., Barsuk, J. H., & Wayne, D. B. (2014). A critical review of simulation-based mastery learning with translational outcomes. *Medical Education, 48*(4), 375–385. doi:10.1111/medu.12391

Michael S. Gordon Center for Simulation and Innovation in Medical Education. (n.d.). Next generation Harvey: The cardiopulmonary patient simulator. Retrieved from http://www.gcrme.miami.edu/harvey_features.php

Naismith, L. M., & Cavalcanti, R. B. (2015). Validity of cognitive load measures in simulation-based training: A systematic review. *Academic Medicine, 90*(11 Suppl.), S24–S35. doi:10.1097/ACM.0000000000000893

National League for Nursing. (2015). *A vision for teaching with simulation.* Retrieved from http://www.nln.org/docs/default-source/about/nln-vision-series-(position-statements)/vision-statement-a-vision-for-teaching-with-simulation.pdf?sfvrsn=2

National League for Nursing. (2019). *Hallmarks of excellence.* Retrieved from http://www.nln.org/professional-development-programs/teaching-resources/hallmarks-of-excellence

Pappano, L. (2018, October 31). Training the next generation of doctors and nurses. *The New York Times.* Retrieved from https://www.nytimes.com/2018/10/31/education/learning/next-generation-of-caregivers.html

Park, C. S., & Murphy, T. F. (2018). *Healthcare simulationist code of ethics.* Retrieved from http://www.ssih.org/Code-of-Ethics

Parsons, J. R., Crichlow, A., Ponnuru, S., Shewokis, S., Goswami, P. A., Griswold, V., & Griswold, S. (2018). Filling the gap: Simulation-based crisis resource management training for emergency medical residents. *Western Journal of Emergency Medicine, 19*(1), 205–210. doi:10.5811/westjem.2017.10.35284

Pinar, G., & Peksoy, S. (2016). Simulation-based learning in healthcare ethics education. *Creative Education, 7*(1), 131–138. doi:10.4236/ce.2016.71013. Retrieved from http://file.scirp.org/pdf/CE_2016012816291545.pdf

Quality and Safety Education for Nurses Institute. (2012). QSEN competencies. Retrieved from http://www.qsen.org/competencies/pre-licensure-ksas/

Reedy, G. B. (2015). Using cognitive load theory to inform simulation design and practice. *Clinical Simulation in Nursing, 11*(8), 355–360. doi:10.1016/j.ecns.2015.05.004

Rodgers, D. L. (2007). *High-fidelity patient simulation: A descriptive white paper report.* [White Paper.] Charleston, WV: Healthcare Simulation Strategies.

Rutherford-Hemming, T., Alfes, C. M., Breymier, T. L. (2019). A systematic review of the use of standardized patients as a simulation modality in nursing education. *Nursing Education Perspectives, 40*(2), 84–90. doi:10.1097/01.NEP.0000000000000401

Sarfati, L., Ranchon, F., Vantard, N., Schwiertz, V., Larbre, V., Parat, S, … Rioufol, C. (2018) Human-simulation-based learning to prevent medication error: A systematic review. *Journal of Evaluation in Clinical Practice, 25*(1), 11–20. doi:10.1111/jep.12883

Schön, D. A. (1983). *The reflective practitioner: How professionals think in action.* New York, NY: Basic Books.

Schön, D. A. (1987). *Educating the reflective practitioner: Toward a new design for teaching and learning in the professions.* Hoboken, NJ: Wiley.

Strevens, C., Grimes, R., & Phillips, E. (2016). *Legal education: Simulation in theory and practice.* London, UK: Routledge.

Sweller, J. (1988). Cognitive load during problem solving: Effects on learning. *Cognitive Science, 12*(2), 257–285. doi:10.1207/s15516709cog1202_4

United States Medical Licensing Examination. (2012). *2013 USMLE bulletin of information.* Philadelphia, PA: Federation of State Medical Boards (FSMB) and National Board of Medical Examiners (NBME). Retrieved from http://www.usmle.org/pdfs/bulletin/2013bulletin.pdf

US Bureau of Labor Statistics. (2019). *Occupational outlook handbook, registered nurses.* Washington, DC: US Bureau of Labor Statistics. Retrieved from http://www.bls.gov/ooh/healthcare/registered-urses.htm

Walsh, C., Lydon, S., Byrne, D., Madden, C., Fox, S., & O'Connor, P. (2018). The 100 most cited articles on healthcare simulation: A bibliometric review. *Simulation in Healthcare, 13*(3), 211–220. doi:10.1097/SIH.0000000000000293

World Health Organization. (2013). *Transforming and scaling up health professions' education and training: World Health Organization guidelines 2013.* Retrieved from https://apps.who.int/iris/bitstream/handle/10665/93635/9789241506502_eng.pdf?sequence=1

"Experience tells you what to do; confidence allows you to do it."

–Stan Smith

Developing Clinical Competence and Confidence

2

Pamela Andreatta, EdD, PhD, MFA, MA, FSSH
Jody R. Lori, PhD, CNM, FACNM, FAAN

OBJECTIVES

- Discuss the relationship between confidence and competence and how simulation can close the gap between the two.

- Understand how simulation can be used to motivate and build confidence in clinical performance.

- Discuss the value of simulation-based methods for acquiring and maintaining competence.

- Describe the ways simulation can be used to build self-assessment skills.

- Discuss instructional considerations for simulation-based methods that support the acquisition and maintenance of clinical competence and confidence.

The purpose of any instruction is to effect change in learners' knowledge, skills, or attitudes that subsequently alters their behaviors. The underpinnings for all human learning lay in several psychological, biological, physical, and environmental constructs. For example, the learner's self-concept of his or her ability to learn (psychological), health status (biological), and any disability (physical) influence learning.

Educators may choose to make accommodations to support these individual influences, but the primary role of an educator is to create an environment that facilitates learning. The environment in which instruction takes place significantly affects learning and can have an impact on the benefits of simulation-based instruction—experiential, situated, multimodal, on-demand, safe, and so on. This is covered in more detail in Chapter 3.

The desired learning outcome of simulation-based instruction in healthcare is to change (improve) learners' behavior in applied clinical practice. Two primary factors that influence behavior in applied practice are:

- Confidence in one's ability to perform what is required

- Competence to correctly perform what is required

Simulation-based instruction supports both these factors. In particular, it can significantly improve the acquisition and maintenance of competence beyond current training systems. This chapter discusses each of these factors independently and then examines the influence of their interaction on learning and instruction.

Confidence

For the purpose of this discussion, *confidence* is defined as learners' conscious and subconscious beliefs about their ability to successfully perform what is required to achieve a favorable outcome in a clinical context.

Conceptually, confidence is related to these theoretical constructs (among others):

- Self-efficacy (Bandura, 1977)

- Self-awareness (Duval & Silvia, 2002)

- Perceptual integration (Stemme, Deco, & Lang, 2011)

- Critical-thinking skills (Dumitru, 2012)

- Motivation to learn (Dweck & Leggett, 1988; Keller, 2008; Pintrich, 1999, 2003, 2004)

- Self-regulation (Bandura, 1991; Carver, 2006)

These theories explore various individual state and trait characteristics that influence a learner's self-perception of ability to perform in a specific context. They examine various individual factors that contribute to the learning process; however, they are difficult to address through instruction alone. Two advantages of simulation-based methods are that they may help learners gain confidence by improving their ability to more accurately self-assess, and they motivate learners to continue through the learning process by increasing the expectancy factor associated with motivation (Judge & Bono, 2001; Nadler, Lawler III, Steers, & Porter, 1977; Vroom, 1964).

Self-Assessment

The ability of learners to self-assess is key to developing both confidence and competence. An inability to self-assess can lead to overconfidence, which impedes further learning and can adversely affect patient and clinician safety. Simulation-based methods help learners gain confidence by improving their ability to more accurately self-assess.

Self-assessment is defined as a process by which learners observe and evaluate their own progress toward performance objectives (Andrade & Valtcheva, 2009). Learners compare the results of their performances against explicit standards, criteria, or objectives and seek to improve, maintain, or advance their abilities depending on the quality of their performance. The ability to identify one's own performance strengths and weaknesses is essential to promote learning and achievement as well as to inform an accurate perception of confidence.

Unfortunately, humans do not have an inherent ability to self-assess. Moreover, techniques for self-assessment are rarely taught in the health sciences. For example, the preponderance of evidence suggests that physicians have a limited ability to accurately self-assess (Davis et al., 2006). Research has demonstrated inaccuracy in self-assessment (Dunning, Heath, & Suls, 2004; Nemec, 2010). While hindsight bias may also be a natural problem in the area of self-assessment using simulation, without a recorded experience, this bias would be more problematic (Motavalli & Nestel, 2016). Healthcare simulation often records the case for video playback, which may decrease some inaccuracies in self-assessment.

Without the mechanisms to accurately self-assess, learners are far less likely to succeed at self-regulated learning, which is learner-centered instruction that supports independent engagement with the learning processes. With self-regulated learning, instructional methods facilitate access to content, instructional events, and social engagements that support the learning process, but the pacing and sequencing of the instruction is left for the learner to decide. Self-regulated learning environments have several advantages—perhaps most notably the ability of learners to access course material at any time and as often as they want. However, there are also disadvantages, such as learners being ill-prepared for this level of independent control over their learning processes.

Educators can help learners develop the ability to self-assess by providing explicit standards with straightforward performance metrics. In addition, educators can offer timely and specific feedback about how learners performed compared to the standards and recommend activities to help learners improve performance (Cunningham, Wright, & Baird, 2015). Nestel, Bello, and Kneebone (2013) propose seven feedback principles that support self-regulation in simulation-based instruction:

- Defining good performance
- Facilitating self-assessment
- Delivering high-quality feedback information
- Encouraging teacher and peer dialogue
- Encouraging positive motivation and self-esteem
- Providing opportunities to close the gap between actual and desired performance
- Using feedback to improve teaching

Feedback about performance can be provided by educators, independent assessors, peers, or through metrics issued by the performance context directly. The latter is a significant incentive for simulation-based instruction because it helps learners develop the ability to self-assess by comparing their subjective interpretation to objective metrics provided by the simulator itself. As learners further develop their ability to self-assess, their confidence level tends to correlate more closely with their performance. This in turn encourages continued engagement (motivation) with the content domain.

Motivation

Motivation is an internal state that directs an individual's goal-oriented behavior. Learners choose to pursue what motivates them. Through that choice, they direct their attention (Wickens, 1991; Young & Stanton, 2002). Motivational factors include the intensity of the internal state (weak–strong) and the direction of the state (negative–positive). For example, one learner may be highly motivated to achieve objective A, whereas another might wish to achieve the same objective but desire objective B even more. Likewise, one learner may strongly want to avoid the recriminations of failure, whereas other learners may not care whether they fail or not.

Numerous factors affect an individual's predisposition to engage in the learning process:

- **Biological:** Thirst, hunger, pain, fatigue, etc.
- **Affective:** Anxious, depressed, calm, happy, etc.
- **Cognitive:** Interest, desire to solve problems, etc.
- **Conative:** Dreams, desires to control life, etc.
- **Behavioral:** Rewards, fame, fortune, kudos, etc.
- **Spiritual:** Humanistic need to grow, self-actual, God-fearing, etc.

The degree to which motivation can be influenced by instruction depends on whether the motivating patterns are a trait or state for an individual.

Techniques to Support Learner Motivation

- Help learners understand the value of what they are being asked to do in both the short and long term.

- Inform learners about what exactly needs to be accomplished and the standard of performance.

- Set short-term objectives with sequentially increased complexity.

- Provide written and verbal acknowledgment of effort and outcomes.

- Use formative assessment to help learners advance and use summative assessment judiciously.

- Capitalize on the arousal value of surprise, suspense, discovery, curiosity, and exploration by occasionally doing the unexpected.

- Use familiar examples in unique and unexpected contexts when applying concepts and principles.

- Reinforce previous learning by including concepts in subsequent activities.

- Minimize unpleasant consequences of learner involvement or the learning environment.

- Encourage a bit of fun!

Motivational patterns include traits (stable) and states (unstable)—each of which may be either innate or learned. Examples of innate traits include curiosity, anxiety, and sexual attraction, whereas examples of learned traits include aspiration of power, need to achieve, and desire for affiliation. Innate states include hunger, thirst, fear, etc., whereas learned states include factors such as test anxiety, overconfidence, stage fright, etc.

Further complicating the motivational soup is an individual's attribution of successes or failures— that is, the learner's personal agency (Bandura, 2001). Learners may have an intrinsic, extrinsic, or mixed motivation orientation (locus of control; Rotter, 1954):

- **Intrinsic motivation orientation:** Learners with an intrinsic orientation (internal locus of control) are motivated by internal factors and rewards. They compare their current performance against their previous performance. These learners are frequently satisfied with unobservable rewards.

- **Extrinsic motivation orientation:** Learners with an extrinsic orientation (external locus of control) are motivated by external factors and rewards and compare their performance to that of others. These learners are motivated by observable rewards.

- **Mixed motivation orientation:** Learners with a mixed orientation may be intrinsically motivated in some contexts and extrinsically motivated in others.

Attribution theory describes how learners explain their successes and failures to themselves (Weiner, 2010). Similar to the concept of motivational orientation, attribution refers to learners' beliefs about the amount of control they have over performance outcomes and whether those outcomes are due to internal factors or external factors. Learners who believe they do not have control may attribute performance outcomes to their innate ability (internal) or luck (external). Learners who believe they do have control over performance outcomes may attribute results to their efforts (internal) or the difficulty of the performance task (external).

Expectancy has also been shown to influence motivation. Simulation-based methods can motivate learners to continue through the learning process by increasing expectancy factors associated with motivation. These factors include awareness of choices and application of skills, knowledge, abilities, personalities, as well as the acquisition of these experiences (Judge & Bono, 2001; Nadler et al., 1977; Vroom, 1964).

The expectancy-value theory of achievement motivation (Fishbein & Ajzen, 1975; Wigfield & Eccles, 2000) supports the organization of these multiple factors into a simple model:

> This theory postulates that learners will be motivated by their perceptions of the likelihood that their efforts will lead to the necessary performance in a desired area and that their performance will be rewarded. In this model:

- *Value* is described as the present or future worth of an outcome to an individual.

- *Expectancy* is described as an individual's sense of confidence or efficacy that an outcome will be successful.

- *Motivation* can thus be viewed as a product of learners' expectancy of achievement if they engage in the learning process and the value placed on the learning outcomes.

Motivating other people to engage in a learning process (instruction) is difficult because motivation is an individual thing. What motivates one person might not necessarily motivate another—or worse, it might demotivate another. Ideally, instruction that provides learners with a moderate challenge has the greatest likelihood of supporting motivation. This is because a moderate challenge increases the expectancy factor without decreasing the value factor, and the challenge level of activities is within the educator's control. Some techniques that can support learner motivation are included in the sidebar on page 26.

Confidence Continuum

Motivation and the ability to self-assess influence learner confidence, but confidence is dynamic. It varies depending on workload, learning curves, and acquired expertise.

Figure 2.1 illustrates the relationships between confidence and expertise. As shown in the figure:

- Novices do not possess much confidence in their abilities in an instructional domain.

- Learners at an intermediate performance level may be quite confident in their abilities—but this confidence is likely the result of not knowing what they don't know. For example, an intra-operative study of stress levels for residents and attending surgeons showed that attending surgeons experienced significantly greater stress than their more junior trainees because they were able to perceive what was actually occurring during the case as well as the potential for error (Goldman, McDonough, & Rosemond, 1972).

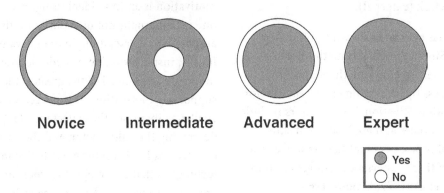

FIGURE 2.1   Perceived learner performance confidence at sequential levels of expertise.

- Advanced learners tend to be confident, although a minimal number remain reticent until they achieve the level of domain expert.

- Most expert performers are confident in their abilities to perform in their domain of expertise and have demonstrated the ability to accurately self-assess their abilities.

The overconfidence of intermediate performers is an area of study in clinical education, primarily because of the potential risks to both patient and clinician safety. Although numerous educational studies measure confidence changes as indicative of a successful outcome, further studies evaluating the uses of retrospective self-assessment suggest the existence of a gap between intermediate and advanced learners in their ability to self-assess and therefore their perceived confidence (Bhanji, Gottesman, de Grave, Steinert, & Winer, 2012; Hewson, Copeland, & Fishleder, 2001; Levinson, Gordon, & Skeff, 1990). Although confidence

is necessary for learners to perform in a given context, it is not sufficient for assessing their abilities to perform in a domain of interest. Assessment of whether or not learners can perform competently is necessary. Fortunately, this is where simulation adds value to healthcare.

Competence

Confidence is one's own belief about one's abilities. Competence is one's actual ability to successfully perform what is required to achieve a favorable outcome in a clinical context.

The American Nurses Association (ANA, 2014) defines a *competency* as "an expected level of performance that integrates knowledge, skills, abilities, and judgment" (p. 2). Knowledge, skills, ability, and judgment are defined as follows (ANA, 2014, p. 4):

- *Knowledge* encompasses thinking, understanding of science and humanities, professional standards of practice, and insights gained from context, practical experiences, personal capabilities, and leadership performance.

- *Skills* include psychomotor, communication, interpersonal, and diagnostic skills.

- *Ability* is the capacity to act effectively. It requires listening, integrity, knowledge of one's strengths and weaknesses, positive self-regard, emotional intelligence, and openness to feedback.

- *Judgment* includes critical thinking, problem solving, ethical reasoning, and decision-making.

Educators play a critical role in acquisition of competence (Sadeghi, Oshvandi, & Moradi, 2019). As health profession educators or professionals, it is our responsibility to create processes for ensuring competency in our health workforce

(ANA, 2014). Figure 2.2 illustrates examples of performance competencies required in clinical practice.

Determining competence requires performance-based assessment in the clinical contexts of interest, which is easier said than done. Clinical contexts are rarely amenable to measuring the performance of multiple clinicians in the process of attending to the needs of multiple patients. Additionally, performance metrics for clinical care task completion, reasoning, and decision-making are for the most part poorly defined and rely on subjective and culturally determined parameters. In a chicken/egg-type analogy, the variability of the clinical context confounds the specification of performance metrics, which in turn challenges performance in the clinical context. Simulation provides an opportunity to control some of the contextual variability by establishing parameters for clinicians even as patient characteristics remain variable.

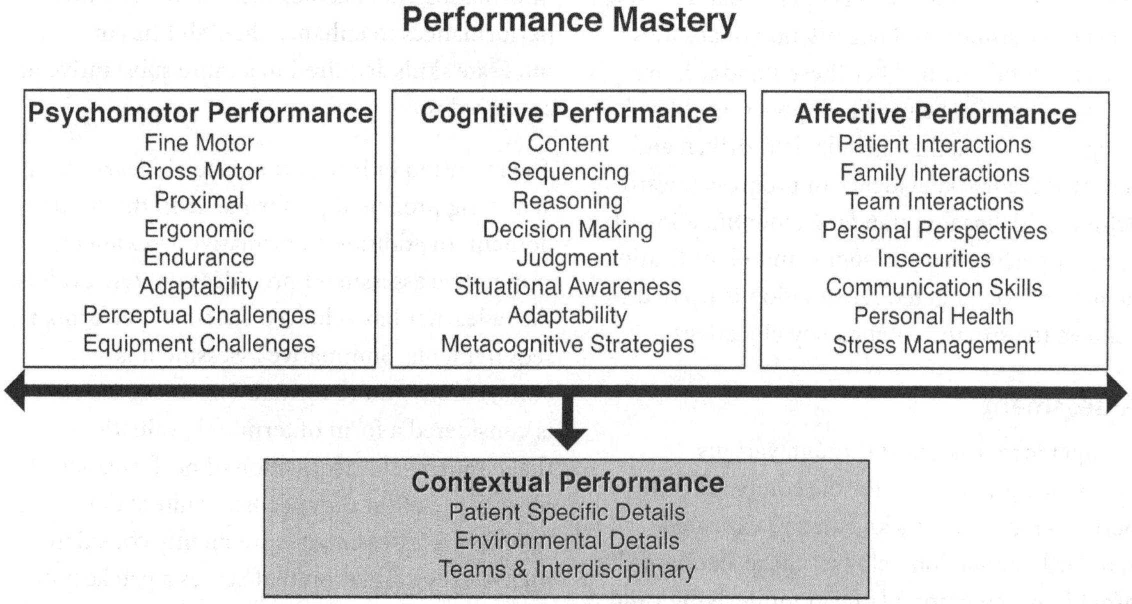

Performance Mastery

Psychomotor Performance	Cognitive Performance	Affective Performance
Fine Motor	Content	Patient Interactions
Gross Motor	Sequencing	Family Interactions
Proximal	Reasoning	Team Interactions
Ergonomic	Decision Making	Personal Perspectives
Endurance	Judgment	Insecurities
Adaptability	Situational Awareness	Communication Skills
Perceptual Challenges	Adaptability	Personal Health
Equipment Challenges	Metacognitive Strategies	Stress Management

Contextual Performance
Patient Specific Details
Environmental Details
Teams & Interdisciplinary

FIGURE 2.2 Examples of performance requirements in clinical practice.

Repetitive performance measurements by experts in a domain of interest define performance metrics in the given domain (Cizek & Bunch, 2007; Hambleton, Jaeger, Plake, & Mills, 2000; McKinley, Boulet, & Hambleton, 2005). The apprenticeship model of clinical training necessitates that instructors prioritize ethical and optimal patient care over performance repetition for learners. Simulation provides a foundation from which performance can be measured because the contextual aspects of patient care can be replicated without the essential prioritization of a real patient's needs.

Simulation facilitates the repetitive acquisition of performance data. Simulation also controls for extraneous variables such as comorbidities that might affect performance during actual patient care. Educators need these data to derive and validate the rigorous performance standards that establish the foundation of competency assessment. Simulation facilitates the ability of educators to establish standards of performance and enables them to establish performance curves for the acquisition and degradation of abilities in a content domain. After these standards are defined, they can be used to support multilevel learning contexts that include data-driven and repeated feedback, evidence of progress toward achieving delineated standards, identification of areas of performance strength, and identification of areas where targeted remediation is needed to achieve the specific competency objectives.

Assessment

Competence is assessed through various mechanisms that allow for the comparison of performance against a known and expected standard. Simulation helps set those standards by providing a common platform for deriving valid and reliable performance metrics and associated assessment mechanisms. Assessment is an essential activity for gaining competence.

Formative assessment is an iterative process that provides information to learners and educators about how well the learner is progressing through the instruction. It provides evidence as to the degree to which the learner is acquiring the requisite cognitive, psychomotor, and affective aspects of the content domain. The dependency factor for learning is therefore whether performance objectives are achieved at each sequential step of the learning process. Learners who are given specific feedback about their progress at regular intervals will be better able to identify what they have learned well and what requires improvement before moving to the next level (self-assessment). This affords them the opportunity to spend additional time in those areas in which performance is less than optimal before continuing on. Formative assessment may be formal or informal, but it always includes elements that provide learners with specific information that enables them to modify their performances to enhance their abilities or integrate skills acquired in a more substantive or advanced way.

The intention of instruction is to aid learners in achieving proficient performance in the content domain. In addition to formative assessment, summative assessment provides concrete evidence that a learner has achieved specified performance requirements. Summative assessment is almost always more formal. This is because it is considered a form of terminal evaluation that confirms the acquisition of performance objectives within the specified content domain. Summative assessment is frequently considered a high-stakes evaluation that serves a gatekeeping function. Therefore, the statistical reliability and validity of summative assessment mechanisms are more rigorous than those for formative assessment. Although considerable data must be assembled before simulation-based assessment can serve this summative function, the contextual consistency of simulation is instrumental to collecting these data and establishing accurate contextual performance standards. Thus, simulation-based methods serve to provide immediate feedback about performance against the known standard (formative) as well as inform the development of credentialing and certification requirements.

Acquiring and Maintaining Competence

Learners acquire competence by achieving explicit cognitive, psychomotor, or affective objectives under the guidance and supervision of an instructor. New learning builds upon that which has already been attained, in the same way a house is built upon a foundation. If the foundation is weak (poor prerequisite abilities), the walls of the house will also be weak (poorly learned abilities). Optimal instruction includes explicit learning objectives, specific performance criteria, and assessment opportunities that allow learners to achieve their objectives and to avoid the loss of learning time because of knowledge gaps.

Numerous theoretical constructs describe the acquisition of abilities through instruction. Three have significant relevance for simulation-based learning environments:

- Experiential learning

- Deliberate practice

- Reflective practice

The foundation of experiential learning theory is that experience plays a central role in the cycle of learning. That is, a learner has an experience, the experience promotes observation and reflection, and the observation and reflection transform the experience into abstractions. The learner then actively tests these abstractions, which leads to further experiences. Learning experiences may be formal or informal, directed or flexible, derived from standards, or organic in nature (Kolb, 1984). The common component of all experiential-learning environments is the active engagement of the learner toward assembling, analyzing, and synthesizing perceptual cues stemming from the instructional context. The theoretical supposition is that instructional designs that encourage learners to have a variety of relevant experiences will lead to improved outcomes. Simulation-based instruction presents multiple experiences of different modalities and forms but within the desired content domain. This enables learners to consider the content through different perspectives that subsequently lead to deeper understanding while at the same time ensuring patient safety.

Deliberate practice theory proposes that deep expertise is developed through highly motivated learners engaging in concentrated repetitive practice tied to well-defined objectives (Ericsson, 2004, 2011; Ericsson & Charness, 1994; Ericsson, Nandagopal, & Roring, 2009; Hunt et al., 2014; Taras & Everett, 2017). Learners actively and incrementally refine their performances using feedback and guidance provided by an expert coach until they achieve proficiency. The key features of deliberate practice include:

- Repetition

- Feedback

- Motivation
- Establishing clear challenges at the right level of difficulty

A simulated environment facilitates the iterative performance-feedback loop necessary for developing abilities through deliberate practice. This is especially beneficial for the acquisition of psychomotor skills, high-order cognitive processing and critical thinking, and team-based practice behaviors. Empirical evidence strongly suggests that simulation-based deliberate practice is more effective than learning procedural skills through traditional, clinical-based instruction (Andreatta, Chen, Marsh, & Cho, 2011; Andreatta, Saxton, Thompson, & Annich, 2011; Barsuk, Cohen, McGaghie, & Wayne, 2010; Issenberg, McGaghie, Petrusa, Lee Gordon, & Scalese, 2005; McGaghie, Issenberg, Cohen, Barsuk, & Wayne, 2011; McGaghie, Issenberg, Petrusa, & Scalese, 2006; Wayne et al., 2012).

Reflective practice refers to the process by which learners deliberately think about their own individual experiences to learn from them. Reflection is an important part of professional development during training, and it is associated with self-assessment. Reflection helps learners adjust their performance during practical experiences (in-action) and analyze their performance after its occurrence (on-action; Schön, 1983, 1987). Reflective practice helps learners examine what they did well and what they could improve and identify strategies for strengthening areas of weakness. Ideally, the reflective process includes feedback from multiple sources (instructor, peers, performance outcomes, etc.).

Simulation clearly serves these theoretical models in support of acquiring domain-specific performances associated with competency. But how are these performance criteria maintained over

time so that competency is sustained? Empirical evidence suggests that clinical performance abilities decline after instruction in as few as three weeks without use (Andreatta et al., 2016; Einspruch, Lynch, Aufderheide, Nichol, & Becker, 2007; Hunt, Fiedor-Hamilton, & Eppich, 2008; Latif et al., 2016; Seki, 1987, 1988; Woollard et al., 2006). Fortunately, evidence also suggests that simulation-based activities in support of professional development and maintenance of competency have a positive effect on both clinical performance and clinical outcomes (Andreatta, Perosky, & Johnson, 2012; Barsuk et al., 2015; Killien & Roberts, 2016; Oermann et al., 2011; Sawyer & Gray, 2016).

Simulation-based instruction is necessarily learner-centered. It places the locus of control with the learner. A learner-centered approach encourages individuals to take responsibility for their learning, which is essential for developing the lifelong learning and self-assessment skills required for healthcare providers in every specialty. Not only do these types of post-training activities facilitate the maintenance of individual performance, they also foster the development of interdisciplinary and team-based performance, which results in the types of synergistic competencies desired in healthcare. Much like the acquisition phases of developing competence, feedback—and its team-based correlate, debriefing—facilitates reflective practice during professional practice.

Competence Continuum

Competence is a dynamic construct that depends on acquired and maintained expertise. Figure 2.3 illustrates the relationship between competence and expertise. As shown in the figure:

- Novices generally lack competence in an instructional domain.

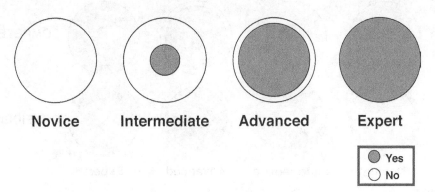

FIGURE 2.3   Expected performance competence at sequential levels of expertise.

- Intermediate learners might perform competently in some areas, but they likely lack sufficient competence to perform most domain-specific skills without supervision. For example, an intermediate-level nurse practitioner might demonstrate sufficient competence in placing an intravenous catheter but struggle placing a central venous catheter.

- Advanced learners generally demonstrate the ability to achieve most performance standards within a domain.

- Experts consistently demonstrate competent performance in a domain.

The Confidence-Competence Connection

Confidence and competence are both dynamic constructs associated with different psychological processes (Cohn, 2019). Therefore, each individual variably develops and maintains them. They are related, however, and this relationship can be used to design programs that individuals and groups can use to support optimal levels of both confidence and competence. Figure 2.4

illustrates the relationship between confidence and competence at sequential levels of learner expertise.

The gap between the confidence to perform in a clinical context and the actual competence of clinicians is an area of concern for learners, instructors, patients, clinicians who work with the learner during the provision of care, the responsible healthcare institution, and society in general. This gap is most pronounced at intermediate levels of domain expertise, where learners have acquired some domain-specific capability but have not acquired sufficient expertise to accurately self-assess their abilities. As described earlier in this chapter, this is largely an interaction effect between learners having poor self-assessment skills while also being unaware of the influences of content they haven't yet learned. Clinical instructors can reduce this gap through simulation-based methods that provide learners with specific feedback about the quality of their performance and help them to accurately self-assess. This benefits learners as they develop professional identities based on factual evidence, which subsequently supports their ability to maintain and expand their competencies.

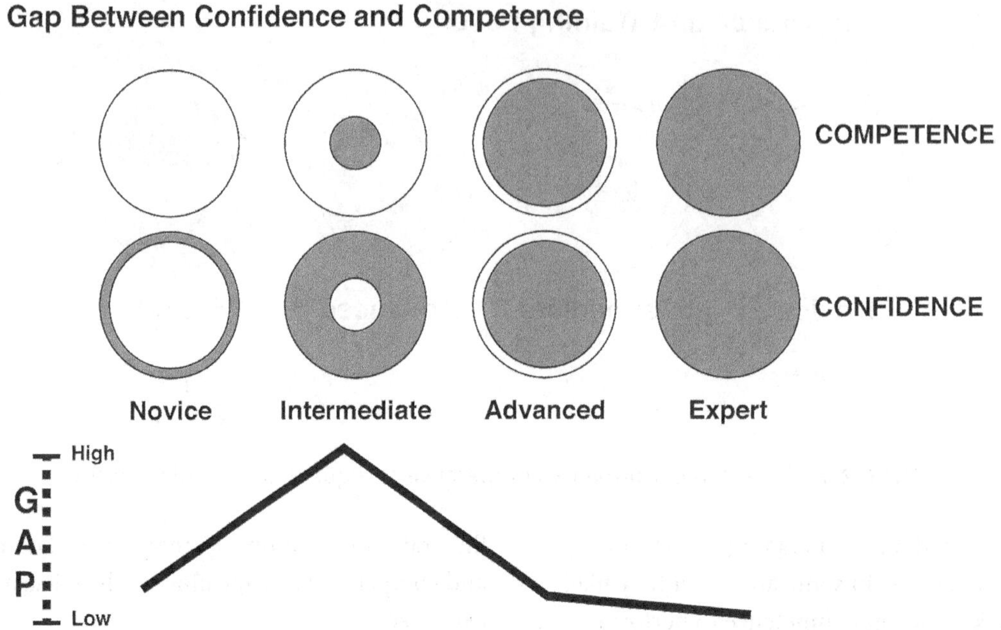

Gap Between Confidence and Competence

FIGURE 2.4 The gap between performance confidence and competence at sequential levels of expertise.

Simulation and Clinical Competency

All instruction optimally includes detailed instructional objectives for each relevant performance area in a content domain (cognitive, psychomotor, affective, system) that collectively lead to the achievement of domain competence. These learning objectives should be explicit and measurable—stating what learners should be able to do, the context in which they should be able to do it, and the expected standard of successful performance. Segmenting and sequencing content in a logical progression so that introductory concepts precede more advanced ones supports the construction and integration of domain-specific information, especially when formative assessment helps learners (and instructors) progress in an organized and efficient manner without exceeding the moderate challenge level that serves learner motivation. This approach helps learners engage with the content domain and progressively acquire competency.

Consulting relevant theoretical underpinnings ensures that optimal instructional activities support learner achievement for each objective. For example, instructional events designed to help learners achieve an objective with significant psychomotor factors benefit from Chapman's eight steps for learning procedural skills and deliberate practice strategies (see sidebar on page 35; Chapman, 1994). Similarly, a cognitive objective requiring complex relational integration, or affective objectives tied to interpersonal relating, benefit from the application of experiential learning theory and reflective practice. Strategically facilitated formative feedback allows learners to benefit from the naïve exploration favored by experiential learning theory while still providing them the opportunity to reflect on their performance through constructive feedback that subsequently informs their performances in succeeding activities.

Eight Steps of Procedural Skills Learning

1. Identify the acceptable skill level.
2. Identify when to perform the procedure.
3. Select the instruments and resources required to complete the procedure.
4. Identify the critical steps of the procedure.
5. Accurately sequence the critical steps.
6. Develop a mental image of performing the procedure.
7. Practice the movements required to perform the skills; use performance feedback.
8. Assess whether performance meets the acceptable level for skill achievement.

Source: Chapman, 1994

Sequencing instructional events in accordance with a natural progression of competency from lesser to more complex within the content domain ensures that learners are working at an appropriate level of challenge.

Simulation-based methods for clinical instruction are widely interpreted by various constituencies of users. Simulation methods are associated with the acquisition of abilities that lead to professional competency but also with maintenance of competency and even expansion of competencies in other areas of practice. Within these various applications, simulation-based activities support:

- Procedural skills

- Physical and clinical assessment skills

- Diagnostic reasoning

- Psycho-social skills and history-taking

- Clinical management

- Team-based practices

- Communication skills (patients, families, colleagues)

- Regulatory and administrative management

- Development and refinement of clinical techniques

In other words, simulation-based methods can be—and are—used for every aspect of clinical practice. However, some uses of simulation in healthcare are more mature than others in terms of equipment, resource specifications, assessment mechanisms, and development of instructional scenarios and events.

Designing simulation-based instruction can be time-consuming. It is both easier and prudent to use resources developed by others if possible. After all, why reinvent the wheel? But caution is merited when criticality of the instructional goal of simulation-based instruction is considered: to facilitate the acquisition and maintenance of clinical competence performed in applied practice. If existing instruction is not designed to achieve the specific competencies required by a learner in a given domain, it will not serve that goal. Therefore, it is essential to thoroughly evaluate any instructional activities designed for other programs to be certain that they also support the development of competencies in the program for which they are being considered. This minimizes the likelihood that a learner successfully completes all required instructional activities without being able to perform competently in applied clinical practice.

As with all types of instruction, the simulation environment itself influences learning. Apart from the effects of learner characteristics discussed in this and other chapters, the selection of models or simulators and setting characteristics affects not only learning within the simulated context but also the transfer of that learning to applied practice. This concept is tied to the concept of fidelity in simulation. Any discussion of competencies derived from simulation-based practices must include the issue of fidelity. This is because the more accurately a simulated context replicates the clinical context, the surer you can be that performance will transfer between the two contexts. A simulated clinical environment that adequately reflects the contextually relevant factors influencing performance of the learning objective maximizes transfer of the acquired abilities to the applied clinical environment (Konkola, Tuomi-Gröhn, Lambert, & Ludvigsen, 2007; Sohn, Doane, & Garrison, 2006; Thomas, 2007). The quality and type of fidelity required for the transfer of these abilities is an active area of research—principally because the costs associated with the space, equipment, materials, and resources required to replicate a clinical context can be quite high.

The term high fidelity is used for simulators designed to replicate clinical contexts with as much visual and functional precision as possible. These tend to be high-technology products driven by expensive computer and graphics systems. The term low fidelity describes simulators that are less technology-driven, although low-fidelity simulators often have equal or greater sensorial precision compared to high-fidelity simulators. Empirical evidence suggests that both types of simulation equipment can lead to favorable or unfavorable performance outcomes. This is because the elements of a simulated context are only as effective as the instructional design that uses them. If you consider the optimal instructional path for learners described earlier in this chapter, an exact replica of a clinical context is not necessary at every step of an instructional sequence. Rather, the concept of contextual fidelity is more appropriate when selecting the resources that will be included in a training program. Contextual fidelity is defined as a simulation activity that has sufficient detail to support the acquisition or maintenance of the skills described by the learning objective to the extent that those skills will support the acquisition of more advanced skills and will transfer to applied uses in clinical contexts.

Simulation-based instruction has many advantages over traditional, apprentice-based healthcare training. However, one disadvantage is that clinically embedded affective elements might be absent in a simulated context. Living patients are integral components of the apprenticeship learning context. This, along with the demands of clinical care at a busy healthcare institution, places extraordinary affective demands on the learner, both including and apart from cognitive and psychomotor demands. Because the apprenticeship-learning context includes these real factors, they must be accommodated during the instructional process if the learner is to be successful. The absence of these affective factors in simulated environments enables learners to focus exclusively on the cognitive and psychomotor competencies associated with the learning objectives for a domain. Learners might face challenges when required to transfer these cognitive and psychomotor competencies to an applied clinical environment, including affective factors that were not accommodated in the learning environment. Arguably, affective overload is one of the most challenging aspects of providing clinical care. Yet, it is largely overlooked as an integral part of healthcare education. Although affective factors are embedded in the apprenticeship model, these factors must be conscientiously considered and built into simulation-based instruction to support transfer from the less stressful learning context (simulation) to the more stressful context (applied patient care; Andreatta, Hillard, & Krain, 2010; Langan-Fox & Vranic, 2011).

Conclusion

Simulation-based instruction that successfully alters behaviors as a result of improvements in learners' knowledge, skills, or attitudes will take into account the psychological, biological, physical, and environmental constructs that affect human learning. Educators who implement simulation-based instruction in a healthcare setting may optimally facilitate changes to learners' behaviors in applied clinical practice as well. Simulation-based instruction supports the development of learner confidence to perform what is required and learner competence to accurately perform what is required. The potential for simulation-based methods to significantly improve the acquisition and maintenance of competence will help clinicians achieve consistent and accurate performance assessments that will ultimately improve quality and safety for patients and clinicians alike.

References

American Nurses Association. (2014). *Professional role competence.* [ANA Position Statement.] Retrieved from https://www.nursingworld.org/practice-policy/nursing-excellence/official-position-statements/id/professional-role-competence/

Andrade, H., & Valtcheva, A. (2009). Promoting learning and achievement through self-assessment. *Theory Into Practice, 48*(1), 12-19. doi:10.1080/00405840802577544

Andreatta, P., Chen, Y., Marsh, M., & Cho, K. (2011). Simulation-based training improves applied clinical placement of ultrasound-guided PICCs. *Supportive Care in Cancer, 19*(4), 539-543. doi:10.1007/s00520-010-0849-2

Andreatta, P., Perosky, J., & Johnson, T. R. (2012). Two-provider technique is superior for bimanual uterine compression to control postpartum hemorrhage. *Journal of Midwifery & Women's Health, 57*(4), 371-375. doi:10.1111/j.1542-2011.2011.00152.x

Andreatta, P., Saxton, E., Thompson, M., & Annich, G. (2011). Simulation-based mock codes significantly correlate with improved pediatric patient cardiopulmonary arrest survival rates. *Pediatric Critical Care Medicine, 12*(1), 33-38. doi:10.1097/PCC.0b013e3181e89270

Andreatta, P. B., Dooley-Hash, S. L., Klotz, J. J., Hauptman, J. G., Biddinger, B., & House, J. B. (2016). Retention curves for pediatric and neonatal intubation skills after simulation-based training. *Pediatric Emergency Care, 32*(2), 71-76. doi:10.1097/PEC.0000000000000603

Andreatta, P. B., Hillard, M., & Krain, L. P. (2010). The impact of stress factors in simulation-based laparoscopic training. *Surgery, 147*(5), 631-639.

Bandura, A. (1977). Self-efficacy: Toward a unifying theory of behavioral change. *Psychological Review, 84*(2), 191-215. doi:10.1037/0033-295X.84.2.191

Bandura, A. (1991). Social cognitive theory of self-regulation. *Organizational Behavior and Human Decision Processes, 50*(2), 248-287. doi:10.1016/0749-5978(91)90022-L

Bandura, A. (2001). Social cognitive theory: An agentic perspective. *Annual Review of Psychology, 52,* 1-26. doi:10.1146/annurev.psych.52.1.1

Barsuk, J. H., Cohen, E. R., McGaghie, W. C., & Wayne, D. B. (2010). Long-term retention of central venous catheter insertion skills after simulation-based mastery learning. *Academic Medicine, 85*(10 Suppl.), S9-S12. doi:10.1097/ACM.0b013e3181ed436c

Barsuk, J. H., Cohen, E. R., Mikolajczak, A., Seburn, S., Slade, M., & Wayne, D. B. (2015). Simulation-based mastery learning improves central line maintenance skills of ICU nurses. *Journal of Nursing Administration, 45*(10), 511-517. doi:10.1097/NNA.0000000000000243

Bhanji, F., Gottesman, R., de Grave, W., Steinert, Y., & Winer, L. R. (2012). The retrospective pre–post: A practical method to evaluate learning from an educational program. *Academic Emergency Medicine, 19*(2), 189-194. doi:10.1111/j.1553-2712.2011.01270.x

Carver, C. S. (2006). Approach, avoidance, and the self-regulation of affect and action. *Motivation and Emotion, 30*(2), 105-110. doi:10.1007/s11031-006-9044-7

Chapman, D. M. (1994). Use of computer-based technologies in teaching emergency procedural skills. *Academic Emergency Medicine, 1*(4), 404-407.

Cizek, G. J., & Bunch, M. B. (2007). *Standard setting: A guide to establishing and evaluating performance standards on tests.* Thousand Oaks, CA: Sage Publications, Inc.

Cohn, E. S. (2019). Asserting our competence and affirming the value of occupation with confidence. *American Journal of Occupational Therapy, 73*(6). doi:7306150010p1–7306150010p10

Cunningham, J., Wright, C., & Baird, M. (2015). Managing clinical education through understanding key principles. *Radiologic Technology, 86*(3), 257-273.

Davis, D. A., Mazmanian, P. E., Fordis, M., Van Harrison, R., Thorpe, K. E., & Perrier, L. (2006). Accuracy of physician self-assessment compared with observed measures of competence: A systematic review. *Journal of the American Medical Association, 296*(9), 1094-1102. doi:10.1001/jama.296.9.1094

Dumitru, D. (2012). Critical thinking and integrated programs: The problem of transferability. *Procedia, 33*, 143-147. doi:10.1016/j.sbspro.2012.01.100

Dunning, D., Heath, C., & Suls, J. M. (2004). Flawed self-assessment: Implications for health, education, and the workplace. *Psychological Science in the Public Interest, 5*(3), 69–106. doi:10.1111/j.1529-1006.2004.00018.x

Duval, T. S., & Silvia, P. J. (2002). Self-awareness, probability of improvement, and the self-serving bias. *Journal of Personality and Social Psychology, 82*(1), 49-61. doi:10.1037/0022-3514.82.1.49

Dweck, C. S., & Leggett, E. L. (1988). A social-cognitive approach to motivation and personality. *Psychological Review, 95*(2), 256-273.

Einspruch, E. L., Lynch, B., Aufderheide, T. P., Nichol, G., & Becker, L. (2007). Retention of CPR skills learned in a traditional AHA Heartsaver course versus 30-min video self-training: A controlled randomized study. *Resuscitation, 74*(3), 476-486. doi:10.1016/j.resuscitation.2007.01.030

Ericsson, K. A. (2004). Deliberate practice and the acquisition and maintenance of expert performance in medicine and related domains. *Academic Medicine, 79*(19 Suppl.), S70-S81.

Ericsson, K. A. (2011). The surgeon's expertise. In H. Fry & R. Kneebone (Eds.), *Surgical education: Theorising an emerging domain* (pp. 107-122). New York, NY: Springer Science + Business Media.

Ericsson, K. A. & Charness, N. (1994). Expert performance: Its structure and acquisition. *American Psychologist, 49*(8), 725-747. doi:10.1037/0003-066X.49.8.725

Ericsson, K. A., Nandagopal, K., & Roring, R. W. (2009). Toward a science of exceptional achievement: Attaining superior performance through deliberate practice. *Annals of the New York Academy of Sciences, 1172*(1), 199-217. doi:10.1196/annals.1393.001

Fishbein, M., & Ajzen, I. (1975). *Belief, attitude, intention, and behavior: An introduction to theory and research.* Reading, MA: Addison-Wesley.

Goldman, L. I., McDonough, M. T., & Rosemond, G. P. (1972). Stresses affecting surgical performance and learning: 1. Correlation of heart rate, electrocardiogram, and operation simultaneously recorded on videotapes. *Journal of Surgical Research, 12*(2), 83-86.

Hambleton, R. K., Jaeger, R. M., Plake, B. S., & Mills, C. (2000). Setting performance standards on complex educational assessments. *Applied Psychological Measurement, 24*(4), 355-366. doi:10.1177/01466210022031804

Hewson, M. G., Copeland, H. L., & Fishleder, A. J. (2001). What's the use of faculty development? Program evaluation using retrospective self-assessments and independent performance ratings. *Teaching and Learning in Medicine, 13*(3), 153-160.

Hunt, E. A., Duval-Arnould, J. M., Nelson-McMillan, K. L., Bradshaw, D. H., Diener-West, M., Perretta, J. S., & Shilkofski, N. A. (2014). Pediatric resident resuscitation skills improve after "rapid cycle deliberate practice" training. *Resuscitation, 85*(7), 945–951. doi:10.1016/j.resuscitation.2014.02.025

Hunt, E. A., Fiedor-Hamilton, M., & Eppich, W. J. (2008). Resuscitation education: Narrowing the gap between evidence-based resuscitation guidelines and performance using best educational practices. *Pediatric Clinics of North America, 55*(4), 1025-1050. doi:10.1016/j.pcl.2008.04.007

Issenberg, S. B., McGaghie, W. C., Petrusa, E. R., Lee Gordon, D., & Scalese, R. J. (2005). Features and uses of high-fidelity medical simulations that lead to effective learning: A BEME systematic review. *Medical Teacher, 27*(1), 10-28.

Judge, T. A., & Bono, J. E. (2001). Relationship of core self-evaluations traits—self-esteem, generalized self-efficacy, locus of control, and emotional stability—with job satisfaction and job performance. *Journal of Applied Psychology, 86*(1), 80-92. doi:10.1037/0021-9010.86.1.80

Keller, J. M. (2008). First principles of motivation to learn and e³-learning. *Distance Education, 29*(2), 175-185. doi:10.1080/01587910802154970

Killien, E., & Roberts, J. (2016). Maintenance of procedural skills competency for pediatric critical care providers. *Critical Care Medicine, 44*(12), 176. doi:10.1097/01.ccm.0000509077.14163.33

Kolb, D. A. (1984). *Experiential learning: Experience as the source of learning and development.* Englewood Cliffs, NJ: Prentice-Hall.

Konkola, R., Tuomi-Gröhn, T., Lambert, P., & Ludvigsen, S. (2007). Promoting learning and transfer between school and workplace. *Journal of Education and Work, 20*(3), 211-228. doi:10.1080/13639080701464483

Langan-Fox, J., & Vranic, V. (2011). Surgeon stress in the operating room: Error-free performance and adverse events. In J. Langan-Fox & C. L. Cooper (Eds.), *Handbook of stress in the occupations* (pp. 33-48). Northampton, MA: Edward Elgar Publishing, Inc.

Latif, R. K., Bautista, A., Duan, X., Neamtu, A., Wu, D., Wadhwa, A., & Akça, O. (2016). Teaching basic fiberoptic intubation skills in a simulator: Initial learning and skills decay. *Journal of Anesthesia, 30*(1), 12-19. doi:10.1007/s00540-015-2091-z

Levinson, W., Gordon, G., & Skeff, K. (1990). Retrospective versus actual pre-course self-assessments. *Evaluation & the Health Professions, 13*(4), 445-452. doi:10.1177/016327879001300406

McGaghie, W. C., Issenberg, S. B., Cohen, E. R., Barsuk, J. H., & Wayne, D. B. (2011). Medical education featuring mastery learning with deliberate practice can lead to better health for individuals and populations. *Academic Medicine, 86*(11), e8-e9. doi:10.1097/ACM.0b013e3182308d37

McGaghie, W. C., Issenberg, S. B., Petrusa, E. R., & Scalese, R. J. (2006). Effect of practice on standardised learning outcomes in simulation-based medical education. *Medical Education, 40*(8), 792-797.

McKinley, D. W., Boulet, J. R., & Hambleton, R. K. (2005). A work-centered approach for setting passing scores on performance-based assessments. *Evaluation & the Health Professions, 28*(3), 349-369.

Motavalli, A., & Nestel, D. (2016). Complexity in simulation-based education: Exploring the role of hindsight bias. *Advances in Simulation, 1*(3). doi:10.1186/s41077-015-0005-7

Nadler, D. A., Lawler III, E. E., Steers, R. M., & Porter, L. W. (1977). Motivation: A diagnostic approach. In L. Porter, G. Bigley, & R. Steers (Eds.), *Motivation and work behavior* (pp. 26-38). New York, NY: McGraw Hill.

Nemec, P. B. (2010). Inaccurate self-assessments. *Psychiatric Rehabilitation Journal, 34*(2), 159-161. doi:10.2975/34.2.2010.159.161

Nestel, D., Bello, F., & Kneebone, R. (2013). Feedback in clinical procedural skills simulations. In D. Boud & E. Molloy (Eds.), *Feedback in higher and professional education: Understanding it and doing it well* (pp. 140-157). New York, NY: Routledge.

Oermann, M. H., Kardong-Edgren, S., Odom-Maryon, T., Hallmark, B. F., Hurd, D., Rogers, N., … Smart, D. A. (2011). Deliberate practice of motor skills in nursing education: CPR as exemplar. *Nursing Education Perspectives, 32*(5), 311-315.

Pintrich, P. R. (1999). The role of motivation in promoting and sustaining self-regulated learning. *International Journal of Educational Research, 31*(6), 459-470.

Pintrich, P. R. (2003). A motivational science perspective on the role of student motivation in learning and teaching contexts. *Journal of Educational Psychology, 95*(4), 667-686. doi:10.1037/0022-0663.95.4.667

Pintrich, P. R. (2004). A conceptual framework for assessing motivation and self-regulated learning in college students. *Educational Psychology Review, 16*(4), 385-407. doi:10.1007/s10648-004-0006-x

Rotter, J. B. (1954). *Social learning and clinical psychology.* Englewood Cliffs, NJ: Prentice-Hall.

Sadeghi, A., Oshvandi, K., & Moradi, Y. (2019). Explaining the inhibitory characteristics of clinical instructors in the process of developing clinical competence of nursing students: A qualitative study. *Journal of Family Medicine and Primary Care, 8*(5), 1664-1670. doi:10.4103/jfmpc.jfmpc_34_19

Sawyer, T., & Gray, M. M. (2016). Procedural training and assessment of competency utilizing simulation. *Seminars in Perinatology, 40*(7), 438-446. doi:10.1053/j.semperi.2016.08.004

Schön, D. (1983). *The reflective practitioner: How professionals think in action.* New York, NY: Basic Books.

Schön, D. (1987). *Educating the reflective practitioner: Toward a new design for teaching and learning in the professions.* Hoboken, NJ: Wiley.

Seki, S. (1987). Accuracy of suture techniques of surgeons with different surgical experience. *The Japanese Journal of Surgery, 17*(6), 465-469.

Seki, S. (1988). Techniques for better suturing. *The British Journal of Surgery, 75*(12), 1181-1184. doi:10.1002/bjs.1800751212

Sohn, Y. W., Doane, S. M., & Garrison, T. (2006). The impact of individual differences and learning context on strategic skill acquisition and transfer. *Learning and Individual Differences, 16*(1), 13-30. doi:10.1016/j.lindif.2005.06.002

Stemme, A., Deco, G., & Lang, E. W. (2011). Perceptual learning with perceptions. *Cognitive Neurodynamics, 5*(1), 31-43. doi:10.1007/s11571-010-9134-9

Taras, J., & Everett, T. (2017). Rapid cycle deliberate practice in medical education: A systematic review. *Cureus, 9*(4), e1180. doi:10.7759/cureus.1180

Thomas, E. (2007). Thoughtful planning fosters learning transfer. *Adult Learning, 18*(3-4), 4-8. doi:10.1177/104515950701800301

Vroom, V. H. (1964). *Work and motivation.* Oxford, UK: Wiley.

Wayne, D. B., Moazed, F., Cohen, E. R., Sharma, R. K., McGaghie, W. C., & Szmuilowicz, E. (2012). Code status discussion skill retention in internal medicine residents: One-year follow-up. *Journal of Palliative Medicine, 15*(12), 1325-1328. doi:10.1089/jpm.2012.0232

Weiner, B. (2010). The development of an attribution-based theory of motivation: A history of ideas. *Educational Psychologist, 45*(1), 28-36. doi:10.1080/00461520903433596

Wickens, C. D. (1991). Processing resources and attention. In D. L. Damos (Ed.), *Multiple task performance* (pp. 3-34). Bristol, PA: Taylor & Francis, Inc.

Wigfield, A., & Eccles, J. S. (2000). Expectancy-value theory of achievement motivation. *Contemporary Educational Psychology, 25*(1), 68-81. doi:10.1006/ceps.1999.1015

Woollard, M., Whitfield, R., Newcombe, R. G., Colquhoun, M., Vetter, N., & Chamberlain, D. (2006). Optimal refresher training intervals for AED and CPR skills: A randomised controlled trial. *Resuscitation, 71*(2), 237-247. doi:10.1016/j.resuscitation.2006.04.005

Young, M. S., & Stanton, N. A. (2002). Malleable attentional resources theory: A new explanation for the effects of mental underload on performance. *Human Factors, 44*(3), 365-375.

"The function of education is to teach one to think intensively and to think critically. Intelligence plus character—that is the goal of true education."

–Martin Luther King, Jr.

Creating an Effective Simulation Environment

Teresa N. Gore, PhD, DNP, FNP-BC, NP-C, CHSE-A, FAAN

3

OBJECTIVES

- Describe the levels and types of fidelity for an effective simulation environment.

- Identify key elements required for an effective simulation environment.

- Articulate how to identify what type and level of fidelity is required based on the objectives of the simulation.

- Synthesize at least two strategies that can be incorporated into a simulation practice.

Simulation can be used in all areas in which patient care is performed or in which educating healthcare providers occurs. In clinical practice environments, simulation can be used in the hiring and onboarding process to evaluate critical thinking and practice, for competency evaluations of experienced healthcare providers, and for testing new procedures and practice sites. In academia, simulation can be used to educate students and clinical faculty or to develop faculty expertise in teaching techniques and strategies.

Simulation is a teaching strategy, not just a technology. The National Council of State Boards of Nursing (NCSBN) conducted a national, longitudinal, randomized controlled study replacing clinical hours with simulation in pre-licensure nursing education at 10 schools of nursing (Hayden, Smiley, Alexander, Kardong-Edgren, & Jeffries, 2014). The study compared a control group in which 10% of clinical time was replaced with simulation with two groups in which 25% and 50% of clinical time was replaced with simulation. Results revealed no statistical differences in the Assessment Technologies Institute Comprehensive Predictor scores, the New Graduate Nurse Performance Survey, the Critical Thinking Diagnostic Scale, or the Global Assessment of Clinical Competency and Readiness for Practice. Therefore, it was determined that simulation can be a substitute for clinical time—if it incorporates International Nursing Association for Clinical Simulation and Learning (INACSL) standards (Hayden et al., 2014).

After the publication of this survey, a group of experts developed NCSBN simulation guidelines (Alexander et al., 2015). These guidelines include a commitment from nursing schools to support the program, have appropriate facilities to conduct simulation, have educational and technical resources and equipment to meet the objectives, have personnel who are qualified and educated to conduct simulation, and have policies and procedures as part of the simulation program. Before conducting simulations, faculty members should be educated on the INACSL standards, simulations based on educational theory (to facilitate the development of clear objectives to be achieved in the simulation), creating a learning environment, facilitation and debriefing methods, evaluating all aspects of the simulation, and providing professional development in using effective simulation.

The environment in which the simulation occurs is critical to the success of the simulation experience. Effective simulation environments require several key elements:

- Planning that includes clear objectives, evidence-based scenarios, and an evaluation plan

- Educators who are experienced in simulation and grounded in the INACSL standards

- Debriefers who are skilled in simulation and facilitation and are experts in relevant clinical content

- Safe learning environment for learners

- Physical fidelity (mannequins, moulage, etc.)

- Environmental fidelity

- Psychological fidelity

This chapter addresses creating the learning environment. Other chapters in the book focus on the details of components such as developing scenarios (Chapter 4), debriefing (Chapter 5), evaluations (Chapter 6), etc.

Fidelity

Both the INACSL standards and the NCSBN guidelines include the use of appropriate fidelity to create a realistic learning experience. *Fidelity* is "the ability to view or represent things as they are to enhance believability. The degree to which a simulated experience approaches reality; as fidelity increases, realism increases. The level of fidelity is determined by the environment, the tools and resources used, and many factors associated with the participants. Fidelity can involve a variety of dimensions" (INACSL Standards Committee, 2016e, p. S42). Fidelity should replicate real situations in ways that are appropriate to the learning objectives. Typically, this means creating an environment that is as close as possible to reality in order for the participants to respond to the simulated situation as they would in a professional interaction with a patient, family, or community (INACSL Standards Committee, 2016d). The fidelity of a scenario can be increased or decreased by the type of mannequins used and/or the environmental factors included. Some environmental factors include olfactory factors, visual factors, and sounds (Rudolph, McIntosh, Simon, & Raemer, 2015; Scheese, 2019).

Creating effective simulation environments can allow learners to see patients holistically. The concept of holism has proven challenging for learners in a traditional clinical setting and even more difficult for educators in a teacher-centered lecture. Creating an effective simulation environment offers a solution to both and allows discovery learning through deliberate practice and guidance. Environmental fidelity is often not addressed until late in the development of the simulation program, however, assuring that effective simulation environments can be the key to developing keen clinical assessment skills. Observational skills may be cultivated through inclusion of cues for the learner to develop effective clinical anticipation skills and to focus the personal patient history. In healthcare simulation, effective simulation environments are referred to and measured as environmental fidelity (Kamp, 2018).

Learning Environments Versus Testing Environments

Simulation is used in both learning environments and testing environments. These environments differ in several important ways. For example, in learning environments, opportunities for variation and personalization of experiences are encouraged. In a testing environment, however, the goal is to standardize all aspects of the experience to evaluate the knowledge, skills, and abilities of all participants.

The simulation learning environment is:

- "An atmosphere that is created by the facilitator to allow for sharing and discussion of participant experiences without fear of humiliation or punitive action. The goals of the simulation learning environment are to promote trust and foster learning" (INACSL Board of Directors, 2011, p. s6).

In contrast, the simulation testing environment is:

- "An atmosphere that is created by the facilitator to allow for formative and summative evaluation to occur. The goals of the simulation testing environment are to create an equivalent activity for all participants in order to test their knowledge, skills, and abilities in a simulated setting" (INACSL Board of Directors, 2011, p. s6).

It is important to establish more rigorous evaluation methods by utilizing valid and reliable tools to objectively evaluate student performance. How can healthcare providers involved in simulation-based education create learning environments that are efficient, effective, and foster the acquisition of educational objectives? The INACSL Standards of Best Practice Committee has developed a standard to guide educators and facilitators on simulation design (INACSL Standards Committee, 2016d).

The use of simulation should begin with activities associated with basic psychomotor skills and scaffolds to include elements of critical thinking and clinical judgment. This evidence-based approach should be used with inexperienced learners to avoid overwhelming them and to promote learning (INACSL Standards Committee, 2016b). Other studies have examined the elements of environmental and psychological fidelity in simulations, specifically, the incorporation of stressors into high-fidelity simulation training scenarios (Damazo & Damazo, 2018).

Studies have shown students prefer higher levels of fidelity when reporting their level of satisfaction and self-efficacy with simulated learning opportunities (Hayden et al., 2014). There is a growing body of literature within nursing and healthcare to evaluate the differences in learner outcomes using low-fidelity and high-fidelity simulation experiences. Initial simulation research measured learner perceptions. More recently, there has been an increase in quantitative studies. Cantrell, Franklin, Leighton, and Carlson (2017), in a review of studies on simulation-based learning experiences, found studies showing no statistically significant differences in learner outcomes or performances when comparing varying levels of fidelity as a teaching strategy as well as other studies that found that the level of fidelity used in simulation increased students' self-perceived improvements and satisfaction, knowledge, competence, self-efficacy, and confidence. They also noted that some studies revealed simulation improved patient care and clinical performance.

Effective simulations require the educator to use varying levels of realism and tools to meet the needs of the learners and the learning experience. Educators need to remember one important aspect: Simulation is limited only by your imagination, so think outside the box. By increasing the realism, learners can forget they are participating in a lab experience and can treat the simulation as a real-life experience. This is referred to as "suspension of disbelief" (Muckler, 2017). Higher levels of fidelity can contribute to learners being able to suspend disbelief. In a study of graduate and undergraduate nursing students, Muckler and Thomas (2019) found three themes that impacted the suspension of disbelief: frame of mind (including the sub-themes of cognitive focus, apprehension, and confidence), environment, and tempo. All learners in the simulation will appreciate your effort and preparedness in allowing them to become immersed in the simulation experience. Through their simulation participation, learners will be exposed to various experiences and learn ways to respond to patient, family, or community needs in a safe manner, incorporating best practices.

Aspects of fidelity can include the physical, the psychological, the culture of the group, and the degree of trust (INACSL Standards Committee, 2016e). The ability of the facilitator to improve the psychological fidelity increases with the facilitator's experience and comfort in simulation (Zigmont, Oocumma, Szyld, & Maestre, 2015). The *facilitator* is "a trained individual who provides guidance, support, and structure at some or all stages of simulation-based learning including prebriefing, simulation, and/ or debriefing" (INACSL Standards Committee, 2016e, p. S42).

Simulated Mannequin Fidelity

Mannequin fidelity is the degree to which the mannequin used for simulation represents the way a patient would appear and respond.

Task trainers represent anatomical human body parts and are used to practice psychomotor skills (see Figure 3.1). Task trainers lack realism in that they represent only a section of a human body or have limited responsive capabilities. A task trainer could provide the appropriate level of fidelity if the educational objective is psychomotor skill acquisition (Lioce et al., 2020).

Static (low-fidelity) mannequins are basic mannequins that lack pulses, heart sounds, and lung sounds and do not realistically mimic human beings (see Figures 3.2 and 3.3). Static mannequins do not have to be controlled or programmed (Palaganas, Maxworthy, Epps, & Mancini, 2015). Learners can use these mannequins to train for tasks such as dressing changes for wound care, urinary catheter insertions, and bathing/linen changes (Lioce et al., 2020).

Mid-fidelity mannequins more realistically mimic reality with pulses, heart sounds, and lung sounds but lack the physiological display of chest rise and fall with breathing, blinking, or automated physiological responses to interventions (Kardong-Edgren, Lungstrom, & Bendel, 2009; Lioce et al., 2020).

High-fidelity mannequins have all the features of a mid-fidelity mannequin and, in addition, mimic reality by blinking, having the chest rise and fall with respirations, and offering physiological responses to interventions (Kardong-Edgren et al., 2009; Lioce et al., 2020).

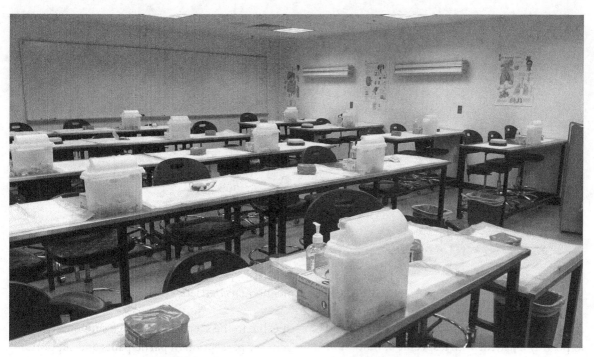

FIGURE 3.1   Task trainer pads for injections.
(Courtesy Dr. Teresa N. Gore, University of South Florida College of Nursing [USFCON])

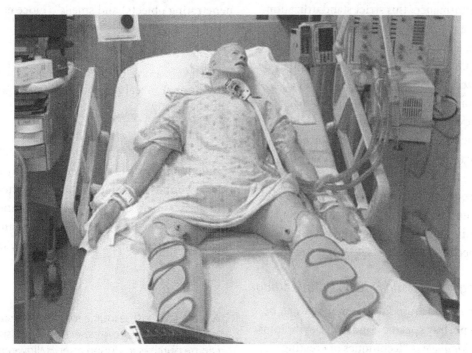

FIGURE 3.2   A static mannequin bed setup for tubes and drains training for a physical
therapy lab. (Courtesy of Dr. Teresa N. Gore, USFCON)

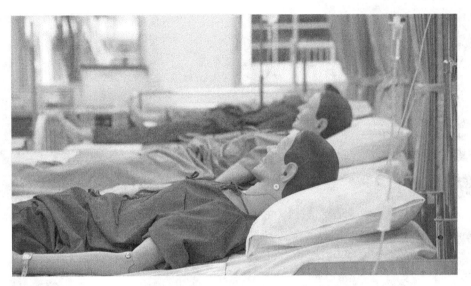

FIGURE 3.3   Static mannequins bed lab.

A *standardized patient* "is an individual trained to portray a patient with a specific condition in a realistic, standardized, and repeatable way and where portrayal/presentation varies based only on learner performance; this strict standardization of performance in a simulated session is what can distinguish standardized patients from simulated patients" (Lioce et al., 2020, p. 49; see Figure 3.4). Standardized patients may be actors, trained citizens from the community, or individuals who possess previous healthcare work experience. Standardized patients are the best choice when communication is the main educational objective. To increase environmental fidelity when using a standardized patient, computer-based programs can generate vital signs or auscultatory sounds for abnormal findings, or moulage can be added to portray specific conditions, symptoms, or illness.

Enhancing Mannequin Fidelity With Moulage

To enhance mannequin fidelity, moulage can be applied to portray specific conditions, symptoms, or illness. *Moulage* is "techniques of creating simulated wounds, injuries, diseases, the aging processes, and other physical characteristics

specific to the scenario; moulage supports the sensory perception of participants and supports the fidelity of the simulation scenario through the use of makeup, attachable artifacts (e.g., penetrating objects) and smells" (Lioce et al., 2020, p. 32).

> The first example of medical moulage was the use of anatomical wax models to study the human body.

Types of moulage frequently used in healthcare simulation include cosmetics, wigs, body art, odors, wounds, bruising, rashes, and other visual assessment cues to draw the attention of the learners (see Figure 3.5). Moulage can assist learners in preparing to provide quality, safe patient care.

> A great low-cost resource for moulage supplies is a Halloween store—especially when supplies can be purchased during after-Halloween sales.

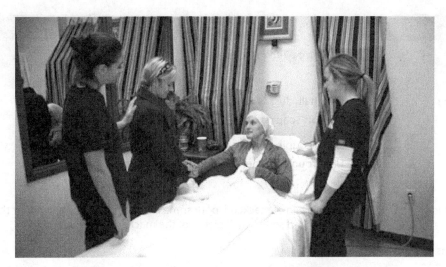

FIGURE 3.4   Standardized patient.
(Courtesy of Dr. Valerie M. Howard, Robert Morris University [RMU], Regional RISE Center)

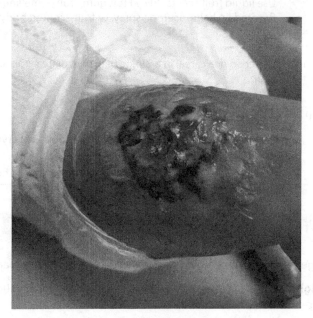

FIGURE 3.5   Spider bite on a child.

Moulage does have its constraining factors including cost, knowledge/imagination, manpower (personnel and time), supplies, and storage. Still, by increasing the fidelity of simulation, moulage can help engage learners in the simulation. Providing clinically appropriate moulage ensures that clinical details are provided for learners and allows them to observe objective-based cues and take the correct action. Moulage also gives learners and educators the opportunity to discuss the clinical reasoning that led to learner actions and the benefits or consequences of those actions. Table 3.1 shows examples of moulage techniques to engage the senses.

Table 3.1	Moulage to Engage the Senses
Sense	*Moulage Techniques*
Visual	
Infected urine	Use chalk dust or vanilla pudding to produce sediment.
	Use soft soap or liquid dish soap to produce cloudy urine.
Hematuria	Add a couple of drops of meat blood for positive urine dipstick.
	Use ground-up cherries for clots.
Olfactory	
Infected amniotic fluid	Open a can of mackerel, pour some of the juice onto a pad under the patient, and spread some small pieces of the mackerel onto pad.
Feces or flatus	Use fecal spray.
Infection	Apply parmesan cheese, limburger cheese, bleu cheese, or Goo Gone gel.
Acetone breath	Use liquid fruit scents, Juicy Fruit gum, fruity-smelling car air freshener, fruit-flavored lip balm, acetone spray, or fruit-scented body spray.
Tactile	
Subcutaneous emphysema (place under skin of mannequin)	Use crisp rice cereal in a Ziploc bag, chocolate syrup and kitty litter, or bubble wrap.
Auditory/Psychological	
	Have a call bell and alarms sound or the sounds of crying children as background noise.
	Present an upset and demanding family member or healthcare team member.

Internet Resources for Moulage

- **Military Moulage Combat Injury Simulation:** http://www.militarymoulage.com/

- **Moulage—Bridging the Gap in Simulation:** http://www.healthysimulation.com/28/moulage-bridging-the-gap-in-simulation/

- **Mad Simulationist's Lab #5 – Moulage 101 (Video Tutorial):** https://youtu.be/oY479ulSwJ4

- **Chez Moulage Recipe Book:** https://static1.squarespace.com/static/5121177ae4b06840010a00c1/t/51487539e4b0d1d31cb2f3a8/1363703097118/Chez_Moulage.pdf

- **Behind the Sim Curtain:** http://wiki.behindthesimcurtain.org/index.php/Main_Page

Aligning Mannequin Fidelity With Learner Objectives

The decision on the level of mannequin fidelity is based on the learner objectives (see Table 3.2). Educators must decide the appropriate level of fidelity to use to achieve SMART (specific, measurable, achievable, realistic, and time-phased) objectives and goals (Doran, 1981; INACSL Standards Committee, 2016b).

Environmental Fidelity

In healthcare simulation, effective simulation environments are gauged in terms of environmental fidelity (Kamp, 2018). *Environmental fidelity* is "the degree to which the simulated environment (manikin, room, tools, equipment, moulage, and sensory props) replicates the reality and appearance of the real environment" (Lioce at al., 2020, p. 16). Some environmental factors include olfactory factors, visual factors, and sounds (Rudolph et al., 2015; Scheese, 2019). For example, a hospital-based scenario could include hospital sounds (call light, alarms, background noises), patient care devices, and equipment. The growth of technology and the internet has greatly increased access to sources of material to create low-level environmental fidelity.

As with other dimensions of fidelity, there are levels of environmental fidelity. *Low-level environmental fidelity* employs pictures of equipment used for patient care rather than actual equipment (see Figure 3.6). For example, if your simulation requires a patient-controlled analgesia pump but none are available, a low-level solution would be to print a life-size colored picture of the pump and paste it to a box, run tubing into the pump, and write the dose in ink.

Mid-level environmental fidelity provides higher fidelity. For example, the simulation could occur in a furnished hospital room with actual equipment (see Figure 3.7).

Table 3.2 Matching Fidelity With Learner Objectives	
Objective – The learner will:	**Type(s) of Mannequin/Trainer**
Correctly insert an intravenous catheter	Task trainer
Correctly insert an IV during an urgent situation (hypertensive crisis)	Mid-fidelity mannequin in a high-fidelity environment High-fidelity mannequin
Use effective communication skills to obtain an accurate history from a patient	Standardized patient
Use varying techniques to communicate with a family member under situational stress	Standardized patient
Recognize and correctly respond to a patient's deteriorating condition—for example, the first five minutes of a code	High-fidelity mannequin in a high-fidelity environment

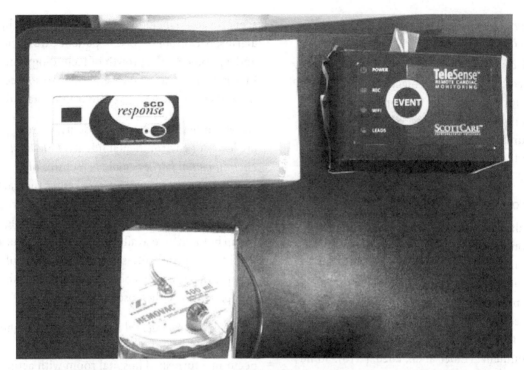

FIGURE 3.6 Using pictures to depict the actual equipment represents low-level environmental fidelity.

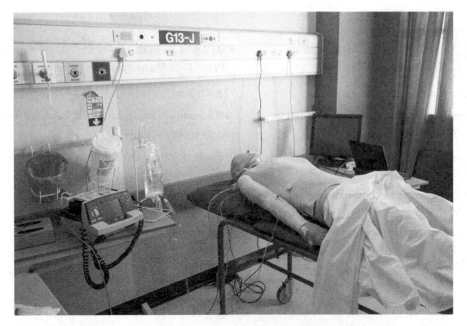

FIGURE 3.7 A mannequin with functioning IV equipment.

A mid-level fidelity environment with mannequins and props can be used to teach concepts such as infections control and isolation precautions. One example of a prop that reflects mid-level fidelity is a product called GlitterBug—a lotion or powder that can be applied to hands, mannequins, or surfaces. Upon application, GlitterBug becomes transparent but reveals unclean or contaminated areas under a black light. GlitterBug offers an excellent way to teach the concepts of infection control and isolation precautions. For example, prior to beginning a simulation scenario, the facilitator can apply GlitterBug to work surfaces and other common areas of contamination, including the mannequin. At the end of the simulation, a black light is used to reveal the contaminated areas on the mannequin, bed, clothing, light switches, handles, faucet, paper towel dispenser, and the learners. Seeing this contamination can be a "light bulb" moment for learners and help them understand that even if they performed everything correctly, it takes only one person *not* following evidence-based infection control practices to contaminate everything.

High-level environmental fidelity portrays an actual patient setting with appropriate working equipment, as in a real-world setting. This level of fidelity can be applied to community settings as well as hospital or clinic settings. Figure 3.8 shows the use of high-level environmental fidelity and moulage to increase the realism of the simulation.

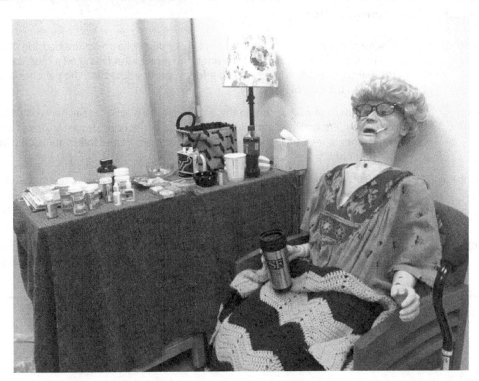

FIGURE 3.8 Community setting with a focus on safety and conducting a functional geriatric assessment. (Courtesy of Dr. Teresa N. Gore, USFCON)

Psychological Fidelity

Successful simulation requires educators to provide a trusting, psychologically safe learning environment. *Psychological fidelity* refers to "the extent to which the simulated environment evokes the underlying psychological processes necessary in the real-world setting. The degree of perceived realism, including psychological factors such as emotions, beliefs, and self-awareness of participants in simulation scenarios" (Lioce et al., 2020, p. 38). Incorporating interference or stressors into the simulation has been shown to increase the level of realism perceived by learners and prepares them for patient care in the real world. Interference and stressors increase the sense of urgency, potentially leading to a quicker response to patient changes by participants (Damazo & Damazo, 2018). The experience of the facilitator is a critical element in the use of psychological fidelity. The ability of the facilitator to improve psychological fidelity increases with the facilitator's experience and comfort in simulation (Zigmont et al., 2015).

There are developmental, spiritual, sociocultural, and psychological dimensions of psychological fidelity. Table 3.3 includes examples of ways to increase psychological fidelity across these various dimensions.

Table 3.3   Improving Psychological Fidelity

Dimension	Improving Fidelity
Developmental	Place a shopping bag of children's toys and a diaper bag near the bedside of a 27-year-old roofer who was admitted for a fractured femur after falling off a roof. This prompts the learner to explore family needs—for example, addressing the patient's anxiety related to the care of his family.
Spiritual	Place a tattoo of a faith icon on the arm of or rosary beads in the hand of a 42-year-old female patient with a recent diagnosis of breast cancer post-mastectomy. This prompts the learner to recognize the need for spiritual support and follow through with a call for consultation.
Sociocultural	Place dirty clothes and a sleeping bag with fecal and ammonia odor in a backpack at the bedside of a 53-year-old homeless patient. This prompts the learner to explore financial resources related to interventions, such as contacting a homeless shelter or social worker.
Psychological	Place a football jersey at the bedside of a 22-year-old male patient post-op knee surgery. This prompts the learner to explore how the patient feels about the loss of his ability to participate in the sport.

Source: Howard, Leighton, & Gore, 2018

Increasing Environmental Fidelity Through Sound

To increase environmental fidelity, computer-based programs or other audio tools can be used to generate vital signs or auscultatory sounds for abnormal findings. Examples of resources for sound effects include:

- **Voice Changer Solutions for Your Medical Simulation Lab:** http://www.healthysimulation.com/1263/voice-changers-in-your-sim-lab/

- **Audio Micro Hospital Sound Effects:** https://www.audiomicro.com/sound-effects/emergency/hospital

- **Pond5 Hospital Royalty-Free Sound Effects:** https://www.pond5.com/sound-effects/1/hospital.html

- **Hospital Sound Effects/Hospital Ambience:** https://www.youtube.com/watch?v=3LUuyDdWOy4

- **Hospital Emergency Room 1 (Ambience, Emergency, Medical):** https://www.youtube.com/watch?v=qR9YzVqO9Zg

- **Hospital Background Intensive Care Unit Sound:** https://www.youtube.com/watch?v=raWMup_kisk

- **Hospital Sound Effects:** https://www.zapsplat.com/sound-effect-category/hospital/

- **SoundBible:** https://soundbible.com/

Developing a Safe Learning Environment

Regardless of the level of fidelity used in a simulation, the facilitator must intentionally create a safe learning environment, which is:

> A learning environment where it is clarified that learners feel physically and psychologically safe to make decisions, take actions, and interact in the simulation. A learning environment of mutual respect, support, and respectful communication among leaders and learners; open communication and mutual respect for thought and action encouraged and practiced. (Lioce et al., 2020, p. 41)

To develop a safe learning environment requires educator buy-in as well as orientation to the simulation environment for both the learners and educators. Educators are seen as the experts in their specialties. However, when educators are placed in the simulation lab for a scenario the first time, their inexperience with simulation makes them feel more novice and out of their comfort zone (INACSL Standards Committee, 2016a). This environment is unfamiliar to the educators as compared to the patient setting. In human patient care, educators cannot allow the learners to make errors and learn the consequences of the actions or inactions. Therefore, even for experienced educators, using simulation is a new skill that must be developed.

To facilitate educator development, educators should undertake simulation education to learn evidence-based or best practices for the best learner outcomes.

To create a safe learning environment, all learners should be oriented to the equipment, surroundings, environment, and fidelity of all equipment to be used in the simulation. Orientation for learners should occur prior to any requirement to perform and address any equipment that is not high-fidelity or working the same as it would in the real environment. An example of this would be an IV pump that is actual patient equipment but is off and instead has a piece of tape on the display screen as a visual cue of the rate of infusion. Orientation may be required for assessment findings also. An example is applying anti-embolism stockings stuffed with cushioning or towels to a mannequin's lower legs to depict edema. This could be confusing to the learners in the simulation because without explanation they might assume it is just the stockings and not edema.

Being familiar and comfortable with the simulation scenario themselves can help educators provide a safe environment for learners. After the simulation has been developed, educators should rehearse with simulation personnel or other simulation educators to determine the flow and accuracy of the simulation and note any deficiencies prior to learners participating. Peer review scenarios to ensure the incorporation of evidence-based practices, accuracy, and appropriateness for the level of the learner—and to ensure the objectives can be accomplished within the time frame stated.

As with any new activity, learners will face a learning curve. The learners should be oriented to the lab and equipment along with the expectations. Learners need to understand this is not "play time" but a chance to practice the role of a healthcare professional providing evidence-based care to a human. The more suspension of disbelief that occurs, the more immersed the learner can become in the simulation. Educators must explain clear expectations of the performance as well as the behaviors that are allowed and others that will not be tolerated. Learners' first simulation experience should be formative as a learning experience before they are subjected to any testing, such as skills validation or summative performance.

Learners must also understand the need for professional integrity. For everyone to feel safe, the simulation information must remain confidential, and learners should understand that no information should be shared and that they must maintain legal, ethical, and/or institutional regulations (INACSL Standards Committee, 2016c). Educators need to explain the relationship between the Health Insurance Portability and Accountability Act and academic integrity in the simulation setting. Learners must understand that by discussing the simulation experience with others not directly involved in the same simulation session, they are sharing privileged information. One intervention that can assist with maintaining the academic integrity of the simulation is to have the learners sign a confidentiality agreement (see Figure 3.9) after offering a detailed explanation of the need for self-discovery of a problem.

School of Nursing
Professional Integrity and Confidentiality for Simulated Clinical Experiences

Professional integrity, including confidentiality of the performances, scenario content, and experience, is expected to be upheld. Professional integrity is expected for all components and participants in the simulation environment. Failure of the participants to maintain professional integrity related to simulation could undermine the benefits of the simulated clinical experience.

Privileged information of any kind can bias an individual's performance and interfere with the group's dynamics, thereby interfering with learning outcomes. Sharing of events and individual performances occurring during the simulation sessions with those not involved in the event may decrease the safe environment of the simulation setting. Sharing of events and correct action in the simulation with those not involved in the event may negatively alter future participants' learning outcomes. Failure to comply with this is an act of academic dishonesty. Please refer to X and the academic dishonesty section of the course syllabus.

I, _____, promise to adhere to the X
     (Print Name)
University School of Nursing Professional Integrity and Confidentiality for Simulated Clinical Experiences statement. I will not provide or share any information after completion of a simulated clinical experience, ask for information about the simulated clinical experience prior to participating in a simulated clinical experience, and/or provide any cues or hints to other students until all students have participated in the simulation experience. Failure to comply with this is an act of academic dishonesty. Refer to X University Academic Dishonesty Policy for details.

_____   _____
    Date   Student Signature

_____   _____
   Course   Witness Signature

FIGURE 3.9 Sample confidentiality agreement.

Educational Objectives

Scenarios need to be evidence-based. An effective simulation environment is one intentionally linked to the educational objectives. As shown earlier in Table 3.2, educators should select the type of mannequin and degree of fidelity based on the goals, outcomes, and objectives of the simulation, not just the type of equipment and fidelity available (INACSL Standards Committee, 2016d). Objectives determine the focus of the simulation and specify what the learner will be able to perform when the simulation is complete. The objectives guide all simulation planning, including cues for fidelity, the scenario end point, debriefing, and evaluation. Objectives must be clear and measurable to guide the educator to consistent and reliable evaluation of outcomes.

Planning and Preparing for the Simulation Experience

Educators should begin simulation planning and development by reviewing the learning objectives. What must the learner do to demonstrate competence? An example of a simulation observation template is shown in Template 3.1. After the goal and objectives are determined, educators need to determine the level of fidelity required (mannequin, environment, psychological). Ideally, this process should begin at least four weeks prior to each simulation.

Simulation centers should develop checklists for simulation that staff and facilitators use for scenario preparation to ensure that an appropriate level of fidelity is created and consistency is maintained between learning sessions. Checklists are also helpful in ensuring the many details are brought together.

Developing a clinically specific simulator setup list of moulage, learners, props, and equipment available in the simulation lab enables educators to clearly and consistently communicate their needs while providing examples that will stimulate their imagination. This tool helps simulation staff ensure that clinically significant cues are in place for the learner. These tools and other simulation documents may be archived in an online faculty simulation course to increase faculty access and use. A sample simulation setup request form is shown in Template 3.2.

Rubric Formative Simulation Center Observation
NGR 6002C Advanced Health Assessment
Semester _____ Year_____
SP Case 2

1.
2.
3.
4.
* = critical element
This is a checklist for observing students during Simulation Center encounters with the Standardized Patients. Support your scoring with Feedback.

Student: **Faculty Observer:**

Elements and Samples of Behavior	Poss Pts	S	U	Comments
Must verify patient's name and DOB	1			All or nothing

TEMPLATE 3.1   Simulation observation template.

USF Health Simulation Request Form (DUE 8 WEEKS PRIOR TO SIM DATE)

Simulation Scenario/Lab Title:

Faculty Requesting: Date of Request:

USF
HEALTH

Simulation/Lab Request Form

Location of Simulation (select one)	CACL	CAMLS	Nursing Lab
Time required for simulation:			
Time required for debrief:			
Simulation			
Dates			
Times			
Days of Week			
Number of simulation sessions requesting			
Course Name and Number			
Number of Total Students			
Maximum of Students in each simulation			
Minimum of Students in each simulation			
Description of simulation			
B Line or Video Recording			

TEMPLATE 3.2   Sample simulation setup request form.

Online educator simulation courses can be developed in any electronic classroom management system such as Blackboard, Canvas, or WebCT for academic institutions and an intranet system for healthcare institutions. They serve as a wonderful repository for moulage recipes, faculty-accessible scenarios, documents used in simulations such as patient files, simulation framework, simulation education updates, forms, and simulation policies and procedures.

Educators should plan to arrive early for their scheduled simulation and check the simulation environment for simulation cues and clinical accuracy. Photographing the setup and moulage of each scenario is also recommended. Photographs provide visual cues to stage the simulation consistently every time, thereby increasing the reliability and validity and potentially improving outcomes. This is especially true for courses with a large number of learner groups in which the same simulation is conducted over a period of time, requiring the scenario to be set up multiple times. These photographs can be digitally stored, printed, or kept with the scenario.

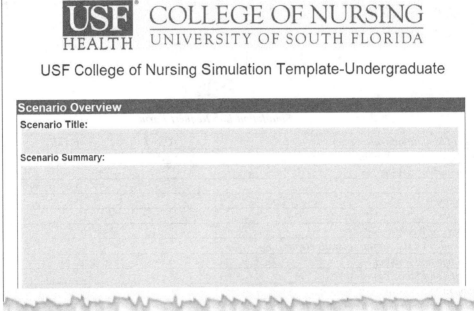

TEMPLATE 3.3   Undergraduate simulation template.

Planning, managing, and organizing moulage and props can be challenging. Stacking plastic boxes with lids and inventory lists for each scenario may provide a manageable solution. Creating a basic moulage kit is a great starting point. This kit should include basic makeup such as blue, brown, and black non-shimmering eye shadows or powders, which may be used as eye shadow or to simulate cyanosis or bruising. Be sure to check with the simulator manufacturer regarding what products may damage or permanently stain the simulator. Application tips can usually be found on the manufacturer's webpage. Kits range from basic to extensive for wounds or replication of trauma victims. Suggested resources to include in a simulation kit are listed in the accompanying sidebar.

Simulation Kit Resources

- **Simulaids:** https://simulaids.com
- **Moulage Concepts:** https://moulageconcepts.com
- **Image Perspectives (The Injury Simulation People!):** www.moulage.net/index.html
- **Bound Tree:** https://boundtree.com

Planning a Simulation

1. Review the learning objectives.
2. Identify what the learner must do to demonstrate competence.
3. Determine the level of fidelity required.
4. Assemble a preparation checklist.
5. Generate or fill out a simulation request form.
6. Peer review the scenario.
7. Rehearse.
8. Arrive early.
9. Photograph the setup.

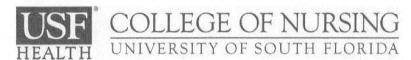

USF College of Nursing Simulation Template-Graduate

Scenario Overview

Scenario Title:

Scenario Summary:

TEMPLATE 3.4 Graduate simulation template.

Standardized Patient Case #

Disciplines: Case Code: SP stats:
Reviewer:

Presenting Problem:

Author(s):

Patient name:

Case Objectives:

Vital Signs should be included on the "Scenario" page

TEMPLATE 3.5   Online educator simulation courses scenario template.

Evaluation

Evaluating the simulation is an important step in maintaining and improving the quality of the simulation experience, determining whether the objectives of the simulation were met, and providing opportunities for improvements in the environmental fidelity of the simulation. This evaluation should include feedback on the simulation environment, props, moulage, content, and more. Typically, simulations require several rounds of minor adjustments before everyone involved deems them "perfect." Chapter 6 provides details on evaluating simulations.

Conclusion

Simulation educators can create effective simulation environments for the purposes of educating students (undergraduate or graduate-level), practitioners from all disciplines and experience levels, faculty, and healthcare providers who wish to continue professional development or want to be lifelong learners. We provide in Templates 3.3, 3.4, and 3.5 examples of scenarios that incorporate what has been presented in this chapter.

Increasing the depth to which learners can become immersed in the simulation environment through strategies that facilitate the suspension of disbelief increases the potential for learning.

Through incorporation of psychological factors throughout the simulation and the use of mannequins and moulage, suspension of disbelief can be achieved, allowing learners to find the relevance in the simulation.

The use of simulation is limited only by one's imagination. So, dream big, reach for the stars, and improve healthcare one provider at a time.

References

Alexander, M., Durham, C. F., Hooper, J. I., Jeffries, P. R., Goldman, N., Kardong-Edgren, S., . . . Tillman, C. L. (2015). NCSBN simulation guidelines for prelicensure nursing programs. *Journal of Nursing Regulation, 6*(3), 39-42. doi:10.1016/S2155-8256(15)30783-3

Cantrell, M. A., Franklin, A., Leighton, K., & Carlson, A. (2017). The evidence in simulation-based learning experiences in nursing education and practice: An umbrella review. *Clinical Simulation in Nursing, 13*(12), 634-667. doi:10.1016/j.ecns.2017.08.004

Damazo, R. J., & Damazo, B. J. (2018). Leading artistry in simulation: Moulage and more. In C. Foisy-Doll & K. Leighton (Eds.), *Simulation champions: Courage, caring, and connection* (pp. 378-396). Philadelphia, PA: Wolters Kluwer.

Doran, G. T. (1981). There's a S.M.A.R.T. way to write management's goals and objectives. *Management Review, 70*(11), 35-36.

Hayden, J. K., Smiley, R. A., Alexander, M., Kardong-Edgren, S., & Jeffries, P. R. (2014). The NCSBN national simulation study: A longitudinal, randomized controlled study replacing clinical hours with simulation in prelicensure nursing education. *Journal of Nursing Regulation, 5*(2), S1–S64. Retrieved from https://www.ncsbn.org/JNR_Simulation_Supplement.pdf

Howard, V., Leighton, K., & Gore, T. (2018). Simulation in healthcare education. In R. Nelson & N. Staggers (Eds.), *Health informatics: An interprofessional approach* (2nd ed., pp. 557-576). St. Louis, MO: Elsevier.

International Nursing Association for Clinical Simulation and Learning Board of Directors. (2011). Standards of best practice: Simulation. Standard I: Terminology. *Clinical Simulation in Nursing, 7*(4S), s3-s7. doi:10.1016/j.ecns.2011.05.005

International Nursing Association for Clinical Simulation and Learning Standards Committee. (2016a). INACSL standards of best practice: Simulation. Facilitation. *Clinical Simulation in Nursing, 12*(S), S16-S20. doi:10.1016/j.ecns.2016.09.007

International Nursing Association for Clinical Simulation and Learning Standards Committee. (2016b). INACSL standards of best practice: Simulation. Outcomes and objectives. *Clinical Simulation in Nursing, 12*(S), S13-S15. doi:10.1016/j.ecns.2016.09.006

International Nursing Association for Clinical Simulation and Learning Standards Committee. (2016c). INACSL standards of best practice: Simulation. Professional integrity. *Clinical Simulation in Nursing, 12*(S), S30-S33. doi:10.1016/j.ecns.2016.09.010

International Nursing Association for Clinical Simulation and Learning Standards Committee. (2016d). INACSL standards of best practice: Simulation. Simulation design. *Clinical Simulation in Nursing, 12*(S), S5-S12. doi:10.1016/j.ecns.2016.09.005

International Nursing Association for Clinical Simulation and Learning Standards Committee. (2016e). INACSL standards of best practice: Simulation. Simulation glossary. *Clinical Simulation in Nursing, 12*(S), S39-S47. doi:10.1016/j.ecns.2016.09.012

Kamp, F. (2018). Making simulation center rooms more realistic. In C. Foisy-Doll & K. Leighton (Eds.), *Simulation champions: Courage, caring, and connection* (pp. 382-383). Philadelphia, PA: Wolters Kluwer.

Kardong-Edgren, S., Lungstrom, N., & Bendel, R. (2009). VitalSim versus SimMan: A comparison of BSN student test scores, knowledge retention, and satisfaction. *Clinical Simulation in Nursing, 5*(3), e105-e111. doi:10.1016/j.ecns.2009.01.007

Lioce, L. (Ed.), Lopreiato, J. (Founding Ed.), Downing, D., Chang, T. P., Robertson, J. M., Anderson, M., . . . the Terminology and Concepts Working Group. (2020). *Healthcare simulation dictionary* (2nd ed.). AHRQ Publication No. 20-0019. Rockville, MD: Agency for Healthcare Research and Quality. Retrieved from https://doi.org/10.23970/simulationv2

Muckler, V. C. (2017). Exploring suspension of disbelief during simulation-based learning. *Clinical Simulation in Nursing, 13*(1), 3-9. doi:10.1016/j.ecns.2016.09.004

Muckler, V. C., & Thomas, C. (2019). Exploring suspension of disbelief among graduate and undergraduate nursing students. *Clinical Simulation in Nursing, 35*, 25–32. doi: https://doi.org/10.1016/j.ecns.2019.06.006

Palaganas, J. C., Maxworthy, J. C., Epps, C. A., & Mancini, M. E. (Eds.). (2015). *Defining excellence in simulation programs*. Philadelphia, PA: Wolters Kluwer.

Rudolph, J. W., McIntosh, C. A., Simon, R., & Raemer, D. B. (2015). Helping learners "buy in" to simulation. In J. C. Palaganas, J. C. Maxworthy, C. A. Epps, & M. E. Mancini (Eds.), *Defining excellence in simulation programs* (pp. 579-580). Philadelphia, PA: Wolters Kluwer.

Scheese, C. H. (2019). Operations and management of environment, personnel, and nonpersonnel resources. In L. Wilson & R. A. Wittman-Price (Eds.), *Review manual for the Certified Healthcare Simulation Educator (CHSE) Exam* (2nd ed., pp. 297–322). New York, NY: Springer Publishing.

Zigmont, J., Oocumma, N., Szyld, D., & Maestre, J. J. (2015). Educator training and simulation methodology courses. In J. C. Palaganas, J. C. Maxworthy, C. A. Epps, & M. E. Mancini (Eds.), *Defining excellence in simulation programs* (pp. 546-557). Philadelphia, PA: Wolters Kluwer.

"See it, feel it, believe it, achieve it!"

−R. Byrne

Creating Effective, Evidence-Based Scenarios

4

Valerie M. Howard, EdD, MSN, RN, CNE, FAAN

Simulation is an experiential teaching methodology. As such, its use in a healthcare or academic setting should be guided by sound educational principles (Clapper, 2010; International Nursing Association for Clinical Simulation and Learning [INACSL] Standards Committee, 2016a). Because simulation offers a standardized, controlled environment for applied learning opportunities, it is ideal for conveying knowledge needed to handle low-occurrence, high-risk situations in the clinical setting.

When implementing simulation either within an academic or service setting, you must first develop a scenario. A *clinical scenario* is defined as:

> a detailed outline of a clinical encounter that includes: the participants in the event, briefing notes, goals and learning objectives, participant instructions, patient information, environmental conditions, manikin, or standardized patient preparation, related equipment, props, and tools or resources for assessing and managing the simulated experience. (Lioce et al., 2020, p. 10)

Therefore, a simulation is a planned educational experience developed by a facilitator or educator to help the learner meet learning objectives. The scenario guides the learning opportunities for the participants. Solid educational practices consist of active learning, providing appropriate feedback, facilitating learner-educator interaction, and fostering diverse and collaborative learning.

To be effective, simulation scenarios need to be valid and reliable. *Simulation validity* is "the degree to which a test or evaluation tool accurately measures the intended concept of interest" (INACSL Standards Committee, 2016f, p. s45). *Simulation reliability* is "the consistency of a simulation activity, or the degree

OBJECTIVES

- Identify educational theories to guide simulation scenario development.

- Utilize the best clinical evidence when developing simulation scenarios.

- Demonstrate the critical elements of scenario development.

to which a simulation activity measures in the same way each time it is used under the same conditions with the same participants" (Lioce et al., 2020, p. 46).

The key to successful implementation of a simulation scenario lies in careful planning to map out the scenario details (Howard, Englert, Kameg, & Perozzi, 2011; Jeffries, 2012; Waxman, 2010). The scenario-development process should include participant preparation, pre-briefing materials, patient information with descriptions of the scenario, learning objectives, environmental conditions, related equipment and props to enhance realism, roles and expectations of participants, standardized patient scripts, a progression outline for the actual simulation implementation, a standardized debriefing process, and evaluation criteria (Alinier, 2011; INACSL Standards Committee, 2016a; Jeffries, 2007). Outcomes of a positive simulation experience can include knowledge attainment, improved skill performance, learner satisfaction, and increased self-confidence, among others.

The first step in the scenario planning process is to choose a topic for the simulation scenario. Topics for simulation scenarios can be generated

in multiple ways. For example, scenarios in an academic setting can be developed to:

- Align with course content and objectives
- Provide opportunities to practice skills that do not occur often in a clinical situation
- Enhance student performance in areas where feedback from clinical agencies suggests it may be lacking
- Address additional training needed as a result of emerging healthcare trends or new policies or regulations
- Address needs identified from evaluation data from standardized tests, such as the National Council Licensure Examination (NCLEX) for registered nurses (RNs), to provide application of knowledge

In clinical settings, such as hospitals or ambulatory care settings, scenarios can be developed to:

- Teach new competencies
- Evaluate ongoing competencies of clinical professionals

Generating Ideas for Simulation Scenarios

- Course objectives
- Essential learning outcomes
- High-risk, low-occurrence situations
- Results of standardized tests
- Learner performance in the clinical setting
- Healthcare trends
- Journal articles
- Policy and regulations
- Competency evaluation
- System assessment and improvement

- Improve efficiency

- Assess a process for the potential for latent errors

- Test workflow design

Relevant Educational Theories and Models

When designing any educational modality, educational theories and models should guide development (Clapper, 2010; Kaakinen & Arwood, 2009). The same holds true for simulation.

Multiple learning theories can be used to guide the educational process, such as novice to expert (Benner, 1984), the adult learning theory (Knowles, 1984), situated learning (Lave & Wenger, 1991), and the interactive model of clinical judgment development (Lasater, 2007). However, two theories in particular uniquely align with simulation—Kolb's experiential learning theory (Kolb, 1984) and the National League for Nursing (NLN) Jeffries simulation theory (Jeffries, 2007; see Table 4.1).

The ability to transfer theoretical knowledge and apply this in a practice setting leads to the acquisition of knowledge, according to experiential learning theory (Kolb, 1984). Service industry professions such as nursing and medicine have long accepted this notion by incorporating clinical experiences along with didactic lecture. The learners need to be able to apply these abstract classroom concepts during a practical learning experience in order to enhance cognitive development. According to experiential learning theory, learning is enhanced when learners are actively involved in gaining knowledge through experience with problem solving and decision-making, and active reflection is integral to the learning process (Dewey, 1938; Kolb, 1984). Education is a result of experience (Dewey, 1938). The process of reflection is a cognitive process that can be enhanced through a structured learning activity. Kolb's theory has been used many times in service industries to explain the necessity for incorporating practice into the curriculum, such as through a nursing student's clinical experiences and simulation. The debriefing experience after the simulation experience directly mirrors the importance of reflection as an integral part of the learning process. It is during this experience that learners cognitively and purposefully think about the learning experience, and the abstract principles learned in the classroom become concrete as a result of their application.

Table 4.1 Educational Theories and Models Linked to Simulation	
Theory	**Theorist**
Novice to expert	Benner, 1984
Experiential learning theory	Kolb, 1984
Adult learning theory	Knowles, 1984
Situated learning	Lave & Wenger, 1991
Interactive model of clinical judgment development	Lasater, 2007
NLN/Jeffries simulation theory	Jeffries, 2015

The NLN, in partnership with the Laerdal Corporation, developed a simulation framework based upon empirical and theoretical literature (Jeffries, 2007). This framework, known as the NLN/Jeffries simulation framework, was updated in 2015 to the NLN/Jeffries simulation theory after a thorough synthesis of the literature, discussions with simulation educators and leaders, and minor edits to the concepts. The theory is useful in designing, implementing, and evaluating simulations (see Figure 4.1; Jeffries, Rodgers, & Adamson, 2015). The design of the simulation experience is characterized by a dynamic interaction between the facilitator and participant, including educational strategies that are experiential, interactive, collaborative, learner centered, and conducted in an environment of trust. Outcomes of simulation experiences can be measured at the system, patient, or participant level (Jeffries et al., 2015). Although the framework was initially developed for the academic setting in 2007, each component can be applied to scenario development in the service or hospital setting. For example, the *teacher* in the academic setting is equivalent to the *nurse educator* or *staff development personnel* in the hospital setting. According to the INACSL standards, the more appropriate term would be *facilitator.* "A facilitator assumes responsibility and oversight for managing the entire simulation-based experience" (see Table 4.2; INACSL Standards Committee, 2016b, p. S16).

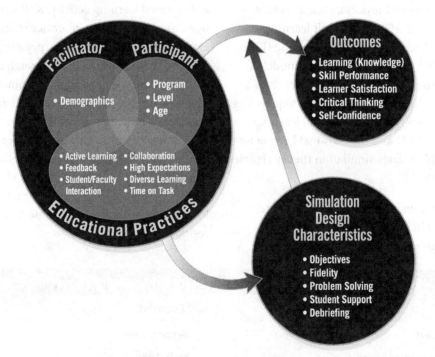

FIGURE 4.1   NLN/Jeffries Simulation Theory.

Table 4.2 Terms		
Terms Used in NLN/Jeffries Simulation Framework for Nursing Education or Academic Setting	**Terms Used in the Service, Hospital, or Clinical Setting**	**INACSL Standard I Terminology That Can Be Used Interchangeably in Any Setting**
Teacher	Nurse educator Staff development specialist	Facilitator
Student	Learner	Participant

Within each component, variables exist that should be addressed when designing simulations. For example, educators need to be facilitators of learning in this learner-centered environment. In addition, educators may need support with technology and simulation design. Within the simulation environment, the roles of the learners within the scenario should be clearly defined. Learners are expected to be self-motivated and responsible for their own learning. Educational practices consist of active learning, providing appropriate feedback, facilitating student-faculty interaction (or learner-educator interaction), and fostering diverse, collaborative learning. A time frame for each scenario should be established. Objectives should be clearly defined. With the exception of the pre-briefing, learners should receive relatively little information at the start of the scenario so that the details of the scenario are not exposed prior to the scenario being run. For example, the participants may be informed that they will be providing care for a cardiac patient, without providing the details that the patient is experiencing an acute myocardial infarction. Building on this concept, the participants should be informed of the need to intervene appropriately, without providing the details that they will need to administer oxygen or specific medications. The participants have the opportunity to analyze the situation and ask appropriate questions to gather more data during the scenario. Debriefing may be the most powerful tool used following the simulation experience, allowing participants to reflect and analyze their performance critically, and adequate time should be allotted for this activity. Finally, the outcomes of a simulated experience can be those of knowledge attainment, improved skill performance, learner satisfaction, and increased self-confidence, among others. Utilizing the NLN/Jeffries simulation theory can maximize the amount of learning that occurs, and it is described in more detail throughout subsequent sections of this chapter.

In addition, INACSL developed standards of best practice for simulation in 2011, with published revisions every three years, that can guide scenario development (Sittner et al., 2015). The standards were developed with input from simulation experts and address the following topics: simulation design, outcomes and objectives, facilitation, debriefing, participant evaluation, professional integrity, simulation enhanced IPE, and operations. Many of these standards address elements related to scenario development and will be referenced accordingly.

Preplanned Simulation Scenarios for Purchase

Many organizations offer preplanned scenarios for purchase. Examples include:

- Simulation Learning System (Elsevier Publishing Company)
- Program for Nursing Curriculum Integration (CAE Healthcare)
- Real Nursing Simulations (Pearson Publishing Company)
- Lippincott's Clinical Simulations (Lippincott Publishing Company)
- Simulation Innovation Resource Center (NLN)
- Nursing Scenarios (Laerdal Corporation and NLN)

Although these scenarios can save time and resources, educators must ensure that the preplanned scenario objectives correlate with a program's objectives and with the level of the learner.

Kolb's experiential learning theory, the NLN/Jeffries simulation theory, and the INACSL standards provide a sound basis to guide simulation research and training. A conceptual framework should be utilized when designing simulation experiences and research studies (Paige & Daley, 2009).

Scenario Development

Proper planning is paramount to successful implementation of a simulation scenario for education and training purposes. The scenario development process can be broken down into three distinct phases. The constructs of the NLN/Jeffries simulation theory can provide guidance in each phase.

- Phase I: Planning and Pre-briefing
- Phase II: Scenario Implementation
- Phase III: Debriefing and Evaluation

Phase I: Planning and Pre-briefing

Often called the "pre-scenario" phase, the planning phase incorporates all the activities that must occur before the scenario is actually implemented. During this phase, the facilitator must allot enough time to both plan and pilot test the scenario prior to participation by the learners.

Because of the level of detail needed to plan a scenario, using a standardized planning form or template can be helpful (Howard, Ross, Mitchell, & Nelson, 2010; INACSL Standards Committee, 2016a; iRIS, n.d.; Waxman, 2010). These tools help ensure all aspects of scenario development are considered and that the simulation experience can be replicated in the future (thus providing a standardized educational experience for all learners).

Although templates developed at several organizations are publicly available, one example of a scenario planning template is included at the end of this chapter in Figure 4.10. Each element of this particular template is discussed in detail. A note about the use of scenario templates: Although the example provided in this chapter follows the NLN/Jeffries simulation framework and is used by the Robert Morris University Regional RISE Center, there are many standard templates available on the internet. You can find examples in the INACSL Standards of Best

Practice: Simulation Design (2016a), in the NLN Simulation Innovation Resource Center, on many simulation vendor websites, and in other resources such as MedEdPortal and the Society for Simulation in Healthcare's SimConnect. It is important to find a template that applies to your situation and that can be modified to meet your own organization's needs.

Initial Elements

A scenario planning template should have clearly identifiable information, such as the name of the simulation course and the simulation focus, listed first. To help make sure the most up-to-date evidence is being used for development and implementation, clinical content experts should review each scenario to ensure the activities mirror clinical standards of care (INACSL Standards Committee, 2016a; Reibel, Cason, & Screws, 2019; Waxman, 2010). This ensures that the scenario content closely mirrors the best practices of the clinical setting—a goal for simulation experiences. Standards and guidelines for clinical treatment of conditions should be reviewed, and current references should be included in the template. Although there is no evidence that establishes a specific time limit for each scenario, the time limit should be specified, in addition to indicating the time needed for the debriefing experience. This is helpful for planning and scheduling in the simulation center.

A trained facilitator should conduct simulation scenarios and use different types of facilitation methods to guide the learning activities for the participants to assist them in meeting the scenario objectives (INACSL Standards Committee, 2016b). The methods of facilitation should be based upon the level of the learner and determined prior to implementing the scenario.

Facilitation methods and cueing are based upon the level of the learner, the outcomes, and the goal for the simulation (Lewis et al., 2019). For example, if the scenario is being used for evaluative purposes, the facilitator would refrain from prompting in order to maintain a controlled testing environment for the participant. Alternatively, a more fully engaged facilitation method might be needed for less experienced participants in order to guide them to attain the educational objectives. Although any degree of facilitation may be used, identifying the level prior to implementing the scenario is important to ensure standardized conditions for learning within the simulation room (INACSL Standards Committee, 2016b; Waxman, 2010).

To maximize successful performance, the scenario should be developed at a level appropriate for the learner (INACSL Standards Committee, 2016a). In other words, facilitators and educators must assess the level of the learner before developing the scenario in order to effectively build upon prior learning. Prerequisite knowledge should be addressed, and any pre-scenario learning activities (pre-briefing) for the participant should be identified. The purpose of pre-briefing is to set the stage for the scenario, identify expectations, and establish ground rules and guidelines (INACSL Standards Committee, 2016a, McDermott, 2016). This enables participants to adequately prepare to meet the challenges of the scenario and intervene effectively with the patient. The scenario description is a one- to two-paragraph summary of the scenario and can help guide future facilitators in your institution when choosing scenarios. Figure 4.2 shows the initial elements portions of a scenario planning template.

Course: NURS 4031 Transition to Professional Practice

Scenario Topic/Name: Alcohol Withdrawal Syndrome

Developed by Kameg, K., Howard, V., Perozzi, K., & Englert, N.

Robert Morris University, School of Nursing & Health Sciences

Template adapted from J. Sarasnick, MSN, RN

References Used:

Adams, B., & Ferguson, K. (2017). Pharmacologic management of alcohol withdrawal syndrome in intensive care units. *AACN Advanced Critical Care, 28*(3), 233–238.

Foertsch, M. J., Winter, J. B., Rhoades, A. G., Martin, L. T., Droege, C. A., & Ernst, N. E. (2019). Recognition, assessment, and pharmacotherapeutic treatment of alcohol withdrawal syndrome in the intensive care unit. *Critical Care Nursing Quarterly, 42*(1), 12–29.

Halter, M. J. (2018). *Varcarolis' foundations of psychiatric mental health nursing: A clinical approach* (8th ed.). St. Louis, MO: Elsevier.

Higgins-Biddle, J. C., & Babor, T. F. (2018). A review of the Alcohol Use Disorders Identification Test (AUDIT), AUDIT-C, and US AUDIT for screening in the United States: Past issues and future directions. *The American Journal of Drug and Alcohol Abuse, 44*(6), 578–586.

Linder, L. M., Robert, S., Mullinax, K., & Hayes, G. (2018). Thiamine prescribing and Wernicke's encephalopathy risk factors in patients with alcohol use disorders at a psychiatric hospital. *Journal of Psychiatric Practice, 24*(5), 317–322.

Parsons, G. (2018). Prevalence, identification and harms of alcohol use disorders. *Prescriber, 29*(11), 19–23.

Thursz, M., Gual, A., Lackner, C., Mathurin, P., Moreno, C., Spahr, L., ... Cortez-Pinto, H. (2018). EASL clinical practice guidelines: Management of alcohol-related liver disease. *Journal of Hepatology, 69*(1), 154–181.

Estimated Scenario Time: 30 minutes

Estimated Debriefing Time: 30 minutes

Instructors of the Course:

Simulation Facilitator:

Facilitation Prompting: Partial

Student level: Senior BSN Students

Prerequisite Knowledge/Pre-scenario Learning Activity:

1. Successful completion of NURS 4020 Advanced Management of the Adult II

2. Successful completion of NURS 4025 Nursing Care of Psychiatric Clients

3. Read Chapter 22 of Halter, M. J. (2018). *Varcarolis' foundations of psychiatric mental health nursing: A clinical approach* (8th ed.). St. Louis, MO: Elsevier.

Scenario Description

Helene is a 70-year-old female admitted to the hospital for acute gastritis. On the second day of admission, she becomes anxious and jittery and begins to hallucinate. Her husband, George, brings these behaviors to the attention of the nurse. During the scenario, the nursing student will have the opportunity to provide nursing care for a client experiencing symptoms of acute alcohol withdrawal.

FIGURE 4.2   Scenario planning template: Initial elements

Development of Objectives

The development of educational objectives can address the three domains of learning: cognitive, affective, and psychomotor. Educational objectives should be written as clearly and concisely as possible. These objectives guide the experience and provide assistance in determining the outcomes from the experience. Objectives should be measurable (or observable) and use verbs based upon Bloom's Taxonomy of Learning (Bloom et al., 1956). Because simulation requires application of knowledge, the objectives should be written at Bloom's Taxonomy level of "application" or higher. Participant objectives should address the domains of learning, be congruent with the program outcomes and learner level, incorporate evidence-based practice, and be achievable within the recommended time frame (INACSL Standards Committee, 2016c). The Centers for Disease Control and Prevention (2018) suggests that objectives for healthcare education should be S.M.A.R.T.—smart, measurable, achievable, realistic, and time-phased. Childs and Sepples (2006) suggest using the nursing process to design scenario objectives. Figure 4.3 shows objectives that align with the nursing process and address the three domains of learning.

Scenario Planning Template: Objectives

Learning Objectives

Upon completion of this scenario, the participant will be able to:

1. Assess the client who is experiencing signs and symptoms of alcohol withdrawal (Psychomotor Domain).
   - Tremors, diaphoresis, hypertension, tachycardia, hallucinations
   - The Clinical Institute Withdrawal Assessment for Alcohol scale (CIWA-Ar) score
2. Utilize therapeutic communication while caring for the client who is experiencing signs and symptoms of alcohol withdrawal (Affective Domain).
   - Establish rapport with the patient and husband
   - Use open-ended questions, empathy, clarification, etc.
3. Utilize appropriate Nursing Diagnoses to plan care for the client who is experiencing signs and symptoms of alcohol withdrawal (Cognitive Domain).
   - Deficient knowledge
   - Ineffective individual coping
   - Ineffective health maintenance
   - Risk for injury

4. Intervene effectively for the client who is experiencing signs and symptoms of alcohol withdrawal (Psychomotor Domain).
   - Quiet, well-lit room with environmental cues
   - IVF: NSS at 100 mL/hour
   - Thiamine 100mg IV prior to giving any glucose containing IVF
   - Folate 1mg
   - Multivitamin with B-12
   - CIWA-Ar Score: 18 – Lorazepam 0.5-1 mg IV q 15 min prn withdrawal symptoms
5. Evaluate the effectiveness of interventions for the client who is experiencing signs and symptoms of alcohol withdrawal (Cognitive and Psychomotor Domains).
   - Vital signs
   - Level of agitation/anxiety
   - Sedation scale
   - Absence of seizure activity
   - Absence of falls
   - Absence of hallucinations
6. Reflect upon the learning that occurred during the simulation scenario (Affective Domain).
   - Journal
   - Discussions during debriefing
   - Administer post-simulation evaluation survey upon conclusion of experience.

FIGURE 4.3   Scenario planning template: Objectives.

Fidelity and Supplies

Adequate planning also includes matching the appropriate level of fidelity with the objectives, and this leads to the identification of necessary supplies. Situated learning theory stresses the importance of learning within social situations and a social context (Lave & Wenger, 1991), which is why the experience in the simulation lab should closely mimic the reality of the clinical setting. Simulation facilitators should try to replicate the clinical setting as much as possible.

Depending upon the objectives, it may be realistic to use a standardized patient rather than a high fidelity full-body simulator. For example, many scenarios with objectives primarily focusing on therapeutic communication may be best developed using standardized patient simulation techniques. However, a programmable mannequin might be best suited for objectives related to care of a patient experiencing a cardiac arrest due to the invasive nature of the psychomotor skills that need to be performed. Therefore, the type of mannequin, task trainer, or standardized patient should be predetermined using the scenario template (Jeffries, 2007; Waxman, 2010). In addition, any supplies related to the implementation of the scenario should be identified, such as medications, healthcare supplies, and those moulage materials meant to enhance the fidelity or realism of the environment (see Figure 4.4). Detailed information on creating effective simulation environments can be found in Chapter 3.

The Use of Standardized Patients

A *standardized patient* is "an individual trained to portray a patient with a specific condition in a realistic, standardized, and repeatable way and where portrayal/presentation varies based only on learner performance; this strict standardization of performance in a simulated session is what

can distinguish standardized patients from simulated patients" (Lioce et al., 2020, p. 49). Standardized patients are particularly valuable when implementing scenarios focusing upon development of communication skills. When using standardized patients in a simulation scenario, many experts suggest a detailed process to follow when developing the scripts, training the actor, and allowing the standardized patient to participate in the debriefing process (Bosek, Li, & Hicks, 2007). The Association for Standardized Patient Educators (ASPE) adopted Standards of Best Practice in 2017 (Lewis et al., 2017). These standards should be used when developing simulation-based learning experiences incorporating standardized/simulated patients in scenarios.

Patient Information

Just as in the clinical setting, the simulated patient's history and physiologic vital signs play an important part in clinical decision-making. Therefore, when planning the scenario, it is helpful to provide as much information about the patient's history to guide the participant in meeting the objectives. Although some simulation experts may prefer to fully develop a simulated patient's medical record in order to enhance realism, many suggest that just the important details be included in the patient's history in order to guide the decision-making process during the scenario. The facilitator must make a conscious decision to determine which elements of a simulated patient's history are necessary to include to enable the participant to meet the objectives of the scenario. The facilitator must also provide the initial simulator settings for the presenting patient condition. The settings are dependent upon the simulator chosen and the functions provided. Figure 4.5 shows a sample scenario planning template with patient information added.

Scenario Planning Template: Supplies		
Identify Type of Mannequin, Task Trainer, or Standardized Patient		
High-fidelity mannequin for patient **Standardized patient or actor to play the role of spouse**		
Equipment Needed		
PPE gloves	Mask	Goggles
Isolation Gown	Stethoscope	
X SPO$_2$	X ECG Monitor	Defibrillator/Pacer
Lab Reports	X MD Orders	X Medical Records
EMR—SLS#_____	X iPod touch/PDA	Reference Material (book)
Oxygen NC	Oxygen FM	Oxygen Non-Rebreather
X Suction	Tracheostomy	Foley
X IV in Place	IV Start Kit	Crash Cart
X Glucometer	X-rays	12 Lead Type, i.e. NSR
ECG Machine (12 lead)	Blood	Baby Bottle
Ventilator	Vaginal Bleeding	Pediatric Supplies
Diaphoresis	Bloody wound	X ID/Allergy Band
Nasal Secretions	Mouth Secretions	Urine
Other:	Other:	Other:
Medications and IV Fluids: Dosage, Diluents Used, Methods of Delivery		
1. NSS 1 liter bag 2. Thiamine 100mg IV 3. Folate IV 4. Multivitamin/B12 for IV bag 5. Lorazepam 1mg IV q15 minutes for symptoms of alcohol withdrawal—Monitor sedation scale		

FIGURE 4.4   Scenario planning template: Supplies.

Scenario Planning Template: Patient Information

Simulated Patient History

Name: Helene Bender

Age: 70

Weight: 140 lb.   Height: 5'6"

Gender: Female

Past Medical History: Gastritis

Medications: Pepcid 20mg qd

Allergies: PCN

MD: Dr. Molnar

Simulation Setting: Inpatient Unit—Medical Surgical Floor

Background of presenting illness: Mrs. Bender was admitted 2 days ago for severe epigastric distress and heme positive emesis while at home. Her hemoglobin/hematocrit (H/H) were 10.9 gr/dL / 35%. An endoscopy performed yesterday revealed gastritis, and she was placed on IV Protonix. She was admitted to monitor H/H and epigastric symptoms.

Initial Vital Signs for Mannequin

Temperature	99.0° F
SPO$_2$	94%
Heart Rate	120
NIBP	150/90
ABP	
CVP/PA	
ECG Rhythm	Sinus Tachycardia
Sweating	Yes
Pulses normal, weak, or absent Pedal, dorsal, femoral, carotid, brachial	Pulses normal
Respirations shallow, labored, or normal	30—labored

FIGURE 4.5 Scenario planning template: Patient information.

Embedded Participants and Roles

An *embedded participant* is:

> an individual who is trained or scripted to play a role in a simulation encounter in order to guide the scenario, and may be known or unknown to the participants; guidance may be positive or negative, or a distractor based on the objectives, level of the participants, and the needs of the scenario. (Lioce et al., 2020, p. 16)

Embedded participants can play the roles of family members, neighbors, or healthcare providers. In order for the embedded participant to function effectively, the role must be described with a background story and a script for potential responses to questions provided (see Figure 4.6). The embedded participant can ask critical-thinking questions, such as "How does that medication work?" or "Why is my loved one acting so funny?" Although it is impossible to anticipate every action of a scenario, the preparation of a script to provide answers to potential questions or situations can assist all involved in the simulation scenario (Waxman, 2010). Often, the facilitator plays the role of the patient via the simulator voice function and the voice of other members of the healthcare team via telephone. Because the facilitator might be playing different roles based upon the resources available in the simulation lab, a script is especially helpful to guide the conversations. Trained actors can be used to play the additional roles in the scenario, but this requires additional cost for payment of services. Therefore, many simulation facilities use retired healthcare professionals, students, or faculty members to play these roles. Keep in mind that the use of embedded participants works best when the participant does not know the real identity of the person, because this can create role confusion. For example, using a faculty member to play the role of an embedded participant may create additional performance anxiety for the student in a simulation scenario because of the fear of unintended evaluation or judgment on the part of the faculty member.

Scenario Planning Template: Embedded Participants and Roles

XX	Primary Nurse
	Secondary Nurse
XX	Family Member: George (husband)
	Family Member
XX	MD or NP
	Ancillary Personnel (type)

continues

(cont.)

Scripts

Helene

Initially:

What is climbing on the wall?

Why am I shaking?

Where am I?

Where's my purse? I need to leave to go to Bingo.

Helene's Responses to Alcohol Withdrawal Assessment Scoring Guidelines (CIWA-Ar)

Nausea/Vomiting: 0

Anxiety: 4

Paroxysmal Sweats: 1

Tactile Disturbance: 0

Visual Disturbance: 4

Tremors: 2

Agitation: 3

Orientation and Clouding of Sensorium: 2

Auditory Disturbances: 3

Headache: 1

Helene Bender's Responses to CAGE Questionnaire

Following Lorazepam administration:

Helene: I'm feeling much more relaxed. What happened? Why am I in the hospital?

RN: *Helene, I am concerned about your drinking. When was your last drink, and how much did you drink?*

Helene: Oh, honey, I'm not sure. I think I had a few drinks with my friends at lunch the day before I came in. Then my stomach started to bother me. I thought it was from the crab cakes.

RN: *Have you ever experienced something similar to this before?*

Helene: No.

RN: *C: Have you ever felt you should cut down on your drinking?*

Helene: Well, sometimes George tells me this, but he is so conservative and strait-laced. All my friends drink like I do. I have to have drinks with them when we go out to lunch.

George: I am concerned about her. I just see her drinking more and more.

RN: *A: Have people annoyed you by criticizing your drinking?*

Helene: George is always the first to get on my nerves about my drinking. And, sometimes, my friends agree with him. Do you believe it? What kinds of friends are these?

RN: *G: Have you ever felt bad or guilty about your drinking?*

Helene: Well, only when my friends make a comment. But I've tried to quit several times.

RN: *E: Have you ever had an eye-opener, a drink first thing in the morning to steady your nerves or get rid of a hangover?*

Helene: I usually have a shot of whiskey in my coffee. It calms my nerves in the morning and helps me to think clearly. Then, my luncheons usually start around 12 noon, so I will have whatever is on the menu, spiked, of course.

RN expected actions:

Educate on complications of alcohol abuse/dependence

Utilize therapeutic communication

Contact MD with repeat CIWA-Ar score

MD Script

"What are the vital signs and CIWA-Ar score for Mrs. Bender?"

"I'm giving you a verbal order for Lorazepam 0.5-1 mg IV q15 minutes X 4 prn symptoms of agitation and hallucinations. Give her thiamine 100mg IV X 1. Also, start IVF NSS at 100mL/hour and add MVI, B12, folate 100mg. Call me after she has received these medications. Perform the CAGE assessment when you can."

After CAGE Questionnaire:

"Okay. Continue the CIWA-Ar protocol and the Ativan order. I will order a psychiatric consultation to discuss substance abuse."

George Bender (Helene's husband)

George has been the loving and enabling husband of Helene for 50 years. He is aware of her alcohol use but has not made the determination that it is detrimental to her health. He is caring and very concerned and scared about her initial state of withdrawal. He asks many questions of the primary nurse and does everything within his power to calm Helene down, yet his over-attentiveness begins to contribute to the anxiety of the situation. He tries to respond to the questions asked of Helene during the CIWA-Ar and CAGE assessments. The primary nurse should reinforce that Helene should be the one responding to the questions.

During the course of the scenario, George can ask or state:

"Why is she acting so funny?"

"Why are you giving her those medications? Do they have any side effects?"

"She usually has a drink around noon time each day."

"She is quite a socialite and attends many functions during the week."

FIGURE 4.6   Scenario planning template: Embedded participants and roles

Patient Report

Immediately before beginning a simulation, the facilitator may read a patient report to provide the framework and background history for the impending scenario (see Figure 4.7). This report sets the context for the participant and is the beginning of the scenario implementation phase. It is best to mirror the patient report to that which the learner may receive in the real-life clinical situation.

Scenario Planning Template: Patient Report

Mrs. Bender is a 70-year-old female admitted with acute epigastric distress and Heme positive emesis (coffee ground) 2 days ago. Her admitting hemoglobin and hematocrit (H/H) was 10.9 gm/dL / 35%. She had an EGD yesterday that revealed a small gastric ulcer, and she was placed on IV Protonix. She continues to be monitored for her H/H and signs of epigastric pain. VS have been stable with trends: Temp 98.4°; BP 120/76; Pulse 90; RR 16. It is admission day 3 at 10 a.m. Her husband, George, is at the bedside today and has just called for the nurse. As you enter the room, George states that his wife is "acting funny."

FIGURE 4.7   Scenario planning template: Patient report.

Phase II: Scenario Implementation

The next step in the scenario-development process is to design how the scenario will be implemented. This includes a pre-briefing phase and an implementation phase.

The purpose of the pre-briefing phase is four-fold:

- To set the stage for the scenario (INACSL Standards Committee, 2016a; McDermott, 2016)

- To identify expectations (INACSL Standards Committee, 2016a; McDermott, 2016)

- To establish ground rules and guidelines (INACSL Standards Committee, 2016a; McDermott, 2016)

- To establish a sense of trust and respect

Following the structured pre-briefing, learners participate in the scenario to provide care for the simulated patient. However, this process should be documented in advance using the scenario template so the simulator can be programmed, and responses to interventions by participants can be anticipated.

As with the planning phase, the simulation's learning objectives guide the implementation phase. This is shown in Figure 4.8, in which the learning objectives established in Figure 4.3 appear in the scenario planning template to guide the simulation facilitator.

When developing the scenario implementation phase, the facilitator must try to anticipate the actions of participants and plan accordingly. However, as mentioned, it is impossible to predict every action that might occur during a simulation. Therefore, facilitators must maintain a high level of flexibility and use proper facilitation methods in order to cue the participant toward meeting the objectives. However, cueing should be minimized during sessions in which simulation is used for summative evaluation as this could result in an inaccurate evaluation or give one participant an unfair advantage over another.

Phase III: Planning for Debriefing and Evaluation

The period immediately after the simulation experience is commonly referred to as the debriefing phase. It is one of the most important aspects of the scenario and is where the majority of the learning occurs (Decker, Gore, & Feken, 2011; INACSL Standards Committee, 2016d; Jeffries et al., 2015). A debriefing session should follow all simulation experiences. This session should be conducted by a debriefer trained to create "an environment that is conducive to learning and supports confidentiality, trust, open communication, self-analysis, feedback, and reflection" (INACSL Standards Committee, 2016d, p. S22).

Scenario Implementation Phase

Opening State and Objectives

Assess the client who is experiencing signs and symptoms of alcohol withdrawal

- Tremors, diaphoresis, hypertension, tachycardia, hallucinations
- CIWA-Ar Score

Utilize therapeutic communication while caring for the client who is experiencing signs and symptoms of alcohol withdrawal.

- Establish rapport with the patient
- Use of open-ended questions, empathy, clarification, etc.

Initial VS/Physiologic Parameters:

BP: 150/90; Temp: 99.0° F; Pulse 120; RR 30; Patient states: "I feel so nervous. Please get that crawly thing off the wall now! Where's my purse? I need to leave to go to bingo."

Anticipated Interventions:

Upon entering the room, the student acting in the role of the primary nurse notes that Mrs. Bender's vital signs are abnormal and that she is having hallucinations. The student should explore the patient's alcohol use and should utilize the CIWA-Ar tool and calculate a score. During this period, the student must utilize therapeutic communication techniques to develop a therapeutic environment of trust.

Next State and Objectives

Intervene effectively for the client who is experiencing signs and symptoms of alcohol withdrawal.

- Quiet, well-lit room with environmental cues
- IVF: NSS at 100 mL/hour
- Thiamine 100mg IV prior to giving any glucose containing IV fluid
- Folate 1mg
- Multivitamin with B-12
- CIWA-Ar Score: 18 – Lorazepam 0.5-1 mg IV q 15 min prn withdrawal symptoms

Vital Signs/Physiologic Parameters: No change

Anticipated Interventions: After calculating the CIWA-Ar score (18), the student telephones the MD on call to obtain orders to treat the acute alcohol withdrawal symptoms. The MD orders IVF, thiamine, folate, multivitamin, and Lorazepam as listed previously. The student should provide a quiet, well-lit room and ensure that the environmental cues (clock, calendar) are within the patient's view in order to provide frequent reorientation. The student will then initiate the IVF and medication regimen, assuring appropriate nursing considerations and assessments are in place prior to initiation. The student must continue to provide therapeutic communication techniques with both the patient and the husband, George. The student nurse provides brief and concise patient education regarding the signs and symptoms of acute alcohol withdrawal and the need for immediate intervention.

Final State and Objectives

Evaluate the effectiveness of interventions for the client who is experiencing signs and symptoms of alcohol withdrawal.

- VS
- Level of agitation/anxiety
- Sedation scale
- Absence of seizure activity
- Absence of falls
- Absence of hallucinations

Vital Signs/Physiologic Parameters:

Following medication administration: VS: 98.6°F, 92, 14 130/80; CIWA-Ar = 2

Patient's diaphoresis resolves and patient states, "I'm starting to feel sleepy. What just happened?"

Anticipated Interventions: Following medication and IVF administration, the student nurse re-evaluates the VS and patient's level of sedation. The student nurse must continue to educate both Helene and George about side effects of the medications and the need for frequent reorientation and assessment for seizure activity. The student nurse also explores the patient's alcohol use and administers the CAGE questionnaire.

FIGURE 4.8   Scenario planning template: Implementation.

A debriefing session can begin with a set of standard questions to be used in all scenarios, followed by specific questions that pertain to the actual scenario and reflect evidence-based clinical practice. The questions should be developed in advance per the scenario planning template so that the learning experience is standardized for all participants (see Figure 4.9). Adequate time should be allotted for this activity. Chapter 5 discusses methods for debriefing.

Objective 6: Reflect upon the learning that occurred during the simulation scenario (Affective Domain)

Journal

- Discussions during debriefing
- Administer post-simulation evaluation survey upon conclusion of experience.

Debriefing Questions

1. What worked well during the scenario?

2. If you had the opportunity to participate in the same scenario again, what would you do differently?

3. What was the primary problem?

4. What were your priorities of care?

5. State observations of each objective, state point of view about observation, then elicit learners' points of view.

6. Please provide the rationales for the interventions you performed.

7. How will you use this information in the real-life clinical setting?

Evidence-Based Clinical Questions

Question	What are the signs and symptoms of Alcohol Withdrawal Syndrome (AWS)?
Answer	Symptoms of light or moderate AWS may include hypertension, tachycardia, tremors, hyperreflexia, irritability, anxiety, headache, nausea, and vomiting. If left untreated, these symptoms may progress to more severe forms of AWS characterized by delirium tremens, seizures, coma, cardiac arrest, and death (Halter, 2018; Thursz et al., 2018).
Rationale and Reference	AWS is a complex neurologic disorder that develops after a reduction in or cessation of chronic alcohol consumption that alters neurotransmitter conduction. This is primarily driven by downregulation of gamma-aminobutyric acid (GABA) leading to autonomic excitation and psychomotor agitation (Foertsch, 2019).
Question	**When do symptoms of alcohol withdrawal (AWD) appear?**
Answer	The classic sign of alcohol withdrawal is tremulousness that begins 6 to 8 hours after alcohol cessation. Psychotic and perceptual disturbances may begin in 8 to 10 hours. Withdrawal seizures may occur within 12 to 24 hours after alcohol cessation (Halter, 2018; Thursz et al., 2018).
Rationale and Reference	Alcohol is a CNS depressant. Upon abrupt cessation of alcohol intake, an individual may experience CNS activation, causing the symptoms of alcohol withdrawal.

Question	**What is the purpose for administering nutritional supplements (MVI, folate, thiamine) for the treatment of AWS? Why must the thiamine be given prior to any glucose-containing fluids?**
Answer	Patients with alcohol dependence are often thiamine deficient. Thiamine deficiency is associated with the development of Wernicke's encephalopathy and Wernicke-Korsakoff syndrome.
Rationale and Reference	Thiamine administration has a low risk of adverse effects and can prevent the development of these conditions. In particular, thiamine should be given before administration of IV fluids containing glucose, as the IV administration of glucose may precipitate acute thiamine deficiency (Linder, Robert, Mullinax, & Hayes, 2018). Multivitamins containing or supplemented with folate should be given routinely, and deficiencies of potassium, magnesium, glucose, and phosphate should be corrected as needed.
Question	**What is the purpose of the CAGE questionnaire and Alcohol Use Disorders Identification Test (AUDIT)?**
Answer	Both are screening instruments used to assess alcohol consumption, drinking patterns, and alcohol-related problems. The CAGE Questionnaire is a 4-item screen. A score of 2 or more is significant; however, even a score of 1 requires further assessment. The AUDIT is a 10-item screening tool developed by the World Health Organization. A score of 8 or more is considered to indicate hazardous or harmful alcohol use (Halter, 2018; Higgins-Biddle & Babor, 2018).
Rationale and Reference	Both the CAGE questionnaire and the AUDIT have been validated in numerous studies as indicators of the need for further investigation of alcohol use (Higgins-Biddle & Babor, 2018).
Question	**What is the CIWA-Ar tool, and why is this used?**
Answer	The CIWA-Ar scale (The Clinical Institute Withdrawal Assessment for Alcohol scale) is used widely as a means to gauge the severity of alcohol withdrawal. The CIWA-Ar is a numeric scale with numbers being assigned to severity of symptoms such as anxiety, nausea, headache, and several other parameters.
Rationale and Reference	The CIWA-Ar score is used to guide treatment parameters with benzodiazepines (Parsons, 2018; Thursz et al., 2018).
Question	**What are common side effects of benzodiazepines, and why are they used for treatment of alcohol withdrawal?**
Answer	Common side effects include an exacerbation of the therapeutic effects of sedation and somnolence. Benzodiazepines enhance GABA transmission and are effective in treating the CNS excitation that accompanies alcohol withdrawal.
Rationale and Reference	The initial therapeutic goal in patients with AWS is control of agitation and autonomic stimulation. Rapid and adequate control of autonomic stimulation reduces the incidence of clinically important adverse events. Benzodiazepines are recommended as the primary agents for managing AWS. Current evidence does not clearly indicate that a specific benzodiazepine is superior to others. Agent selection should be based on patient-specific factors such as renal and hepatic metabolism, duration of action, and clearance. Careful monitoring of sedation scale is key following administration (Adams & Ferguson, 2017; Foertsch et al., 2019).

FIGURE 4.9   Scenario planning template: Debriefing and evaluation.

Simulation can be used for summative or formative evaluation purposes. When developing a scenario, facilitators and educators should determine and indicate whether participants will be evaluated, and if so, what type of instrument will be used. This information should be documented in the scenario planning template to ensure standardization of the experience. The participants should also be informed if the simulation is a summative evaluation and instruments with established reliability and validity should be used (INACSL Standards Committee, 2016e). Chapter 6 discusses the evaluation phase in more detail.

The NLN offers several reliable instruments:

- Student Satisfaction and Self-Confidence in Learning Scale (SCLS)

- Simulation Design Scale (SDS)

- Educational Practices Questionnaire (EPQ)

All three of these instruments offer adequate psychometrics for use in educational research (Franklin, Burns, & Lee, 2014). Another useful tool is the Debriefing Assessment for Simulation in Healthcare (DASH) tool. This tool is used to evaluate the quality of the debriefing session. It has demonstrated evidence of good reliability and validity (Brett-Fleegler et al., 2012).

In addition to educators evaluating learners after the simulation, learners should evaluate the simulation experience as a whole. This promotes continuous improvement of the scenario (Howard et al., 2010).

After the scenario has been developed, it is important to test it before running it with learners. During the test, simulation center staff play the different roles. The purpose of the test is to determine whether all the equipment needed is listed, whether the objectives are clear, and whether any other changes should be made before introducing it to learners. Do not underestimate the importance of this practice session; be sure to allot an adequate amount of time for it.

As in a real-life clinical setting, scenarios should be updated periodically as practice standards change. Most simulation experts suggest at least an annual review of all scenario content within your facility. The scenario review process can be one part of the quality improvement plan for your simulation program or facility.

Conclusion

Developing an effective, evidence-based scenario requires significant planning. Adequate time should be allotted to this activity. Proper planning ensures that all the details related to the scenario have been addressed and can assist the facilitator in a smooth scenario implementation for learners. Ultimately, with adequate time, planning, clinical evidence, practice, and mentoring, the most novice simulation educators can obtain the skills necessary to develop and implement a successful simulation scenario. The right tools can help, too—like the scenario planning template discussed in this chapter. Figure 4.10 contains the complete template.

Complete Alcohol Withdrawal Syndrome (AWS) Scenario

Developed by Kameg, K., Howard, V., Perozzi, K., & Englert, N.
Robert Morris University
School of Nursing & Health Sciences
Template adapted from J. Sarasnick, MSN, RN

Scenario Planning Template: Initial Elements

Course: NURS 4031 Transition to Professional Practice

Scenario Topic/Name: Alcohol Withdrawal Syndrome

Developed by Kameg, K., Howard, V., Perozzi, K., & Englert, N.

Robert Morris University, School of Nursing & Health Sciences

Template adapted from J. Sarasnick, MSN, RN

References Used:

Adams, B., & Ferguson, K. (2017). Pharmacologic management of alcohol withdrawal syndrome in intensive care units. *AACN Advanced Critical Care*, *28*(3), 233–238.

Foertsch, M. J., Winter, J. B., Rhoades, A. G., Martin, L. T., Droege, C. A., & Ernst, N. E. (2019). Recognition, assessment, and pharmacotherapeutic treatment of alcohol withdrawal syndrome in the intensive care unit. *Critical Care Nursing Quarterly*, *42*(1), 12–29.

Halter, M. J. (2018). *Varcarolis' foundations of psychiatric mental health nursing: A clinical approach* (8ᵗʰ ed.). St. Louis, MO: Elsevier.

Higgins-Biddle, J. C., & Babor, T. F. (2018). A review of the Alcohol Use Disorders Identification Test (AUDIT), AUDIT-C, and US AUDIT for screening in the United States: Past issues and future directions. *The American Journal of Drug and Alcohol Abuse*, *44*(6), 578–586.

Linder, L. M., Robert, S., Mullinax, K., & Hayes, G. (2018). Thiamine prescribing and Wernicke's encephalopathy risk factors in patients with alcohol use disorders at a psychiatric hospital. *Journal of Psychiatric Practice*, *24*(5), 317–322.

Parsons, G. (2018). Prevalence, identification and harms of alcohol use disorders. *Prescriber*, *29*(11), 19–23.

Thursz, M., Gual, A., Lackner, C., Mathurin, P., Moreno, C., Spahr, L., ... Cortez-Pinto, H. (2018). EASL clinical practice guidelines: Management of alcohol-related liver disease. *Journal of Hepatology*, *69*(1), 154–181.

Estimated Scenario Time: 30 minutes

Estimated Debriefing Time: 30 minutes

Instructors of the Course:

Simulation Facilitator:

Facilitation Prompting: Partial

Student level: Senior BSN Students

Prerequisite Knowledge/Pre-scenario Learning Activity:

1. Successful completion of NURS 4020 Advanced Management of the Adult II

2. Successful completion of NURS 4025 Nursing Care of Psychiatric Clients

3. Read Chapter 22 of Halter, M. J. (2018). *Varcarolis' foundations of psychiatric mental health nursing: A clinical approach* (8ᵗʰ ed.). St. Louis, MO: Elsevier.

Scenario Description

Helene is a 70-year-old female admitted to the hospital for acute gastritis. On the second day of admission, she becomes anxious and jittery and begins to hallucinate. Her husband, George, brings these behaviors to the attention of the nurse. During the scenario, the nursing student will have the opportunity to provide nursing care for a client experiencing symptoms of acute alcohol withdrawal.

Scenario Planning Template: Objectives

Learning Objectives

Upon completion of this scenario, the participant will be able to:

1. Assess the client who is experiencing signs and symptoms of alcohol withdrawal (Psychomotor Domain).
   - Tremors, diaphoresis, hypertension, tachycardia, hallucinations
   - The Clinical Institute Withdrawal Assessment for Alcohol scale (CIWA-Ar) score

2. Utilize therapeutic communication while caring for the client who is experiencing signs and symptoms of alcohol withdrawal (Affective Domain).
   - Establish rapport with the patient and husband
   - Use open-ended questions, empathy, clarification, etc.

3. Utilize appropriate Nursing Diagnoses to plan care for the client who is experiencing signs and symptoms of alcohol withdrawal (Cognitive Domain).
   - Deficient knowledge
   - Ineffective individual coping
   - Ineffective health maintenance
   - Risk for injury

4. Intervene effectively for the client who is experiencing signs and symptoms of alcohol withdrawal (Psychomotor Domain).
   - Quiet, well-lit room with environmental cues
   - IVF: NSS at 100 mL/hour
   - Thiamine 100mg IV prior to giving any glucose containing IVF
   - Folate 1mg
   - Multivitamin with B-12
   - CIWA-Ar Score: 18 – Lorazepam 0.5-1 mg IV q 15 min prn withdrawal symptoms

5. Evaluate the effectiveness of interventions for the client who is experiencing signs and symptoms of alcohol withdrawal (Cognitive and Psychomotor Domains).
   - Vital signs
   - Level of agitation/anxiety
   - Sedation scale
   - Absence of seizure activity
   - Absence of falls
   - Absence of hallucinations

6. Reflect upon the learning that occurred during the simulation scenario (Affective Domain).
   - Journal
   - Discussions during debriefing
   - Administer post-simulation evaluation survey upon conclusion of experience.

Scenario Planning Template: Supplies

Identify Type of Mannequin, Task Trainer, or Standardized Patient

High-fidelity mannequin for patient
Standardized patient or actor to play the role of spouse

	Equipment Needed				
	PPE gloves		Mask		Goggles
	Isolation Gown		Stethoscope		
X	SPO$_2$	X	ECG Monitor		Defibrillator/Pacer
	Lab Reports	X	MD Orders	X	Medical Records
	EMR—SLS#_____	X	iPod touch/PDA		Reference Material (book)
	Oxygen NC		Oxygen FM		Oxygen Non-Rebreather
X	Suction		Tracheostomy		Foley
X	IV in Place		IV Start Kit		Crash Cart
X	Glucometer		X-rays		12 Lead Type, i.e. NSR
	ECG Machine (12 lead)		Blood		Baby Bottle
	Ventilator		Vaginal Bleeding		Pediatric Supplies
	Diaphoresis		Bloody wound	X	ID/Allergy Band
	Nasal Secretions		Mouth Secretions		Urine
	Other:		Other:		Other:

Medications and IV Fluids: Dosage, Diluents Used, Methods of Delivery

1. NSS 1 liter bag
2. Thiamine 100mg IV
3. Folate IV
4. Multivitamin/B12 for IV bag
5. Lorazepam 1mg IV q15 minutes for symptoms of alcohol withdrawal—Monitor sedation scale

Scenario Planning Template: Patient Information

Simulated Patient History

Name: Helene Bender
Age: 70
Weight: 140 lb.   Height: 5'6"
Gender: Female
Past Medical History: Gastritis
Medications: Pepcid 20mg qd
Allergies: PCN
MD: Dr. Molnar
Simulation Setting: Inpatient Unit—Medical Surgical Floor

Background of presenting illness: Mrs. Bender was admitted 2 days ago for severe epigastric distress and heme positive emesis while at home. Her hemoglobin/hematocrit (H/H) were 10.9 gr/dL / 35%. An endoscopy performed yesterday revealed gastritis, and she was placed on IV Protonix. She was admitted to monitor H/H and epigastric symptoms.

Initial Vital Signs for Mannequin	
Temperature	99.0° F
SPO$_2$	94%
Heart Rate	120
NIBP	150/90
ABP	
CVP/PA	
ECG Rhythm	Sinus Tachycardia
Sweating	Yes
Pulses normal, weak, or absent Pedal, dorsal, femoral, carotid, brachial	Pulses normal
Respirations shallow, labored, or normal	30—labored

Scenario Planning Template: Embedded Participants and Roles

XX	Primary Nurse
	Secondary Nurse
XX	Family Member: George (husband)
	Family Member
XX	MD or NP
	Ancillary Personnel (type)

Scripts

Helene

Initially:

What is climbing on the wall?

Why am I shaking?

Where am I?

Where's my purse? I need to leave to go to Bingo.

Helene's Responses to Alcohol Withdrawal Assessment Scoring Guidelines (CIWA-Ar)

Nausea/Vomiting: 0

Anxiety: 4

Paroxysmal Sweats: 1

Tactile Disturbance: 0

Visual Disturbance: 4

Tremors: 2

Agitation: 3

Orientation and Clouding of Sensorium: 2

Auditory Disturbances: 3

Headache: 1

Helene Bender's Responses to CAGE Questionnaire

Following Lorazepam administration:

Helene: I'm feeling much more relaxed. What happened? Why am I in the hospital?

RN: *Helene, I am concerned about your drinking. When was your last drink, and how much did you drink?*

Helene: Oh, honey, I'm not sure. I think I had a few drinks with my friends at lunch the day before I came in. Then my stomach started to bother me. I thought it was from the crab cakes.

RN: *Have you ever experienced something similar to this before?*

Helene: No.

RN*: C: Have you ever felt you should cut down on your drinking?*

Helene: Well, sometimes George tells me this, but he is so conservative and strait-laced. All my friends drink like I do. I have to have drinks with them when we go out to lunch.

George: I am concerned about her. I just see her drinking more and more.

RN: *A: Have people annoyed you by criticizing your drinking?*

Helene: George is always the first to get on my nerves about my drinking. And, sometimes, my friends agree with him. Do you believe it? What kinds of friends are these?

RN: *G: Have you ever felt bad or guilty about your drinking?*

Helene: Well, only when my friends make a comment. But I've tried to quit several times.

RN: *E: Have you ever had an eye-opener, a drink first thing in the morning to steady your nerves or get rid of a hangover?*

Helene: I usually have a shot of whiskey in my coffee. It calms my nerves in the morning and helps me to think clearly. Then, my luncheons usually start around 12 noon, so I will have whatever is on the menu, spiked, of course.

RN expected actions:

Educate on complications of alcohol abuse/dependence

Utilize therapeutic communication

Contact MD with repeat CIWA-Ar score

MD Script

"What are the vital signs and CIWA-Ar score for Mrs. Bender?"

"I'm giving you a verbal order for Lorazepam 0.5-1 mg IV q15 minutes X 4 prn symptoms of agitation and hallucinations. Give her thiamine 100mg IV X 1. Also, start IVF NSS at 100mL/hour and add MVI, B12, folate 100mg. Call me after she has received these medications. Perform the CAGE assessment when you can."

After CAGE Questionnaire:

"Okay. Continue the CIWA-Ar protocol and the Ativan order. I will order a psychiatric consultation to discuss substance abuse."

George Bender (Helene's husband)

George has been the loving and enabling husband of Helene for 50 years. He is aware of her alcohol use but has not made the determination that it is detrimental to her health. He is caring and very concerned and scared about her initial state of withdrawal. He asks many questions of the primary nurse and does everything within his power to calm Helene down, yet his over-attentiveness begins to contribute to the anxiety of the situation. He tries to respond to the questions asked of Helene during the CIWA-Ar and CAGE assessments. The primary nurse should reinforce that Helene should be the one responding to the questions.

During the course of the scenario, George can ask or state:

"Why is she acting so funny?"

"Why are you giving her those medications? Do they have any side effects?"

"She usually has a drink around noon time each day."

"She is quite a socialite and attends many functions during the week."

Scenario Planning Template: Patient Report

Mrs. Bender is a 70-year-old female admitted with acute epigastric distress and Heme positive emesis (coffee ground) 2 days ago. Her admitting hemoglobin and hematocrit (H/H) was 10.9 gm/dL / 35%. She had an EGD yesterday that revealed a small gastric ulcer, and she was placed on IV Protonix. She continues to be monitored for her H/H and signs of epigastric pain. VS have been stable with trends: Temp 98.4°; BP 120/76; Pulse 90; RR 16. It is admission day 3 at 10 a.m. Her husband, George, is at the bedside today and has just called for the nurse. As you enter the room, George states that his wife is "acting funny."

Scenario Planning Template: Implementation

Opening State and Objectives

Assess the client who is experiencing signs and symptoms of alcohol withdrawal

- Tremors, diaphoresis, hypertension, tachycardia, hallucinations
- CIWA-Ar Score

Utilize therapeutic communication while caring for the client who is experiencing signs and symptoms of alcohol withdrawal.

- Establish rapport with the patient
- Use of open-ended questions, empathy, clarification, etc.

Initial VS/Physiologic Parameters:

BP: 150/90; Temp: 99.0° F; Pulse 120; RR 30; Patient states: "I feel so nervous. Please get that crawly thing off the wall now! Where's my purse? I need to leave to go to bingo."

Anticipated Interventions:

Upon entering the room, the student acting in the role of the primary nurse notes that Mrs. Bender's vital signs are abnormal and that she is having hallucinations. The student should explore the patient's alcohol use and should utilize the CIWA-Ar tool and calculate a score. During this period, the student must utilize therapeutic communication techniques to develop a therapeutic environment of trust.

Next State and Objectives

Intervene effectively for the client who is experiencing signs and symptoms of alcohol withdrawal.

- Quiet, well-lit room with environmental cues
- IVF: NSS at 100 mL/hour
- Thiamine 100mg IV prior to giving any glucose containing IV fluid
- Folate 1mg
- Multivitamin with B-12
- CIWA-Ar Score: 18 – Lorazepam 0.5-1 mg IV q 15 min prn withdrawal symptoms

Vital Signs/Physiologic Parameters: No change

Anticipated Interventions: After calculating the CIWA-Ar score (18), the student telephones the MD on call to obtain orders to treat the acute alcohol withdrawal symptoms. The MD orders IVF, thiamine, folate, multivitamin, and Lorazepam as listed previously. The student should provide a quiet, well-lit room and ensure that the environmental cues (clock, calendar) are within the patient's view in order to provide frequent reorientation. The student will then initiate the IVF and medication regimen, assuring appropriate nursing considerations and assessments are in place prior to initiation. The student must continue to provide therapeutic communication techniques with both the patient and the husband, George. The student nurse provides brief and concise patient education regarding the signs and symptoms of acute alcohol withdrawal and the need for immediate intervention.

Final State and Objectives

Evaluate the effectiveness of interventions for the client who is experiencing signs and symptoms of alcohol withdrawal.

- VS
- Level of agitation/anxiety
- Sedation scale
- Absence of seizure activity
- Absence of falls
- Absence of hallucinations

Vital Signs/Physiologic Parameters:

Following medication administration: VS: 98.6°F, 92, 14 130/80; CIWA-Ar = 2

Patient's diaphoresis resolves and patient states, "I'm starting to feel sleepy. What just happened?"

Anticipated Interventions: Following medication and IVF administration, the student nurse re-evaluates the VS and patient's level of sedation. The student nurse must continue to educate both Helene and George about side effects of the medications and the need for frequent reorientation and assessment for seizure activity. The student nurse also explores the patient's alcohol use and administers the CAGE questionnaire.

Scenario Planning Template: Debriefing and Evaluation

Objective 6: Reflect upon the learning that occurred during the simulation scenario (Affective Domain)

Journal

- Discussions during debriefing
- Administer post-simulation evaluation survey upon conclusion of experience.

Debriefing Questions

1. What worked well during the scenario?

2. If you had the opportunity to participate in the same scenario again, what would you do differently?

3. What was the primary problem?

4. What were your priorities of care?

5. State observations of each objective, state point of view about observation, then elicit learners' points of view.

6. Please provide the rationales for the interventions you performed.

7. How will you use this information in the real-life clinical setting?

Evidence-Based Clinical Questions	
Question	**What are the signs and symptoms of Alcohol Withdrawal Syndrome (AWS)?**
Answer	Symptoms of light or moderate AWS may include hypertension, tachycardia, tremors, hyperreflexia, irritability, anxiety, headache, nausea, and vomiting. If left untreated, these symptoms may progress to more severe forms of AWS characterized by delirium tremens, seizures, coma, cardiac arrest, and death (Halter, 2018; Thursz et al., 2018).
Rationale and Reference	AWS is a complex neurologic disorder that develops after a reduction in or cessation of chronic alcohol consumption that alters neurotransmitter conduction. This is primarily driven by downregulation of gamma-aminobutyric acid (GABA) leading to autonomic excitation and psychomotor agitation (Foertsch, 2019).
Question	**When do symptoms of alcohol withdrawal (AWD) appear?**
Answer	The classic sign of alcohol withdrawal is tremulousness that begins 6 to 8 hours after alcohol cessation. Psychotic and perceptual disturbances may begin in 8 to 10 hours. Withdrawal seizures may occur within 12 to 24 hours after alcohol cessation (Halter, 2018; Thursz et al., 2018).
Rationale and Reference	Alcohol is a CNS depressant. Upon abrupt cessation of alcohol intake, an individual may experience CNS activation, causing the symptoms of alcohol withdrawal.
Question	**What is the purpose for administering nutritional supplements (MVI, folate, thiamine) for the treatment of AWS? Why must the thiamine be given prior to any glucose-containing fluids?**
Answer	Patients with alcohol dependence are often thiamine deficient. Thiamine deficiency is associated with the development of Wernicke's encephalopathy and Wernicke-Korsakoff syndrome.
Rationale and Reference	Thiamine administration has a low risk of adverse effects and can prevent the development of these conditions. In particular, thiamine should be given before administration of IV fluids containing glucose, as the IV administration of glucose may precipitate acute thiamine deficiency (Linder, Robert, Mullinax, & Hayes, 2018).
	Multivitamins containing or supplemented with folate should be given routinely, and deficiencies of potassium, magnesium, glucose, and phosphate should be corrected as needed.

Question	What is the purpose of the CAGE questionnaire and Alcohol Use Disorders Identification Test (AUDIT)?
Answer	Both are screening instruments used to assess alcohol consumption, drinking patterns, and alcohol-related problems. The CAGE Questionnaire is a 4-item screen. A score of 2 or more is significant; however, even a score of 1 requires further assessment. The AUDIT is a 10-item screening tool developed by the World Health Organization. A score of 8 or more is considered to indicate hazardous or harmful alcohol use (Halter, 2018; Higgins-Biddle & Babor, 2018).
Rationale and Reference	Both the CAGE questionnaire and the AUDIT have been validated in numerous studies as indicators of the need for further investigation of alcohol use (Higgins-Biddle & Babor, 2018).
Question	What is the CIWA-Ar tool, and why is this used?
Answer	The CIWA-Ar scale (The Clinical Institute Withdrawal Assessment for Alcohol scale) is used widely as a means to gauge the severity of alcohol withdrawal. The CIWA-Ar is a numeric scale with numbers being assigned to severity of symptoms such as anxiety, nausea, headache, and several other parameters.
Rationale and Reference	The CIWA-Ar score is used to guide treatment parameters with benzodiazepines (Parsons, 2018; Thursz et al., 2018).
Question	What are common side effects of benzodiazepines, and why are they used for treatment of alcohol withdrawal?
Answer	Common side effects include an exacerbation of the therapeutic effects of sedation and somnolence. Benzodiazepines enhance GABA transmission and are effective in treating the CNS excitation that accompanies alcohol withdrawal.
Rationale and Reference	The initial therapeutic goal in patients with AWS is control of agitation and autonomic stimulation. Rapid and adequate control of autonomic stimulation reduces the incidence of clinically important adverse events. Benzodiazepines are recommended as the primary agents for managing AWS. Current evidence does not clearly indicate that a specific benzodiazepine is superior to others. Agent selection should be based on patient-specific factors such as renal and hepatic metabolism, duration of action, and clearance. Careful monitoring of sedation scale is key following administration (Adams & Ferguson, 2017; Foertsch et al., 2019).

References

Adams, B., & Ferguson, K. (2017). Pharmacologic management of alcohol withdrawal syndrome in intensive care units. *AACN Advanced Critical Care, 28*(3), 233-238. doi:10.4037/aacnacc2017574

Alinier, G. (2011). Developing high-fidelity healthcare simulation scenarios: A guide for educators and professionals. *Simulation and Gaming, 42*(1), 9–26. http://dx.doi.org/10.1177/1046878109355683

Benner, P. (1984). *From novice to expert: Excellence and power in clinical nursing practice.* Upper Saddle River, NJ: Prentice-Hall.

Bloom, B., Englehart, M., Furst, E., Hill, W., & Krathwohl, D. (1956). *Taxonomy of educational objectives: The classification of educational goals.* New York, NY: Longmans, Green & Co.

Bosek, M. S., Li, S., & Hicks, F. D. (2007). Working with standardized patients: A primer. *International Journal of Nursing Education Scholarship, 4*(1), ISSN (online). doi:10.2202/1548-923X.1437

Brett-Fleegler, M., Rudolph, J., Eppich, W., Monuteaux, M., Fleegler, E., Cheng, A., & Simon, R. (2012). Debriefing assessment for simulation in healthcare: Development and psychometric properties. *Simulation in Healthcare, 7*(5), 288-294. doi:10.1097/SIH.0b013e318262022

Centers for Disease Control and Prevention. (2018). *Writing SMART objectives.* Retrieved from http://www.cdc.gov/healthyyouth/evaluation/pdf/brief3b.pdf

Childs, J. C., & Sepples, S. (2006). Clinical teaching by simulation: Lessons learned from a complex patient care scenario. *Nursing Education Perspectives, 27*(3), 154-158.

Clapper, T. C. (2010). Beyond Knowles: What those conducting simulation need to know about adult learning theory. *Clinical Simulation in Nursing, 6*(1), e7-e14. doi:10.1016/j.ecns.2009.07.003

Decker, S., Gore, T., & Feken, C. (2011). Simulation. In T. Bristol & J. Zerwehk (Eds.), *Essentials of e-learning for nurse educators* (pp. 277-294). Philadelphia, PA: F. A. Davis.

Dewey, J. (1938). *Experience and education.* New York, NY: Kappa Delta Pi.

Foertsch, M. J., Winter, J. B., Rhoades, A. G., Martin, L. T., Droege, C. A., & Ernst, N. E. (2019). Recognition, assessment, and pharmacotherapeutic treatment of alcohol withdrawal syndrome in the intensive care unit. *Critical Care Nursing Quarterly, 42*(1), 12-29. doi:10.1097/CNQ.0000000000000233

Franklin, A. E., Burns, P., & Lee, C. S. (2014). Psychometric testing on the NLN Student Satisfaction and Self-Confidence in Learning, Simulation Design Scale, and Educational Practices Questionnaire using a sample of pre-licensure novice nurses. *Nurse Education Today, 34*(10), 1298-1304. doi:10.1016/j.nedt.2014.06.011

Halter, M. J. (2018). *Varcarolis' foundations of psychiatric mental health nursing: A clinical approach* (8th ed.). Philadelphia, PA: Saunders.

Higgins-Biddle, J. C., & Babor, T. F. (2018). A review of the Alcohol Use Disorders Identification Test (AUDIT), AUDIT-C, and USAUDIT for screening in the United States: Past issues and future directions. *The American Journal of Drug and Alcohol Abuse, 44*(6), 578-586. doi:10.1080/00952990.2018.1456545

Howard, V. M., Englert, N., Kameg, K., & Perozzi, K. (2011). Integration of simulation across the undergraduate curriculum: Student and faculty perspectives. *Clinical Simulation in Nursing, 7*(1), e1-e10. doi:10.1016/j.ecns.2009.10.004

Howard, V. M., Ross, C., Mitchell, A. M., & Nelson, G. M. (2010). Human patient simulators and interactive case studies: A comparative analysis of learning outcomes and student perceptions. *Computers, Informatics, and Nursing, 28*(1), 42-48. doi:10.1097/NCN.0b013e3181c04939

International Nursing Association for Clinical Simulation and Learning Standards Committee. (2016a). INACSL standards of best practice: Simulation. Simulation design. *Clinical Simulation in Nursing, 12*(S), S5-S12. doi:10.1016/j.ecns.2016.09.005

International Nursing Association for Clinical Simulation and Learning Standards Committee. (2016b). INACSL standards of best practice: Simulation. Facilitation. *Clinical Simulation in Nursing, 12*(S), S16-S20. doi:10.1016/j.ecns.2016.09.007

International Nursing Association for Clinical Simulation and Learning Standards Committee. (2016c). INACSL standards of best practice: Simulation. Outcomes and objectives. *Clinical Simulation in Nursing, 12*(S), S13-S15. doi:10.1016/j.ecns.2016.09.006

International Nursing Association for Clinical Simulation and Learning Standards Committee. (2016d). INACSL standards of best practice: Simulation. Debriefing. *Clinical Simulation in Nursing, 12*(S), S21-S25. doi:10.1016/j.ecns.2016.09.008

International Nursing Association for Clinical Simulation and Learning Standards Committee. (2016e). INACSL standards of best practice: Simulation. Participant evaluation. *Clinical Simulation in Nursing, 12*(S), S26-S29. doi:10.1016/j.ecns.2016.09.005

International Nursing Association for Clinical Simulation and Learning Standards Committee. (2016f). INACSL standards of best practice: Simulation. Simulation glossary. *Clinical Simulation in Nursing, 12*(S), S39–S47. http://dx.doi.org/10.1016/j.ecns.2016.09.012

iRIS. (n.d.). *Simulation authoring software.* Retrieved from http://www.irissimulationauthoring.com/

Jeffries, P. R. (2005). A framework for designing, implementing, and evaluating simulations used as teaching strategies in nursing. Nursing Education Perspectives, 26(2), 96-103.

Jeffries, P. R. (2007). *Simulation in nursing education: From conceptualization to evaluation* (1st ed.). New York, NY: National League for Nursing.

Jeffries, P. R. (2012). *Simulation in nursing education, from conceptualization to evaluation* (2nd ed.). New York, NY: National League for Nursing.

Jeffries, P. R., Rodgers, B., & Adamson, K. (2015). NLN Jeffries simulation theory: Brief narrative description. *Nursing Education Perspectives, 36*(5), 292-293.

Kaakinen, J., & Arwood, E. (2009). Systematic review of nursing simulation literature for use of learning theory. *International Journal of Nursing Education Scholarship, 6*(1), ISSN (online). doi:10.2202/1548-923X.1688

Knowles, M. S. (1984). *The adult learner: A neglected species* (3rd ed.). Houston, TX: Gulf Publishing Co.

Kolb, D. A. (1984). *Experiential learning: Experience as the source of learning and development.* Englewood Cliffs, NJ: Prentice-Hall.

Lasater, K. (2007). High-fidelity simulation and the development of clinical judgment: Students' experiences. *Journal of Nursing Education, 46*(6), 269-276.

Lave, J., & Wenger, E. (1991). *Situated learning: Legitimate peripheral participation.* Cambridge, UK: Cambridge University Press.

Lewis, K. A., Ricks, T. N., Rowin, A., Ndlovu, C., Goldstein, L., & McElvogue, C. (2019). Does simulation training for acute care nurses improve patient safety outcomes: A systematic review to inform evidence-based practice. *Worldviews on Evidence-Based Nursing, 16*(5), 389-396.

Lewis, K. L., Bohnert, C. A., Gammon, W. L., Hölzer, H., Lyman, L., Smith, C., ...Gliva-McConvey, G. (2017). The Association of Standardized Patient Educators (ASPE) standards of best practice (SOBP). *Advances in Simulation, 2*, 10. doi:10.1186/s41077-017-0043-4

Linder, L. M., Robert, S., Mullinax, K., & Hayes, G. (2018). Thiamine prescribing and Wernicke's encephalopathy risk factors in patients with alcohol use disorders at a psychiatric hospital. *Journal of Psychiatric Practice, 24*(5), 317-322. doi:10.1097/PRA.0000000000000326

Lioce, L., Lopreiato, J., Downing, D., Chang, T. P., Robertson, J. M., Anderson, M., ... The Terminology and Concepts Working Group. (2020). *Healthcare simulation dictionary* (2nd ed.). Rockville, MD: Agency for Healthcare Research and Quality. AHRQ Publication No. 20-0019. doi: https://doi. org/10.23970/simulationv2

McDermott, D. S. (2016). The prebriefing concept: A Delphi study of CHSE experts. *Clinical Simulation in Nursing, 12*(6), 219-227. doi:10.1016/j.ecns.2016.02.001

Paige, J. B., & Daley, B. J. (2009). Situated cognition: A learning framework to support and guide high-fidelity simulation. *Clinical Simulation in Nursing, 5*(3), e97-e103. doi:10.1016/j.ecns.2009.03.120

Parsons, G. (2018). Prevalence, identification and harms of alcohol use disorders. *Prescriber, 29*(11), 19-23. doi:10.1002/psb.1717

Reibel, M. D., Cason, M., & Screws, S. (2019). Creating a simulation experience to promote clinical judgment. *Teaching and Learning in Nursing, 14*(4), 298-302.

Sittner, B. J., Aebersold, M. L., Paige, J. B., Graham, L. L., Schram, A. P., Decker, S. I., & Lioce, L. (2015). INACSL standards of best practice for simulation: Past, present, and future. *Nursing Education Perspectives, 36*(5), 294-298.

Thursz, M., Gual, A., Lackner, C., Mathurin, P., Moreno, C., Spahr, L., ... Cortez-Pinto, H. (2018). EASL clinical practice guidelines: Management of alcohol-related liver disease. *Journal of Hepatology, 69*(1), 154–181. doi:10.1016/j.jhep.2018.03.018

Waxman, K. T. (2010). The development of evidence-based clinical simulation scenarios: Guidelines for nurse educators. *Journal of Nursing Education, 49*(1), 29-35. doi:10.3928/01484834-20090916-07

Key Concepts in Simulation: Debriefing and Reflective Practice

5

Shelly J. Reed, PhD, DNP, APRN, CNE

Reflection is an important strategy for learning through practice experiences. Effective reflection to promote learning is a deliberate process of critically thinking about an experience, leading to insights about how to make future practice changes.

Reflection can (Miraglia & Asselin, 2015):

- Enhance knowledge
- Transform assumptions, values, and beliefs
- Inform clinical practice

Reflection fosters self-dialogue about a situation and the emergence of new insights. Meaningful reflection enables a better look at oneself, allowing self-discovery and promoting critical and creative thinking. Through reflection, the intent to change practice develops. For healthcare providers, reflection also helps to maintain competence and keep abreast of current practices (Asselin, Schwartz-Barcott, & Osterman, 2013; Naicker & van Rensburg, 2018).

Reflection is an important part of Kolb's experiential learning theory (Kolb & Kolb, 2017). This theory places the learner, rather than the educator, in the center of the learning cycle. The cycle consists of four stages:

- Concrete experience
- Reflective observation
- Abstract conceptualization
- Active experimentation

OBJECTIVES

- Understand the importance of the reflective practice of debriefing as a part of simulation.

- Identify debriefing techniques that promote participant learning.

- Differentiate among various debriefing methods, and identify situations in which each might be implemented.

- Gain a basic understanding of available evaluation tools for debriefing.

Learners enter this cycle either where they are placed by outside processes—for example, by an educator—or where they are comfortable entering (Kolb & Kolb, 2005, 2017). Through reflection on their experiences, learners can reconcile what they view and think with what they have experienced (Wang, 2011).

The reflective period following a simulation-based experience is called *debriefing*. The purpose of a debriefing is to assimilate new learning, with the intent to transfer this learning to future clinical situations. During debriefing, reflective thinking is encouraged, and feedback is given on the simulation performance. Participants are encouraged to question, explore emotions, and give feedback to each other (International Nursing Association of Clinical Simulation and Learning [INACSL] Standards Committee, 2016c). Debriefing is also important in other areas of nursing education. It should be used throughout a nursing curriculum to help develop reflective practitioners, which may have a significant effect on learning outcomes (National League for Nursing, 2015).

Debriefing should be a part of every simulation-based experience because learning depends on incorporating what is learned in simulation with prior knowledge. The reflection provided through a debriefing should focus on best practices to promote safe, quality patient care and also to promote the participant's professional role.

INACSL has established standards of best practice to help guide debriefings to achieve learning outcomes (INACSL Standards Committee, 2016a; Levett-Jones & Lapkin, 2014; see the sidebar that follows).

Setting the Stage for Debriefing

Setting the stage for a successful debriefing includes creating learning objectives, preparing for the simulation, creating the debriefing environment, establishing psychological safety, determining the timing and length of the debriefing, and choosing the most effective group size.

Learning Objectives

Like any simulation-based experience, debriefing should begin with the development of clearly defined and measurable objectives designed to achieve expected outcomes (INACSL Standards Committee, 2016b). These objectives will guide the debriefing process and provide a template of what will be needed for the debriefing session.

INACSL Debriefing Guidelines

- The debriefing should be facilitated by persons competent in the debriefing process.
- The debriefing environment should support learning, confidentiality, trust, open communication, self-analysis, feedback, and reflection.
- The individuals who will be conducting the debriefing should attend or observe the simulation-based experience so they can provide the most effective debriefing.
- The debriefing should be structured based on a theoretical framework.
- The debriefing should be congruent with the objectives of the simulation-based experience.

Source: INACSL Standards Committee, 2016a

The objectives for the debriefing should align with the outcomes and objectives for the overall simulation-based experience. Objectives should be learner-centered and identify performance gaps based on expected outcomes (Hall & Tori, 2017; INACSL Standards Committee, 2016a).

The objectives are used to guide the processes and provide a template of what will be needed for the debriefing session. Objectives will differ depending on what type of simulation experience has been provided. For example, objectives for a debriefing after a team training simulation might differ from objectives for debriefing after an instructional simulation. Appropriate objectives for team training might be related to improving team performance or team communication; therefore, during debriefing, these concepts would be a focus of the debriefing conversation. In contrast, for an instructional simulation, an objective may be to learn skills to care for patients with a particular nursing diagnosis, without focusing on team care.

Objectives should not be created as one-size-fits-all. They should be based on the learning level of session participants. The simulation and debriefing objectives for beginning learners should vary from learners who have participated in more advanced clinical and simulation experiences and who are familiar with simulated learning. Experienced healthcare professionals would also have different objectives than novice professionals.

Simulation Preparation

Simulation-preparation activities and the pre-briefing phase can set the stage for enhanced learning during debriefing. Preparation activities include readings such as articles or case scenarios, assignments, worksheets, and so on.

Several of these activities, such as Situation-Background-Assessment-Recommendation (SBAR) assignments, start during the simulation-preparation phase and are added upon during the simulation itself and discussed in the debriefing. Completing simulation-preparation activities shifts the focus of the simulation from the concrete experience of Kolb's experiential learning cycle to one of active experimentation. This allows learners to try out what they learn during the preparation phase and to move more rapidly through the learning cycle (Reed, 2016).

Debriefing Environment and Pre-briefing

The debriefing environment should be conducive to learning and support confidentiality, trust, communication, feedback, and self-refection (INACSL Standards Committee, 2016a). The simulation pre-briefing is the optimal time to set the stage for this kind of environment. Activities to support this during the pre-briefing include:

- Giving permission for participants to make mistakes in the simulation

- Describing the learning objectives for the simulation and debriefing

- Establishing rules for a safe environment (including a discussion of confidentiality)

- Setting ground rules for open communication

Based on a review of the literature, Rutherford-Hemming, Lioce, and Breymier (2019) identified the essential pre-briefing elements as:

- Setting the scene: psychological safety, fiction contract, confidentiality, communication, logistics

- Expectations: facilitator, participant

- Debriefing: purpose, methods, process

- Simulation scenario: backstory information, roles, objectives, evaluation

- Simulation room orientation: modality, equipment

- Preparation time: review of specific case information

The debriefing process is outlined in the prebriefing so that learners will know how to participate when debriefing (Hall & Tori, 2017; Reed, 2016; Zigmont, Kappus, & Sudikoff, 2011).

While the optimal physical debriefing environment has not been empirically established, most debriefing sessions take place in a separate room from the simulation. This facilitates and supports open communication and reflection. The room should ensure privacy and be equipped for video reviews if they are available (Kim & Kim, 2017; Mayville, 2011).

Psychological Safety

Establishing psychological safety is a consistent theme in simulation literature. Establishing a psychologically safe learning relationship and environment leads to deeper discussions in debriefing. Maintaining psychological safety during the debriefing and afterward allows continued reflection and learning beyond the debriefing. Methods to maintain a psychologically safe environment include:

- Setting and posting ground rules (which usually include confidentiality)

- Not grading learners

- Not asking questions that could make learners uncomfortable

- Grouping learners by learning level (Reed, 2016)

During the debriefing, participants should be free to show their lack of knowledge without worrying about being criticized by peers.

Other ways debriefers can help participants feel safe include providing ways for learners to release emotions during the debriefing, limiting participation in the debriefing to the debriefer, and limiting participants to the debriefer and learners who participated in or observed the simulation scenario (Abelsson & Bisholt, 2017; Reed, 2016). For example, supervisors or grading professors might be prohibited from observing performance during simulation or debriefings.

Debriefing Timing and Length

The timing and length of the debriefing are important elements of debriefing success. The debriefing is generally conducted immediately after the simulation to allow better recall of scenario performance (post-simulation debriefing). Participants generally prefer this debriefing approach because the simulation experience is forefront in their minds (Hall & Tori, 2017; Kim & Kim, 2017; Neill & Wotton, 2011).

One study involving medical students compared post-simulation debriefing with "in-simulation" debriefing, in which the simulation was temporarily suspended for a period of instruction and then restarted (also known as "pause and discuss simulations"). The advantage found for in-simulation debriefing is avoiding negative learning, as errors are corrected as they occur in the simulation. Advantages for post-simulation debriefing include learning from mistakes made during the simulation and having time post-scenario to allow a comprehensive review. Medical students reported learning from both types of debriefing, although post-simulation debriefing was rated as more effective overall (Van Heukelom, Begaz, & Treat, 2010).

Thorough debriefing requires adequate time (Reed, 2012). Brackenreg (2004) emphasizes allowing enough time and means to explore the implications and consequences of the simulated experience. A general rule is to spend as much or more time debriefing as was spent performing the scenario (Flanagan, 2008).

Determining the Most Effective Group Size

Although there is minimal evidence available regarding the appropriate size for a debriefing group, Tosterud, Hall-Lord, Petzäll, and Hedelin (2014) found that small groups (between eight and 11 members) provided the best learning conditions with regard to ensuring safety and security. Learners in small groups were also more engaged, as they were unable to withdraw the way members of larger groups (between 38 and 50 members) can if put on the spot. However, relevant learning still occurred among large-group participants (Tosterud et al., 2014). A recurrent theme in this study was that those who spoke out were put in a vulnerable position, characterized by an increased risk of embarrassment, resulting in a stressful and intrusive situation. Reluctance to be exposed was a particular problem in larger debriefing groups. Regardless of the size of the debriefing group, its members should consist of simulation participants and debriefers. Flanagan (2008) recommends limiting observers in debriefing, as they may distract participants and provide unsolicited comments. As mentioned, some debriefers limit the debriefing group exclusively to debriefer(s) and the simulation participants to promote a feeling of safety (Reed, 2016).

Facilitating the Debriefing

Debriefers have a primary role in facilitating the debriefing conversation. Conversational skills such as facilitator skills, demeanor, and debriefing philosophy impact the quality of the conversation.

The debriefer conducts the debriefing and guides learners to interpret the simulation and put it into an accurate perspective (Lasater, 2007). The goal of the debriefing is for participants to analyze and evaluate the simulation through discussion and reflection. The debriefer should not dominate the conversation with questions or lectures. Debriefer behaviors that promote this include (McDonnell, Jobe, & Dismukes, 1997):

- Asking questions that identify issues
- Active listening
- Pausing at least three to four seconds rather than immediately answering
- Promoting group participants to answer first

The INACSL debriefing standard has identified key actions to promote debriefer competence (INACSL Standards Committee, 2016a):

- Acquire debriefer training through a formal course, continuing education offering, or targeted work with an experienced mentor.
- Structure and facilitate the debriefing according to established best practices.
- Seek feedback on debriefs from participants and experienced debriefers.
- Maintain debriefing skills through active engagement in simulation-based experiences.
- Confirm ongoing competence through use of a validated instrument(s).

- Participate in continuing education to maintain and update facilitation skills.

Debriefer Demeanor

In a literature review, Neill and Wotton (2011) identified supportive debriefer demeanor as a theme. INACSL standards note that debriefers should "use verbal and nonverbal supportive demeanor to encourage discussion" (INACSL Standards Committee, 2016a). A study by Ganley and Linnard-Palmer (2012) also emphasized the importance of debriefer demeanor. Students in the study felt unsafe when they were ridiculed, experienced debilitating anxiety, or feared failure or being judged or compared with classmates. Students felt safe when they felt challenged, were able to ask questions, and felt faculty were understanding and supportive. "In short, they wanted a friendly, supportive academic climate where they could learn" (Ganley & Linnard-Palmer, 2012, p. e56).

Debriefer as a Guide

The debriefer should guide the debriefing conversation. To achieve this, Neill and Wotton (2011) suggest the use of probing and cueing—keeping the discussion open-ended, focused on skills, and geared toward finding rationales for actions. Asking difficult questions and guiding learners toward accurate knowledge also promote learning (Abelsson & Bisholt, 2017). Fanning and Gaba (2007) note that the level of guidance by the debriefer should depend on the needs of the learners. Debriefers can guide learners by asking open-ended questions and not giving answers and by using silence to compel debriefing participants to consider what they would do in the situation. Debriefers should ask questions in a tone of discovery to help participants put the pieces together (Reed, 2016). The debriefer should not dominate the conversation with questions or lecture; the goal is for participants to analyze and evaluate the simulation through discussion.

Guiding Debriefer Behaviors

- Keep the discussion open-ended.
- Use probing and cueing questions.
- Focus on skills.
- Ask questions in a tone of discovery.
- Discover rationale behind participant actions.
- Adjust the level of facilitation to the need of the individual/group.
- Use silence to compel participants to answer.
- Use participants' names when calling on them.

Source: Reed, 2016

Intentional Debriefing

In a study by Reed (2016), experienced debriefers expressed that they are intentional in their debriefings, usually in the context of their careful preparation for debriefing—preparation that involves practicing and preparing for the debriefing *before* the simulation. Other ways they were intentional included using statements of curiosity, emphasizing and teaching different topics (including the use of video review when teaching these topics), and planning for future experiences.

Video Review

The use of video review for debriefing has traditionally been considered a gold standard (Levett-Jones & Lapkin, 2014). However, there is no clear evidence to promote the use of video review in every debriefing. Discussion without video review may be better for debriefing instructive simulations. This type of debriefing has been found to have a positive impact on learning and knowledge retention (Chronister & Brown, 2012; Reed, Andrews, & Ravert, 2013). Indeed, simulation literature reviews have found no clear benefit on study outcomes, and further investigation into its use is recommended (Cheng et al., 2014; Dufrene & Young, 2014; Levett-Jones & Lapkin, 2014; Motavalli & Nestel, 2016; Raemer et al., 2011). Moreover, discussion-only debriefing can be easily accomplished in multiple environments, whereas the use of video review requires a video system that may be expensive, prone to failure, and anxiety-provoking (Flanagan, 2008). Video review during debriefing should be used with caution. Playing lengthy or unrelated video segments may distract participants from discussing key issues and accomplishing debriefing objectives (Fanning & Gaba, 2007). In addition, one study found students did not feel safe when they were video recorded (Ganley & Linnard-Palmer, 2012).

Video review can help transfer knowledge to real-world settings (Reed et al., 2013), and video playback may be useful to engage different types of learners (Kolb & Kolb, 2005, 2017). Video review can be appropriate in some situations—for example, if it is used as part of a particular debriefing method or framework or for debriefs that discuss communication, teamwork, or time needed to accomplish a clinical skill or task.

Peer-Led Debriefing

Peer-led debriefing is another option for debriefing simulation. Several studies have shown no differences in outcomes of peer-led debriefings compared to facilitated debriefings. For example, in basic skill scenarios, Ha and Lim (2018) found no difference in knowledge, satisfaction, self-confidence, or experience when comparing peer-led versus educator-led debriefings of basic skill scenarios. Students in another study also perceived peer- and faculty-led debriefing as equally effective (Doherty-Restrepo et al., 2018). Finally, a study that compared facilitated debriefing and peer-led debriefing within surgical teams also showed that peer-led debriefing was equally effective (Boet et al., 2013).

Written Debriefing

Written debriefing has been identified as a way to extend learning beyond the formal debriefing period. Other ways to extend learning include reflective journals and assignments, experience papers directed to outcomes, electronic health record assignments, and student self-assessments (Reed, 2016).

Debriefing Structures and Frameworks

Structured reflection and facilitated reflective group dialogue offer learners the opportunity to reach a deeper level of exploration and arrive at a higher level of thinking (Miraglia & Asselin, 2015). The INACSL standard of practice for debriefing recommends that debriefings be based on a theoretical framework and be structured in a purposeful way (INACSL Standards Committee, 2016a).

The following examples of debriefing models and structures can be used for debriefing simulations. Note that regardless of which model or structure is employed, debriefer training is necessary for effective use.

3D Model of Debriefing: Defusing, Discovering, and Deepening

The 3D Model of Debriefing is based on adult learning theory and Kolb's experiential learning cycle (Zigmont et al., 2011). It includes defusing, discovering, and deepening:

- **Defusing** allows venting of emotions, recapping, clarifying what happened in the scenario, and analyzing what is important to the learner.

- **Discovering** analyzes and evaluates performance, discovers the rationale for specific behaviors, and identifies performance gaps.

- **Deepening** focuses on transferring lessons from simulation to clinical practice. The session then ends with a summary of lessons learned. Zigmont and colleagues (2011) say this framework can be used to enhance learning after real or simulated events.

Debriefing for Meaningful Learning

Debriefing for meaningful learning (DML) guides participants in the debriefing to develop clinical reasoning and to "think like a nurse" (Dreifuerst, 2012). Participants identify the reasons for their actions and behaviors and are supported to translate their thinking into knowledgeable decision-making. The goal is to apply this knowledge in subsequent clinical encounters (Dreifuerst, 2012).

Debriefing With Good Judgment

Debriefing with good judgment is an approach that encourages the debriefer to deliver honest and transparent feedback and lead discussions on improvement, while holding participants in high regard and respect. With the "good judgment" approach, debriefers maintain a stance of curiosity, supply their interpretations of simulation actions (advocacy), and pair this with open-ended questions to understand those actions (inquiry). The debriefing is designed to explore learner thoughts and foster discussion on learning needs as identified by participants and the debriefer (Rudolph, Simon, Rivard, Dufresne, & Raemer, 2007).

Gather, Analyze, and Summarize (GAS)

The GAS debriefing method involves three phases:

- **Gather:** Actively listening to participants to understand what they think and how they feel about the simulation.

- **Analyze:** Providing feedback on performance, facilitating participant reflection, and analyzing actions and performance gaps.

- **Summarize:** Identifying lessons learned.

According to Phrampus & O'Donnell (2013), this tool allows those who facilitate debriefings to rapidly gain the necessary skills while remaining comfortable with the process.

Outcome Present-State Test (OPT) Model

The OPT model of clinical reasoning is a structured debriefing used to situate learning by using cognitive critical-thinking strategies and focusing on outcomes (Kuiper, Heinrich, Matthias, Graham, & Bell-Kotwall, 2008). During debriefing, learners use and complete OPT model worksheets that follow interactions associated with the identified nursing diagnosis. A priority focus called a *keystone issue* is identified and serves as the basis for defining a present state. This is described and compared to the desired outcome state, with students identifying interventions to fill the gaps between the two states (Kuiper et al., 2008).

Plus/Delta Debriefing

Pulse/delta debriefing is a simple model adapted from aviation for use in healthcare settings (Gardner, 2013). Findings can be written on a whiteboard or on paper. Listed in the "plus" area are things that went well. The "delta" area identifies specifically what needs to change and be done better next time. This model is quick, convenient, and easy to use as an after-action review, and it can be performed in five minutes or less. The key is to have team members be specific (Gardner, 2013).

Promoting Excellence and Reflective Learning in Simulation (PEARLS)

PEARLS is described as an integrated conceptual framework for a blended approach to debriefing (Eppich & Cheng, 2015). The PEARLS framework integrates three common educational strategies used during debriefing: learner self-assessment, focused discussion, and direct feedback and/or teaching. The PEARLS debriefing script supports simulation educators by setting the stage for the debriefing and then organizing the debriefing to include initial participant reactions, followed by describing relevant case elements. The PEARLS framework involves the selection of a debriefing approach that analyzes positive and suboptimal areas of performance and a summary of lessons learned. The final area of support is in formulating questions that empower educators to share clearly their honest point of view about events (Eppich & Cheng, 2015). Dube et al. (2019) have built on the original PEARLS to create PEARLS for Systems Integration, which can be used to debrief systems-focused simulations "to identify systems issues and maximize improvements in patient safety and quality" (p. 333).

Evaluating the Debriefing

Formal evaluation of the debriefing session is essential to maximize learning provided by the debriefing experience and help establish debriefing best practices. The INACSL debriefing standard also recommends that the competence of debriefers be validated by the use of an established instrument (INACSL Standards Committee, 2016a).

Many tools not specific to debriefing have been used to evaluate and/or compare debriefings. Some debriefing methods (such as DML) also have associated evaluation tools. In addition, there are several evaluation tools that are specific to debriefing and are not tied to a specific debriefing method or framework. Two of these tools pertain to developing debriefing skills—one assesses the participant experience during debriefing and one identifies learning and engagement behaviors during debriefing.

- **Debriefing Experience Scale (DES):**
  The DES was designed to evaluate the participant experience during debriefing though comparison studies (Reed, 2012). It is composed of 20 items rated in the scale areas of experience and importance. Four

of the scale items relate to processing the experience, five pertain to learning, and 11 items are related to the debriefer. The scale was created by Reed (2012) from a review of simulation literature and feedback from three nursing simulation experts. A two-step factor analysis process resulted in its refinement and the removal of redundant items. The scale's reliability has been established for the scale, with a Cronbach's alpha of .93 for the experience portion and .91 for the importance portion (Reed, 2012).

- **Debriefing Engagement and Learning Behaviors (DELB):** The DELB is a new tool that evaluates engagement and learning behaviors exhibited during debriefing (S. J. Reed, personal communication, February 1, 2019). An observer-completed tool, it results in a behavior-per-minute composite score. Validity of the tool has been established through extensive qualitative processes as well as expert input. Inter-rater reliability (consistency between the ratings of raters) of the tool has also been established. Training is required prior to tool use to maintain inter-rater reliability.

- **Debriefing Assessment for Simulation in Healthcare (DASH):** The DASH tool evaluates debriefers on the quality of the debriefing and provides feedback to allow improvement on DASH-established comportments. It is a behaviorally anchored rating scale that requires a training course for its use. There are two versions of the DASH tool: an observer-completed version and a participant- (learner-) completed version. The scale was developed by a consensus of eight emergency medicine physicians with experience in simulation and debriefing. Reliability and validity of the scale were established through

webinar by physicians, nurses, and other highly educated professionals. Statistical significance was achieved rating the three different videos. DASH has been established as useful for rating expert debriefer behaviors for critical care, medical, and team-based simulation debriefings (Brett-Fleegler et al., 2012).

- **Objective Structured Assessment for Debriefing (OSAD):** The purpose of the OSAD tool is to provide feedback to the debriefer to improve the quality of surgical simulation debriefs (Imperial College of London Patient Safety Translational Research Centre, n.d.). The tool is targeted for surgeons and surgical teams. It was developed from a systematic review of the literature as well as expert opinion of those who frequently serve as debriefers in clinical settings. It includes eight core elements of a high-quality debriefing: approach, learning environment, learner engagement, reaction, reflection, analysis, diagnosis, and application (Imperial College of London Patient Safety Translational Research Centre, n.d.).

Conclusion

Debriefing is an essential component of the simulation experience, helping participants to integrate and make meaning of their simulation learning experiences. Feedback should be given during debriefing in a nonthreatening manner to facilitate improved actions in future events. Many best practices have been identified that promote learning. One is to provide structured debriefing. Many debriefing structures, methods, and frameworks exist. Empirical evidence has not established one structure as better than another. Thus, many factors should inform the choice of debriefing structure, including the type of simulation being debriefed, the learning level and needs of the participants, and the debriefer's comfort and training with a particular structure. Debriefers should be trained and undergo ongoing competency assessments to maintain effective debriefing skills. Research regarding debriefing best practices must continue to help make the most of this important simulation learning modality.

References

Abelsson, A., & Bisholt, B. (2017). Nurse student learning acute care by simulation: Focus on observation and debriefing. *Nurse Education in Practice, 24,* 6-13. doi:10.1016/j.nepr.2017.03.001

Asselin, M. E., Schwartz-Barcott, D., & Osterman, P. A. (2013). Exploring reflection as a process embedded in experienced nurses' practice: A qualitative study. *Journal of Advanced Nursing, 69*(4), 905-914. doi:10.1111/j.1365-2648.2012.06082

Boet, S., Bould, M. D., Sharma, B., Revees, S., Naik., V. N., Triby, E., & Grantcharov., T. (2013). Within-team debriefing versus instructor-led debriefing for simulation-based education: A randomized controlled trial. *Annals of Surgery, 258*(1), 53-58. doi:10.1097/SLA.0b013e31829659e4

Bourke, M. P., & Ihrke, B. A. (2016). Introduction to the evaluation process. In Billings, D., & Halstead, J. (Eds.), *Teaching in nursing: A guide for faculty* (5th ed.). St. Louis: Elsevier. (pp. 385-397).

Brackenreg, J. (2004). Issues in reflection and debriefing: How nurse educators structure experiential activities. *Nurse Education in Practice, 4*(4), 264-270. doi:10.1016/j.nepr.2004.01.005

Brett-Fleegler, M., Rudolph, J., Eppich, W., Monuteaux, M., Fleegler, E., Cheng, A., & Simon, R. (2012). Debriefing assessment for simulation in healthcare: Development and psychometric properties. *Simulation in Healthcare, 7*(5), 288–294. doi:10.1097/SIH.0b013e3182620228

Cheng, A., Eppich, W., Grant, V., Sherbino, J., Zendejas, B., & Cook, D. A. (2014). Debriefing for technology-enhanced simulation: A systematic review and meta-analysis. *Medical Education, 48*(7), 657–666. doi:10.1111/medu.12432

Chronister, C., & Brown, D. (2012). Comparison of simulation debriefing methods. *Clinical Simulation in Nursing, 8*(7), e281-e288. doi:10.1016/j.ecns.2010.12.005

Doherty-Restrepo, J., Odai, M., Harris, M., Yam, T., Potteiger, K., & Montalvo, A. (2018). Students' perception of peer and faculty debriefing facilitators following simulation-based education. *Journal of Allied Health, 47*(2), 107-112.

Dreifuerst, K. T. (2012). Using debriefing for meaningful learning to foster development of clinical reasoning in simulation. *Journal of Nursing Education, 51*(6), 326-333. doi:10.3928/01484834-20120409-02

Dube, M. M., Reid, J., Kaba, A., Cheng, A., Eppich, W., Grant, V., & Stone, K. (2019). PEARLS for systems integration: A modified PEARLS framework for debriefing systems-focused simulations. *Simulation in Healthcare, 14*(5), 333–342.

Dufrene, C., & Young. A. (2014). Successful debriefing— Best methods to achieve positive learning outcomes: A literature review. *Nurse Education Today, 34*(3), 372-376. doi:10.1016/j.nedt.2013.06.026

Eppich, W., & Cheng, A. (2015). Promoting Excellence and Reflective Learning in Simulation (PEARLS): Development and rationale for a blended approach to health care simulation debriefing. *Simulation in Healthcare, 10*(2), 106-115. doi:10.1097/SIH.0000000000000072

Fanning, R. M., & Gaba, D. M. (2007). The role of debriefing in simulation-based learning. *Simulation in Healthcare 2*(2), 115-125. doi:10.1097/SIH.0b013e3180315539

Flanagan, B. (2008). Debriefing: Theory and techniques. In R. Riley (Ed.), *Manual of simulation in healthcare* (pp. 155-170). Oxford, UK: Oxford University Press.

Ganley, B. J., & Linnard-Palmer, L. (2012). Academic safety during nursing simulation: Perceptions of nursing students and faculty. *Clinical Simulation in Nursing, 8*(2), e49-e57. doi:10.1016/j.ecns.2010.06.004

Gardner, R. (2013). Introduction to debriefing. *Seminars in Perinatology, 37*(3), 166-174. doi:10.1053/j.semperi.2013.02.008

Ha, E. H., & Lim, E. J. (2018). Peer-led written debriefing versus instructor-led oral debriefing: Using multimode simulation. *Clinical Simulation in Nursing, 18,* 38-46. doi:10.1016/j.ecns.2018.02.002

Hall, K., & Tori, K. (2017). Best practice recommendations for debriefing in simulation-based education for Australian undergraduate nursing students: An integrative review. *Clinical Simulation in Nursing, 13*(1), 39-50. doi:10.1016/j.ecns.2016.10.006

Imperial College of London Patient Safety Translational Research Centre. (n.d.). *The Observational Structured Assessment of Debriefing tool.* Retrieved from http://www.imperial.ac.uk/patient-safety-translational-research-centre/education/training-materials-for-use-in-research-and-clinical-practice/the-observational-structured/

International Nursing Association for Clinical Simulation and Learning Standards Committee. (2016a). INACSL standards of best practice: Simulation. Debriefing. *Clinical Simulation in Nursing, 12*(S), S21–S25. doi:10.1016/j.ecns.2016.09.008

International Nursing Association for Clinical Simulation and Learning Standards Committee. (2016b). INACSL standards of best practice: Simulation. Outcomes and objectives. *Clinical Simulation in Nursing, 12*(S), S13–S15. doi:10.1016/j.ecns.2016.09.006

International Nursing Association for Clinical Simulation and Learning Standards Committee. (2016c). INACSL standards of best practice: Simulation. Simulation glossary. *Clinical Simulation in Nursing, 12*(S), S39–S47. doi:10.1016/j.ecns.2016.09.012

Kim, M., & Kim, S. (2017). Debriefing practices in simulation-based nursing education in South Korea. *Clinical Simulation in Nursing, 13*(5), 201-209. doi:10.1016/j.ecns.2017.01.008

Kolb, A. Y., & Kolb, D. A. (2005). Learning styles and learning spaces: Enhancing experiential learning in higher education. *Academy of Management Learning & Education, 4*(2), 193-212.

Kolb, A. Y., & Kolb, D. A. (2017). Experiential learning theory as a guide for experiential educators in higher education. *Experiential Learning & Teaching in Higher Education, 1*(1), 7-44.

Kuiper, R., Heinrich, C., Matthias, A., Graham, M. J., & Bell-Kotwall, L. (2008). Debriefing with the OPT model of clinical reasoning during high fidelity patient simulation. *International Journal of Nursing Education Scholarship, 5*(1), 1-14. doi:10.2202/1548-923X.1466

Lasater, K. (2007). High-fidelity simulation and the development of clinical judgment: Students' experiences. *Journal of Nursing Education, 46*(6), 269–276.

Levett-Jones, T., & Lapkin, S. (2014). A systematic review of the effectiveness of simulation debriefing in health professional education. *Nurse Education Today, 34,* e58-e63. doi:10.1016/j.nedt.2013.09.020

Mayville, M. L. (2011). Debriefing: The essential step in simulation. *Newborn & Infant Nursing Reviews, 11*(1), 35-39. doi:10.1053/j.nainr.2010.12.012

McDonnell, L. K., Jobe, K. K., & Dismukes, R. K. (1997). *Facilitating LOS debriefings: A training manual* [NASA technical memorandum 112192]. Retrieved from https://ntrs.nasa.gov/archive/nasa/casi.ntrs.nasa.gov/19970015346.pdf

Miraglia, R., & Asselin, M. E. (2015). Reflection as an educational strategy in nursing professional development: An integrative review. *Journal for Nurses in Professional Development, 31*(2), 62-72. doi:10.1097/NND.0000000000000151

Motavalli, A., & Nestel, D. (2016). Complexity in simulation-based education: Exploring the role of hindsight bias. *Advances in Simulation, 1*(3), 1-7. doi:10.1186/s41077-015-0005-7

Naicker, K., & van Rensburg, G. H. (2018). Facilitation of reflective learning in nursing: Reflective teaching practices of educators. *Africa Journal of Nursing and Midwifery, 20*(2), 1-15. doi:10.25159/2520-5293/3386

National League for Nursing. (2015). *Debriefing across the curriculum.* Retrieved from http://www.nln.org/docs/default-source/about/nln-vision-series-%28position-statements%29/nln-vision-debriefing-across-the-curriculum.pdf?sfvrsn=0

Neill, M. A., & Wotton, K. (2011). High-fidelity simulation debriefing in nursing education: A literature review. *Clinical Simulation in Nursing, 7*(5), e161-e168. doi:10.1016/j.ecns.2011.02.001

Phrampus, P. E., & O'Donnell, J. M. (2013). Debriefing using a structured and supported approach. In A. I. Levine, S. DeMaria, A. D. Schwartz, & A. J. Sim (Eds.), *The comprehensive textbook of healthcare simulation* (pp. 73-84). New York, NY: Springer.

Raemer, D., Anderson, M., Cheng, A., Fanning, R., Nadkarni, V., & Savoldelli, G. (2011). Research regarding debriefing as part of the learning process. *Simulation in Healthcare, 6*(Suppl.), S52-S57. doi:10.1097/SIH.0b013e31822724d0

Reed, S. J. (2012). Debriefing experience scale: Development of a tool to evaluate the student learning experience in debriefing. *Clinical Simulation in Nursing, 8*(6), e211-e217. doi:10.1016/j.ecns.2011.11.002

Reed, S. J. (2016). *Identifying learning acquired during debriefing* (Doctoral dissertation, UNLV). Retrieved from http://digitalscholarship.unlv.edu/thesesdissertations/2724

Reed, S. J., Andrews, C. A., & Ravert, P. R. (2013). Debriefing simulations: Comparison of debriefing with video and debriefing alone. *Clinical Simulation in Nursing, 9*(12), e585-e591. doi:10.1016/j.ecns.2013.05.007

Rudolph, J. W., Simon, R., Rivard, P., Dufresne, R. L., & Raemer, D. B. (2007). Debriefing with good judgment: Combining rigorous feedback with genuine inquiry. *Anesthesiology Clinics, 25*(2), 361-376.

Rutherford-Hemming, T., Lioce, L., & Breymier, T. (2019). Guidelines and essential elements for prebriefing. *Simulation in Healthcare, 14*(6), 409-414.

Tosterud, R., Hall-Lord, M. L., Petzäll, K., & Hedelin, B. (2014). Debriefing in simulation conducted in small and large groups: Nursing students' experiences. *Journal of Nursing Education and Practice, 4*(9), 173-182. doi:10.5430/jnep.v4n9p173

Van Heukelom, J. N., Begaz, T., & Treat, R. (2010). Comparison of postsimulation debriefing versus in-simulation debriefing in medical simulation. *Simulation in Healthcare, 5*(2), 91-97. doi:10.1097/SIH.0b013e3181be0d17

Wang, E. E. (2011). Simulation and adult learning. *Disease-A-Month, 57*(11), 664-678. doi:10.1016/j.disamonth.2011.08.017

Zigmont, J. J., Kappus, L. J., & Sudikoff, S. N. (2011). The 3D model of debriefing: Defusing, discovering, and deepening. *Seminars in Perinatology, 35*(2), 53-58. doi:10.1053/j.semperi.2011.01.003

> "I believe in evidence. I believe in observation, measurement, and reasoning, confirmed by independent observers. I'll believe anything, no matter how wild and ridiculous, if there is evidence for it. The wilder and more ridiculous something is, however, the firmer and more solid the evidence will have to be."
>
> —Isaac Asimov

Evaluating Simulation Effectiveness

6

Katie Anne Haerling, PhD, RN

Educators in the health professions have long used various forms of simulation for teaching and learning. However, until recently, they have given little attention to evaluating the effectiveness of simulation endeavors. This chapter focuses on assessment and evaluation—two essential activities for planning, implementing, and continually improving a successful simulation program.

For many charged with the responsibility of managing or running a simulation program—even those who have established competence and confidence in teaching with simulation—evaluating the effectiveness of simulation endeavors may seem like a daunting task. This chapter seeks to make it less intimidating by:

- Answering the essential question of why we assess and evaluate

- Describing a framework for categorizing simulation evaluation strategies

- Suggesting guidelines and instruments from practice and the literature that may be used for evaluation

- Providing exemplars of simulation evaluation

Why Evaluate?

At first glance, assessment and evaluation seem like interchangeable terms. However, it is important to differentiate between the two:

- *Assessment* refers to the process of gathering information about a simulation participant, activity, or program (INACSL Standards Committee, 2016b).

- *Evaluation* refers to the application of the data collected during the assessment process.

We collect data about simulation participants, activities, and programs (assess) and then apply those data (evaluate) for several purposes. These purposes include (Bourke & Ihrke, 2016; Halstead, 2020):

- Helping participants learn and identify what they have learned (or not learned)

- Identifying actual or potential problems, including shortfalls in participant learning or gaps in a specific simulation activity or program

- Assigning participant scores

- Improving current practices

- Identifying how well or efficiently intended outcomes were achieved

Through this reflective practice of generating knowledge (assessment) and applying that knowledge to make decisions (evaluation), we can keep track of how well we are meeting individual, team, and organizational objectives. This is how we communicate to stakeholders (administrators, funders, etc.) about how simulation endeavors contribute to student learning, the bottom line, and the mission of the organization (W. K. Kellogg Foundation, 2017).

In healthcare education, simulation is used to address several challenges including:

- Expanding enrollments

- Faculty shortages

- Graduates who are underprepared for the workforce

- Limited clinical placement sites

- Reduced opportunities for patient care in existing clinical placement sites due to patient acuity and regulatory constraints

In hospitals and healthcare systems, simulation is used to validate and develop competencies, improve quality of care, decrease risks, and optimize resources. Inadequate evidence exists, however, about whether simulation is successful in addressing these challenges. Therefore, we need to increase efforts to document the efficacy of simulation activities.

Formative and Summative Evaluations

In the context of a simulation program, formative evaluations answer the question "Is this working?" and illuminate opportunities for immediate remediation or improvement. In contrast, summative evaluations answer the question "Did this work?" and illuminate opportunities for future changes.

The INACSL glossary (INACSL Standards Committee, 2016b, p. 41) defines *formative evaluation* and *summative evaluation* as follows:

- **Formative:** "Evaluation wherein the facilitator's focus is on the participant's progress toward goal attainment through preset criteria; a process for an individual or group engaged in a simulation activity for the purpose of providing constructive feedback for that individual or group to improve."

- **Summative:** "Evaluation at the end of a learning period or at a discrete point in time in which participants are provided with feedback about their achievement of outcome through preset criteria; a process for determining the competence of a participant engaged in healthcare activity. The assessment of achievement of outcome criteria may be associated with an assigned grade."

From a universal perspective, the evidence supporting the efficacy of simulation is growing; however, many evaluations about the efficacy of simulation endeavors will be done to meet immediate, local needs. For example, after the purchase of simulation equipment and the early implementation of a simulation program, administrators will likely ask the question "How do we know simulation is working?" This question can have several meanings, but, in general, people want to know how the implementation of simulation activities affects the outcomes they care about, including patient care and the bottom line.

To that end, the focus of a simulation evaluation may range from an individual simulation participant to an entire simulation program or strategy. Likewise, the purpose of a simulation evaluation may range from gathering formative data about an individual participant's satisfaction with a particular activity to gathering summative data about the results of an entire simulation training program to guide future research, practice, and policy (W. K. Kellogg Foundation, 2017).

Kirkpatrick's Framework

Kirkpatrick (1998) suggests a framework to categorize evaluation strategies. This framework is helpful for identifying the scope and purpose of an evaluation. Kirkpatrick's (1998) framework has four levels of evaluation:

- Reaction
- Learning
- Behavior
- Results

These levels categorize different types of simulation evaluations. Table 6.1 shows each level of evaluation, what questions are answered at each level, and examples of strategies that may be used to complete evaluations at each level.

Guidelines for Evaluations at Each Level

Kirkpatrick (1998) identifies guidelines for completing evaluations at each level. Similarities between evaluations at every level include starting with the end in mind (Wiggins & McTighe, 2005) to determine what information you want to gather and identifying a standard or benchmark against which you will compare your results. A strategy for evaluation should be included in the early simulation planning process and not tacked on at the end. It is also important, regardless of the types of evaluation you will be doing, to establish whether the evaluations will be formative or summative, or whether you will use both types of evaluations.

Regardless of what level of evaluation you are doing and whether it is formative or summative, after you have collected your data, you need to communicate your results to stakeholders and make any necessary changes based on these results.

Following are the unique characteristics of each level of evaluation:

- **Reaction:** In addition to standardized response questions, encourage participants to provide written comments. Design the evaluation form and participant experience to encourage maximum participation and honesty.

- **Learning:** Consider using a control group so you can make objective comparisons. Evaluate multiple domains of learning: cognitive, affective, and psychomotor. This may be accomplished using measures such as a multiple-choice exam (cognitive), a written reflection about attitudes or beliefs (affective), and an observation-based performance evaluation (psychomotor).

- **Behavior:** Allow adequate time for behavior change to take place, and consider identifying a control group for comparison. Get a 360-degree view of participants' practice behaviors by seeking input from multiple sources: clinical instructors, preceptors, staff, peers, patients, and the participant. Repeat the evaluation of behavior as appropriate.

- **Results:** Allow adequate time for results to occur. Consider what you will use for your comparison. This may mean taking measurements before and after implementation of a simulation program. Consider doing a cost-benefit analysis, and repeat the evaluation of results as

appropriate in the form of periodic monitoring or tracking.

Highlights and Challenges of Evaluations at Each Level

Evaluations become increasingly more challenging and increasingly more meaningful as you move from level 1 (reaction) to level 4 (results; see Table 6.1). Although it might be easy to ask simulation participants about their satisfaction with a simulation activity, it is much more difficult to measure how simulation-based training affects a participant's behavior and ultimately affects patient and organizational outcomes (results). In parallel, it might be interesting to know how well participants enjoyed a simulation activity, but it is much more important to know the answer to the larger question, "Is simulation working?"

Table 6.1	**Questions and Strategy Examples for Levels of Evaluation**	
Level	**Questions**	**Strategy Example**
Reaction	What were the participants' reactions to the simulation activity? Were they satisfied with the simulation experience? Did the simulation activity improve their confidence?	Surveying participants about their level of satisfaction with the simulation experience
Learning	What did the participants learn from the simulation activity? What domains of learning did the simulation activity contribute to—cognitive? affective? psychomotor? Have participants demonstrated readiness to progress into the clinical environment?	Evaluating participants' demonstrations of critical thinking or technical skills in simulation, or pre- and post-testing participants' knowledge and attitudes
Behavior	How did the simulation activity affect participants' behavior in the actual clinical environment? Did learning that occurred in simulation transfer to actual patient care?	Evaluating the competency of new graduates or residents who were educated using simulation
Results	What were the long-term results of the simulation activity? How were patient or organizational outcomes affected?	Calculating cost-savings (Cohen et al., 2010) or improved patient outcomes (Draycott et al., 2008) that result from simulation-based training

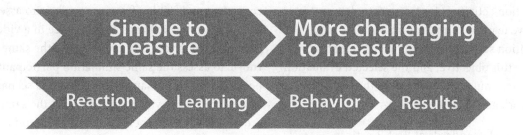

FIGURE 6.1   Continuum of simple to challenging levels of evaluation.

Measuring Progress

Evaluations often involve measuring progress over time. For example, a staff education department faced with complacent or unmotivated learners may be very interested in measuring changes in participant satisfaction with the department's educational offerings. In this case, it may be important to evaluate participants' reactions to simulation activities. Educators are interested in participants' development and learning in the cognitive, affective, and psychomotor domains.

Patient safety advocates are interested in practitioners' behaviors (handwashing, for instance) and the results of these behaviors (Seaton et al., 2019). Data about these behaviors and results are most valuable when they are presented in a context in which change over time may be observed. In these cases, it is valuable to repeat the same evaluation at multiple points in time to document progress.

INACSL Standards of Best Practice: Simulation Participant Evaluation

The INACSL Standards of Best Practice provide guidelines for participant evaluation. These standards focus on the evaluation of the simulation participant rather than the simulation design, facilitation, or other non-participant components of the simulation experience.

An equally important aspect of these standards is the emphasis on selecting the evaluation method in the planning stages of the simulation. While gathering assessment data and making decisions based on this data may be part of the final steps in planning and implementing a simulation, the assessment procedures must align with the objectives of the simulation activity. For example, if the objective of the simulation activity is for learners to demonstrate effective teamwork and communication, the simulation scenario must allow participants to achieve this objective, and the selected evaluation instrument must include criteria that focus on teamwork and communication.

The INACSL Standards of Best Practice: Simulation Participant Evaluation describes specific criteria for formative, summative, and high-stakes simulation participant evaluation. Formative and summative evaluation were defined previously in this chapter. The term *high-stakes evaluation* is used to describe an evaluation "associated with a simulation activity that has a major academic, educational, or employment consequence (such as a grading decision, including pass or fail implications; a decision regarding competency, merit pay, promotion, or certification) at a discrete point in time. High stakes refer to the outcome or consequences of the process" (INACSL, 2016b, p. S41). As shown in Table 6.2, the elements required for each type of evaluation become more and more rigorous as they advance from formative to summative to high-stakes.

Instruments and Methods for Evaluation at Each Level

Ensuring the reliability of the data and the validity of the decisions you are making based on those data are great challenges associated with assessment and evaluation. Looking at reliability, you want to make sure the data are

consistent and stable. If you use a rubric to assess a simulation participant's performance in a video-recorded scenario today and then use the same rubric to assess the same simulation participant's performance in the same video-recorded scenario a week from now, you should arrive at the same score. Likewise, another trained rater should be able to use the rubric you used to assess the same simulation participant's performance in the same video-recorded scenario and assign the same score. These are referred to as *intra-rater* (test-retest) and *inter-rater* reliability, respectively. Other types of reliability that may be explored are internal consistency, alternate forms, and inter-instrument reliability (Park, 2019). Like reliability, it is important to examine the validity of data—or evidence that the assessment procedures are measuring what you want to measure and that the decisions being made based on the assessment data align with the intentions of the evaluation. When simulation-based assessments are being used for high-stakes evaluation or to decide if providers can safely make independent decisions about patient care (readiness assessment), it is even more important to ensure those assessments are providing valid and reliable data (Nabzdyk & Bittner, 2018).

Table 6.3 shows examples of instruments from the literature that may be used to facilitate evaluations at each level. While it may be tempting to develop unique evaluation instruments for specific evaluation needs, consider using an existing instrument that meets your needs.

Table 6.2   Types of Evaluation

Formative Evaluation	Summative Evaluation	High-Stakes Evaluation
"Formative evaluation is conducted to: • Monitor progress toward achieving outcomes. • Provide ongoing formative feedback. • Support participant's clinical competencies. • Identify and close gaps in knowledge and skills. • Assess readiness for real-world experiences. • Facilitate teaching and learning. Requires formally trained facilitators (see INACSL Standard: Facilitation). Use small group ratio, ideally a minimum ratio of one facilitator per three to five students."	"Summative evaluation is conducted: • At a discrete point in time (i.e., at the end of a course or certain time period). • In a safe learning environment. • After orientation to the environment and equipment. • Appropriate level of fidelity necessary to achieve the participant outcomes. • Utilizing a standardized format and scoring methods (i.e., utilizing a standardized scenario that includes information on when to cue, scenario length of time, and other scenario details). • With a video recording of the evaluation to allow review by multiple trained evaluators. Use a theoretically based method to determine passing or cut scores where appropriate. Select a valid and reliable instrument. Provide rater training for observation-based evaluation. Establish interrater reliability when more than one rater required. Inform participants in advance of the evaluation process. Provide summative feedback to participant about achievement of outcomes."	"High-stakes evaluation is conducted: • At the end of the learning process but may occur at other times to assess gaps in knowledge or to identify significant safety issues. • Based on specific participant objectives. • After the consequences and outcomes have been explained to the participants. • With predetermined parameters for terminating the scenario for its completion. • After the simulated-based experience has been pilot tested. • By trained, nonbiased objective raters or evaluators. • By an objective rater or evaluator using a comprehensive tool (i.e., checklist or rubric that clearly outlines desirable and undesirable behaviors). • After the participant has had the opportunity for multiple exposures to simulation-based experiences including evaluations. Use an evaluation tool previously tested with similar populations. Use more than one evaluator for each participant, either directly observed or a video recording."

Source: INACSL, 2016a, p. S27

Table 6.3	Measurement Instruments
Level	**Instrument Examples**
Reaction	Affective:
	Satisfaction and Self-Confidence in Learning Scale (National League for Nursing, 2005)
	Emergency Response Confidence Tool (Arnold et al., 2009)
Learning	Cognitive:
	Multiple choice exam questions such as from the Assessment Technologies Institute (ATI)
	Psychomotor:
	Skills checklists (Perry, Potter, & Elkin, 2012)
	Multiple domains:
	Lasater Clinical Judgment Rubric (Lasater, 2007)
	Sweeny-Clark Simulation Evaluation Rubric (Clark, 2006)
	Clinical Simulation Evaluation Tool (Radhakrishnan, Roche, & Cunningham, 2007)
	DARE2 Patient Safety Rubric (Walshe, O'Brien, Hartigan, Murphy, & Graham, 2014)
Behavior	Creighton Simulation Evaluation Instrument (Todd, Manz, Hawkins, Parsons, & Hercinger, 2008)
Results	Cost/benefit analysis
	Cost savings (Cohen et al., 2010) or improved patient outcomes (Draycott et al., 2008) that result from simulation-based training

Additional Resources for Identifying Existing Instruments

Examples of review articles and instrument websites that may be helpful for identifying possible evaluation instruments include:

- "An Updated Review of Published Simulation Evaluation Instruments," by Adamson, Kardong-Edgren, and Willhaus, in *Clinical Simulation in Nursing* (2013)

- "Assessment of Human Patient Simulation-Based Learning," by Bray, Schwartz, Odegard, Hammer, and Seybert, in *American Journal of Pharmaceutical Education* (2011)

- The Creighton Competency Evaluation Instrument website at https://nursing.creighton.edu/academics/competency-evaluation-instrument

- The Debriefing Assessment for Simulation in Healthcare (DASH) website at https://harvardmedsim.org/debriefing-assessment-for-simulation-in-healthcare-dash/

- "Human Patient Simulation Rubrics for Nursing Education: Measuring the Essentials of Baccalaureate Education for Professional Nursing Practice," by Davis and Kimble, in *Journal of Nursing Education* (2011)

- INACSL Repository of Instruments Used in Simulation Research website at https://www.inacsl.org/resources/repository-of-instruments/

- "A Review of Currently Published Evaluation Instruments for Human Patient Simulation," by Kardong-Edgren, Adamson, and Fitzgerald, in *Clinical Simulation in Nursing* (2010)

- "Tools for Direct Observation and Assessment of Clinical Skills," by Kogan, Holmboe, and Hauer, in *Journal of the American Medical Association* (2009)

- Quality and Safety Education for Nurses (QSEN) Simulation Evaluation website at http://qsen.org/teaching-strategies/simulation/simulation-evaluation/

- "The Contribution of High-Fidelity Simulation to Nursing Students' Confidence and Competence," by Yuan, Williams, and Fang, in *International Nursing Review* (2012)

Methods for Evaluating Participants in Simulation Endeavors

In addition to specific evaluation instruments, it may be helpful to consider general methods for evaluating participants in simulation endeavors. Table 6.4 includes examples of strategies that may be used to reflect participants' experiences, performance, and learning.

Considerations When Selecting an Instrument

Several important questions need to be considered when selecting an evaluation instrument (Halstead, 2020):

- Does the instrument measure what you want to measure?

- Does it measure everything you want to measure, or will you need to add questions or use more than one instrument?

- Is the instrument accessible and understandable to those who will be using it?

Table 6.4   Participant Evaluation Strategies

Method	Uses
360-degree survey of performance	Feedback from multiple sources can provide a more complete picture of participants' performance and/or learning.
Anecdotal faculty notes	Consistent and well-organized notes may reflect participant progress and provide documentation for formative and summative evaluation.
Attitude scales	Frick, Chadha, Watson, Wang, and Green (2009) suggest that participants' perceptions influence their learning. Gathering data about participants' attitudes toward and satisfaction with simulation activities may reflect the efficacy of the activities.
Observation-based evaluations, including short checklists	These evaluations enable educators to observe and rate participant performance systematically.
Reflection papers, blogs, or journals	These types of reflections provide self-reported data about participants' experience in and learning from a simulation activity. Examples from the literature include Marchigiano, Eduljee, and Harvey (2011), who used journaling for the development of critical-thinking skills, and Weller (2004) and McElhinney (2011), who employed unique reflective practices in simulation.
Typical course clinical evaluation tools	These instruments are likely familiar to educators and are typically designed to reflect course or program objectives.

- What type of training will you need to provide to those who will be using it?

- What evidence is there to support the validity and reliability of the results, and how you plan to use them?

> A key consideration when selecting an evaluation strategy or instrument is deciding what you want to measure. For example, should the evaluation reflect the performance of an individual or a team? If you are working with an interprofessional team, are the expectations for each member of the team similar or different? How should this be accounted for in the evaluation?

If you are not satisfied with the answers to these questions for the evaluation instrument you are considering, you might want to modify an existing instrument or design your own. Be warned, however, that designing and validating a new evaluation instrument require a significant investment of time, effort, and expertise in tool development.

Observation-based evaluation instruments are powerful because they have the potential to capture what the person being rated is actually doing—not just what they report they know or how they would act in a hypothetical situation. However, they also have several weaknesses. A key weakness is that the data they produce are influenced not only by the performance of the person being observed but also by variables associated with the person doing the observing and scoring. Rater bias (intentional or not) is a factor that must be considered when selecting an instrument and evaluation strategy. Rater training and careful consideration of how rater

characteristics might influence the ratings they assign will help ensure a more valid and reliable evaluation process.

Evaluation Exemplar: Academic Setting

One exemplar of a multiple-level evaluation of simulation effectiveness is the National Council of State Boards of Nursing (NCSBN) National Simulation Study (Hayden, 2012; Hayden, Smiley, Alexander, Kardong-Edgren, & Jeffries, 2014; NCSBN, 2014). In this study, nursing students were randomized into three study groups. Each group used simulation to replace a percentage of traditional clinical hours—up to 10%, 25%, and 50%, respectively. Students were evaluated throughout their nursing education (phase I and phase II) and into the first year of practice (phase III). This study sought to answer the following research questions (Hayden, 2012; NCSBN, 2013):

- Are there perceived differences in how well learning needs are met in the clinical and simulation environments among the three study groups?

- Are there differences in knowledge among graduating nursing students in the three study groups?

- Are there differences in clinical competency among graduating nursing students in the three study groups?

- Are there differences in clinical competency among the three study groups in each of the core clinical courses?

Table 6.5 shows how each of these questions corresponds with different levels of evaluation and the instruments used.

Table 6.5 Levels of Questions Asked in Phase I and Phase II of the NCSBN National Simulation Study

Question	Evaluation Level	Instruments for Evaluation
Are there perceived differences in how well learning needs are met in the clinical and simulation environments among the three study groups?	Reaction—Level 1	Clinical Learning Environment Comparison Survey
Are there differences in knowledge among graduating nursing students in the three study groups?	Learning—Level 2	ATI Comprehensive Assessment and Review Program
Are there differences in clinical competency among graduating nursing students in the three study groups? Are there differences in clinical competency among the three study groups in each of the core clinical courses?	Behavior—Level 3	Creighton Competency Evaluation Instrument

After graduation, data were collected from the graduates' National Council Licensure Examination results. In addition, graduates were followed for their first year of practice. During that year, investigators sought to evaluate how the learning from simulation translated into the graduates' behavior and outcomes in practice. The findings from this study were incorporated into the NCSBN Simulation Guidelines for Prelicensure Nursing Programs (Alexander et al., 2015) and have had major policy implications throughout the US.

Evaluation Exemplar: Practice Setting

A hypothetical exemplar of a multilevel simulation evaluation in a hospital setting involves an effort to reduce catheter-associated urinary tract infections (CAUTIs) through a simulation-based CAUTI prevention training program. In this exemplar, staff education has been tasked with implementing the hospital-wide training program for nurses and support staff and evaluating the efficacy of the program.

Staff educators are interested in the quality of their programs and have several questions related to evaluation:

- Are staff satisfied with the training they received as part of the CAUTI prevention training program?

- Did staff demonstrate improved knowledge and skill related to CAUTI prevention after participating in the training program?

- How did the CAUTI prevention training program affect participants' behavior in the actual clinical environment?

- How did the CAUTI prevention training program affect hospital CAUTI rates?

Table 6.6 shows how each of these questions corresponds with different levels of evaluation and ideas for instruments that may be used.

Table 6.6 Levels of Questions Asked in the Hypothetical Study		
Question	**Evaluation Level**	**Instruments for Evaluation**
Are staff satisfied with the training they received as part of the CAUTI prevention training program?	Reaction—Level 1	Satisfaction survey distributed to participating staff after completion of the program
Did staff demonstrate improved knowledge and skill related to CAUTI prevention after participating in the training program?	Learning—Level 2	Pre- and post-knowledge exam about CAUTI prevention Lab-based skills check-off for catheter insertion, care, and removal
How did the CAUTI prevention training program affect participants' behavior in the actual clinical environment?	Behavior—Level 3	Peer observation of catheter insertion, care, and removal Self-report survey of behavior in clinical environment
How did the CAUTI prevention training program affect hospital CAUTI rates?	Results—Level 4	Comparing CAUTI rates before and after CAUTI prevention training program or comparing CAUTI rates between units where the program has been implemented and those where it has yet to be implemented

Take a moment to consider education and training needs in your facility. How are these needs being addressed? Is there a formal evaluation process in place to measure their efficacy? This exemplar may be used as a template for evaluating reactions, learning, behavior, and results from education and training programs covering topics ranging from handwashing to complex invasive procedures.

Conclusion

Evaluating the efficacy of simulation endeavors is a complex but necessary step in the process of planning, implementing, and continuously improving a successful simulation program. This chapter has outlined reasons to evaluate simulation endeavors, described a system for categorizing simulation evaluation strategies, and provided guidelines and examples for

completing different types of evaluations. Using these resources and examples will help you and your simulation team take on the challenge of evaluating your simulation endeavors.

References

Alexander, M., Durham, C. F., Hooper, J. I., Jeffries, P. R., Goldman, N., Kardong-Edgren, S., ... Tillman, C. (2015). NCSBN simulation guidelines for prelicensure nursing programs. *Journal of Nursing Regulation, 6*(3), 39-42. Retrieved from https://www.journalofnursingregulation.com/article/S2155-8256(15)30783-3/fulltext

Arnold, J. J., Johnson, L. M., Tucker, S. J., Malec, J. F., Henrickson, S. E., & Dunn, W. F. (2009). Evaluation tools in simulation learning: Performance and self-efficacy in emergency response. *Clinical Simulation in Nursing, 5*(1), e35-e43. doi:10.1016/j.ecns.2008.10.003

Bourke, M. P., & Ihrke, B. A. (2016). Introduction to the evaluation process. In Billings, D., & Halstead, J. (Eds.), *Teaching in nursing: A guide for faculty* (5th ed.). St. Louis: Elsevier. (pp. 385–397).

Clark, M. (2006). Evaluating an obstetric trauma scenario. *Clinical Simulation in Nursing, 2*(2), e75-e77. doi:10.1016/j.ecns.2009.05.028

Cohen, E. R., Feinglass, J., Barsuk, J. H., Barnard, C., O'Donnell, A., McGaghie, W. C., & Wayne, D. B. (2010). Cost savings from reduced catheter-related bloodstream infection after simulation-based education for residents in a medical intensive care unit. *Simulation in Healthcare, 5*(2), 98-102. doi:10.1097/SIH.0b013e3181bc8304

Draycott, T. J, Crofts, J. F., Ash, J. P., Wilson, L. V., Yard, E., Sibanda, T. & Whitelaw, A. (2008). Improving neonatal outcome through practical shoulder dystocia training. *Obstetrics and Gynecology, 112*(1), 14-20. doi:10.1097/AOG.0b013e31817bbc61

Frick, T. W., Chadha, R., Watson, C., Wang, Y., & Green, P. (2009). College students' perceptions of teaching and learning quality. *Educational Technology Research and Development, 57*(5), 705-720.

Halstead, J. A. (2020). Introduction to the evaluation process. In D. M. Billings & J. A. Halstead (Eds.), *Teaching in nursing: A guide for faculty* (6th ed., pp. 437-449). St. Louis, MO: Elsevier.

Hayden, J. (2012). *The National Council of State Boards of Nursing national simulation study.* Presented at 2012 NCSBN Scientific Symposium, Arlington, VA. Retrieved from https://www.ncsbn.org/685.htm

Hayden, J. K., Smiley, R. A., Alexander, M., Kardong-Edgren, S., & Jeffries, P. R. (2014). The NCSBN national simulation study: A longitudinal, randomized controlled study replacing clinical hours with simulation in prelicensure nursing education. *Journal of Nursing Regulation, 5*(2), S1-S64.

International Nursing Association for Clinical Simulation and Learning Standards Committee. (2016a). INACSL standards of best practice: Simulation. Participant evaluation. *Clinical Simulation in Nursing, 12*(S), S26-S29. doi:10.1016/j.ecns.2016.09.009

International Nursing Association for Clinical Simulation and Learning Standards Committee. (2016b). INACSL standards of best practice: Simulation. Simulation glossary. *Clinical Simulation in Nursing, 12*(S), S39-S47. doi:10.1016/j.ecns.2016.09.012

Kirkpatrick, D. L. (1998). *Evaluating training programs: The four levels* (2nd ed.). San Francisco, CA: Berrett-Koehler Publishers.

Lasater, K. (2007). Clinical judgment development: Using simulation to create an assessment rubric. *Journal of Nursing Education, 46*(11), 496-503.

Marchigiano, G., Eduljee, N., & Harvey, K. (2011). Developing critical thinking skills from clinical assignments: A pilot study on nursing students' self-reported perceptions. *Journal of Nursing Management, 19*(1), 143-152. doi:10.1111/j.1365-2834.2010.01191.x

McElhinney, E. (2011). An evaluation of clinical simulation in a virtual world and its impact on practice: An action research project. *Clinical Simulation in Nursing, 7*(6), e258. doi:10.1016/j.ecns.2011.09.050

Nabzdyk, C. S., & Bittner, E. A. (2018). One (not so small) step for simulation-based competency assessment in critical care. *Critical Care Medicine, 46*(6), 1026-1027. doi:10.1097/CCM.0000000000003101

National Council of State Boards of Nursing. (2014). *The NCSBN national simulation study.* Retrieved from https://www.ncsbn.org/jnr_simulation_supplement.pdf

National League for Nursing. (2005). *The student satisfaction and self confidence in learning scale.* Retrieved from http://www.nln.org/docs/default-source/default-document-library/instrument-2_satisfaction-and-self-confidence-in-learning.pdf?sfvrsn=0

Park, Y. S. (2019). Reliability. In R. Yudkowsky, Y. S. Park, & S. M. Downing (Eds.), *Assessment in health professions education* (2nd ed., pp. 33-50). New York, NY: Routledge.

Perry, A. G., Potter, P. A., & Elkin, M. K., (2012). *Nursing interventions & clinical skills* (5th ed.). St. Louis, MO: Mosby.

Radhakrishnan, K., Roche, J. P., & Cunningham, H. (2007). Measuring clinical practice parameters with human patient simulation: A pilot study. *International Journal of Nursing Education Scholarship, 4,* Article 8, 1-11.

Seaton, P., Levett-Jones, T., Cant, R., Cooper, S., Kelly, M. A., McKenna, L., … Bogossian, F. (2019). Exploring the extent to which simulation-based education addresses contemporary patient safety priorities: A scoping review. *Collegian, 26,* 194-203. doi:10.1016/j.colegn.2018.04.006

Todd, M., Manz, J. A., Hawkins, K. S., Parsons, M. E., & Hercinger, M. (2008). The development of a quantitative evaluation tool for simulations in nursing education. *International Journal of Nursing Education Scholarship, 5,* Article 41, 1-17. doi:10.2202/1548-923X.1705

Walshe, N., O'Brien, S., Hartigan, I., Murphy, S., & Graham, R. (2014). Simulation performance evaluation: Inter-rater reliability of the DARE[2]-patient safety rubric. *Clinical Simulation in Nursing, 10*(9), 446-454. http://dx.doi.org/10.1016/j.ecns.2014.06.005

Weller, J. M. (2004). Simulation in undergraduate medical education: Bridging the gap between theory and practice. *Medical Education, 38*(1), 32-38.

Wiggins, G., & McTighe, J. (2005). *Understanding by design.* Alexandria, VA: Association for Supervision and Curriculum Development.

W. K. Kellogg Foundation. (2017). *The W. K. Kellogg Foundation step-by-step guide to evaluation.* Retrieved from https://www.wkkf.org/resource-directory/resource/2017/11/wk-kellogg-foundation-step-by-step-guide-to-evaluation

"Without continual growth and progress, such words as improvement, achievement, and success have no meaning."

–Benjamin Franklin

Simulation as a Continuous Learning System

7

Juli C. Maxworthy, DNP, MSN, MBA, RN, CNL, CPHQ, CPPS, CHSE, FNAP, FSSH
Janice C. Palaganas, PhD, RN, NP, ANEF, FAAN, FSSH

OBJECTIVES

- Understand continuous learning systems.
- Appraise the need for continuous learning systems.
- Understand educational components of continuous learning systems.
- Apply systems integration learning points in healthcare simulation.
- Develop simulation-based interprofessional education to achieve continuous learning health systems.

In July of 2006, the Institute of Medicine (IOM) Roundtable on Evidence-Based Medicine convened a workshop titled "The Learning Healthcare System." This work group sought to "transform the way evidence on clinical effectiveness is generated and used to improve health and healthcare" (IOM, 2007, p. ix). Its work described the development of a learning healthcare system that is "designed to generate and apply the best evidence for the collaborative healthcare choices of each patient and provider; to drive the process of discovery as a natural outgrowth of patient care; and to ensure innovation, quality, safety, and value in healthcare" (IOM, 2007, p. ix).

To achieve this, the work group developed the initial needs for a learning healthcare system. These needs were as follows (IOM, 2007, pp. 4–6):

- *"Adaptation to the pace of change:* continuous learning and a much more dynamic approach to evidence development and application, taking full advantage of developing information technology to match the rate at which new interventions are developed and new insights emerge about individual variation in response to those interventions;

- *Stronger synchrony of efforts:* better consistency and coordination of efforts to generate, assess, and advise on the results of new knowledge in a way that does not produce conflict or confusion;

- *Culture of shared responsibility:* to enable the evolution of the learning environment as a common cause of patients, providers, and researchers and better engage all in improved communication about the importance of the nature of evidence and its evolution;

- *New clinical research paradigm:* drawing clinical research closer to the experience of clinical practice, including the development of new study methodologies adapted to the practice environment and a better understanding of when RCTs are most practical and desirable;

- *Clinical decision support systems:* to accommodate the reality that although professional judgment will always be vital to shaping care, the amount of information required for any given decision is moving beyond unassisted human capacity;

- *Universal electronic health records:* comprehensive deployment and effective application of the full capabilities available in EHRs as an essential prerequisite for the evolution of the learning healthcare system;

- *Tools for database linkage, mining, and use:* advancing the potential for structured, large databases as new sources of evidence, including issues in fostering interoperable platforms and in developing new means of ongoing searching of those databases for patterns and clinical insights;

- *Notion of clinical data as a public good:* advancement of the notion of the use of clinical data as a central common resource for advancing knowledge and evidence for effective care—including directly addressing current challenges related to the treatment of data as a proprietary good and interpretations of the Health Insurance Portability and Accountability Act (HIPAA) and other patient privacy issues that currently present barriers to knowledge development;

- *Incentives aligned for practice-based evidence:* encouraging the development and use of evidence by drawing research and practice closer together, and developing the patient records and interoperable platforms necessary to foster more rapid learning and improve care;

- *Public engagement:* improved communication about the nature of evidence and its development, and the active roles of both patients and healthcare professionals in evidence development and dissemination;

- *Trusted scientific broker:* an agent or entity with the public and scientific confidence to provide guidance, shape priorities, and foster the shift in the clinical research paradigm; and

- *Leadership:* to marshal the vision, strategy, and actions necessary to create a learning healthcare system."

Since that initial meeting in 2006 and the publication of its proceedings, an entire body of work has evolved. There have been significant efforts to improve elements of these initial recommendations.

The Josiah Macy Jr. Foundation spearheaded a number of work groups to further these recommendations. In 2015, the foundation convened experts to explore the role of technology in enhancing health professions education through a continuum. This conference and its recommendations, which serve as the basis of this chapter, were titled "Enhancing Health Professions Education Through Technology: Building a Continuously Learning Health System" (Stuart & Triola, 2015).

During the 2015 conference, the discussion moved from the many ways technology can affect the experiences of educators and individuals within health professions education to ways in which technology—specifically information technologies, data, and analytics—can improve health professions education and healthcare delivery as a whole by helping integrate and align education with practice, promoting ongoing integration and alignment.

Based on these discussions, the work group came to consensus in adopting the concept of a technology-enhanced and fully integrated delivery system, called a *continuous learning system* (CLS). The group also developed a consensus vision statement based on this concept:

> In our vision for the future of health professions education, intelligent use of educational and information technologies supports the linkage between education and delivery systems to create a Continuously Learning Health System. In this system, teachers, learners, and clinical data inform continuous improvement processes, enable lifelong learning, and promote innovation to improve the health of the public. (Stuart & Triola, 2015, p. 30)

The "Enhancing Health Professions Education Through Technology: Building a Continuously Learning Health System" conference report (Stuart & Triola, 2015, p. 32) provides six recommendations for using technology to enhance education and healthcare systems:

- "In health professions education, technology should be used to support the ongoing development of learners from undergraduate levels through clinical practice; enhance interprofessional learning opportunities; and empower every student, faculty member, and clinician to embrace the role of both teacher and lifelong learner.

- Educators in health professions education should be supported to develop skills and expertise in the selection and effective use of educational technologies to complement the teaching-learning process and assessment of outcomes.

- Educational technologies should be used to accelerate the transformation of health professions education to a system that is competency-driven, affordable, and accessible to each learner.

- Technology should be leveraged to bridge the gap between educational and clinical missions, where teaching and learning are embedded within a healthcare delivery system that continuously improves.

- Leaders of health professions education programs should employ technology to analyze community and population data and use those data to continuously inform the design of curriculum content and learning experiences to reflect the contemporary health and healthcare needs of society.

- Educational technologies should be used to facilitate the sharing of content and integration of data across systems and programs, thus promoting the scalability and adoption of efficient and effective educational strategies."

This chapter is structured around these six areas and discusses them as components of a healthcare CLS:

- Integrated learning at all levels

- Educator (or faculty) development

- Realistic simulations of the entire system and healthcare team

- Bridging the education-to-practice gap

- Collecting and analyzing data to continuously inform curriculum design

- Sharing content and the integration of data

Each section discusses the corresponding recommendation as a component of the healthcare system, includes simulation examples for the recommendation, and offers ideas on how simulation can be used as a learning solution in these areas of a continuous healthcare system.

> Healthcare simulation offers powerful advantages to enhance education and healthcare systems.

Integrated Learning at All Levels

Quality healthcare today requires integrated education. Healthcare organizations aim to improve population health and reduce costs, while enhancing patient experiences. Berwick and colleagues have called this the *triple aim* (Berwick, Nolan, & Whittington, 2008). Recently, many organizations have adopted a fourth aim: to improve the experience of healthcare providers (Bodenheimer & Sinsky, 2014). Healthcare organizations around the globe are working to design and create systems to meet the triple (or quadruple) aim, each seeking the most effective model. While we continue to study new methods and models to achieve the triple (or quadruple) aim, one common denominator is evident: the need for continuous integrated education (IOM, 2015). Education must span the entire system to ensure that healthcare professionals become and remain competent in their practice while also dealing with the complexity of healthcare systems (National Academy of Medicine, 2019). This requires the linking of initial and ongoing

interprofessional education to clinical practice. This must occur in the context of the multiple systems that exist within healthcare organizations. It requires the adoption of technologically enhanced and fully integrated health professions education that reflects the care delivery system—in other words, a CLS.

Traditional education is not sustained without practice. Over the last century, academicians have identified the need for massed learning and spaced learning (Ingle, Remstad, Gephart, & Lampsa, 1969; Reed, 1924; Stroud & Ridgeway, 1932):

- **Massed learning** refers to educational activities in which learners practice a task or skill continuously without rest—for example, intense one-week workshop, one semester, etc. Massed learning is associated with the enhanced acquisition of knowledge, skills, attitudes, and other constructive learning gains (KSAOs).

- **Spaced learning** refers to formal or informal educational activities in which individuals are given rest intervals within the practice sessions—for example, recertification, continuous professional development, frequency of types of patient cases, etc. Spaced learning is associated with the retention and improvement of KSAOs.

Traditional health professions education typically involves massed learning but does not consider the need for spaced learning. The result is a decay in KSAOs. This decay affects the confidence and abilities of practitioners as well as their care for patients. It is also often the reason organizations implement efforts to initiate changes in knowledge, procedures, or culture, only to find that these changes are not sustained post-education. The optimal spacing of educational activities depends on the objectives, is largely unstudied, and continues to be an area for future research.

Simulation Support

The fragmented nature of our healthcare system has resulted not only in fragmented education that proliferates siloed approaches but also in training with knowledge decay in the absence of frequent practice. As a result, we are now understanding the need for a focus on CLS—the need to find educational bridges that network the fragments of our healthcare system. Healthcare simulation can bridge these gaps by providing integrated learning experiences that "twin" (provide a simulated data modeling replica of) real systems (Bolton et al., 2018; Bruynseels, Santoni de Sio, & van den Hoven, 2018).

One type of integrated learning simulation is virtual simulation. It can be used to model and project multiple streams of work that occur simultaneously, exploring the patient's continuum of care, points in healthcare that require collaboration, financial modeling, and risk assessments (Bolton et al., 2018; Bruynseels et al., 2018). This virtual "twinning" can simulate processes that occur throughout the system simultaneously and identify areas of concern or nuances if current systems activities continue as is and how those areas of concern would change as a result of changes made within the system. For example, if there are delays in housekeeping and patient room turnovers, virtual simulation can show the impact of these delays throughout the system, including cost impact, and can program an additional housekeeper to show the outcomes of additional staffing and no delays in room turnover. Non-healthcare industries use virtual simulation for business modeling. For example, many business schools have implemented semester-long simulations in which

teams invent companies and manage them over time. The Association for Business Simulation and Experiential Learning (ABSEL, 2019) provides a platform for business educators to collaborate globally to create innovative virtual environments for learners. Healthcare industries have begun to adopt this form of simulation to study patient safety and healthcare costs. For example, virtual simulations can simulate the impact of disaster events on a system and allow health professions to experience virtually, through avatars, how to best collaborate during low-frequency, high-risk (as well as high-frequency, high-risk) events.

Patient safety depends on individuals from different professions and departments working together. A critical aspect of capturing the realistic complexities of healthcare practice is the creation of education that includes the entire team. Healthcare simulation is perhaps the best platform for interprofessional education because you can engineer any simulation to include any profession potentially involved in that case. It is also flexible enough to allow the creation of learning opportunities relevant to all professions involved. Interprofessional simulations can also be expanded to just-in-time simulations or simulations and debriefings of a high-risk case provided just before engaging in the actual case. Finally, periodic interprofessional simulations allow for refreshed learning and new learning as new systems issues are discovered. This promotes a culture of lifelong learning and interprofessional education at all levels, in which everyone is a teacher and a learner. Chapter 9 discusses interprofessional simulations in more detail.

The impact of one's involvement in a patient's case extends beyond one's interactions with that patient. For example, prehospital intubation, if done incorrectly, may have implications throughout a patient's hospital stay. The complexities of patient care often depend on a good transfer of care from department to department. For this reason, continuum-of-care simulations, or simulations that start in one setting (e.g., prehospital) and continue into the next settings (e.g., flight team to emergency department to operating room) enable individuals to reflect on their care as it extends beyond their time with a patient. These simulations also allow practitioners to practice and review clinical transition report hand-offs and transfers of care to ensure that important information is carried forward with the patient, providing safer care. In addition, continuum-of-care simulations allow multiple teams to be involved and enable them to participate in a team debriefing as well as a larger systems-care debriefing. This supports individualized learning, team learning, and collaborative learning, with consideration for efficiency and effectiveness of delivery.

Longitudinal simulations allow for learning opportunities that are not bound by time. Longitudinal simulations provide the opportunity for learners to gain a better understanding of patient care; they can interact with the patient over time as they would over time in that patient's care and understand the impact of their care in relation to patient outcomes.

Longitudinal simulations are simulations that fast-forward in time. For example, longitudinal simulations work well in the area of wound care. In such a simulation, a care team might treat a patient's wound. Then, while the care team is debriefing, the simulation team might use moulage to make the wound appear better or worse, depending on how the care team treated it. The care team then conducts a second visit with the "wounded" patient to begin another cycle of simulation and debriefing. Some physical therapy schools also use this type of simulation.

Examples

The following examples demonstrate simulation activities that integrate learning at all levels:

- **Business and systems modeling:** ABSEL (2019) has an annual meeting that draws educators, designers, and gamers to share best practices in providing experience-based learning opportunities to their students. They also simulate business models to test new strategies. Data simulation can show impact along the healthcare continuum (Murray, Ryan, & Reisinger, 2011).

- **Healthcare systems modeling and simulation:** The Society for Simulation in Healthcare (SSH) has an affinity group dedicated to systems modeling and simulation that uses a systems engineering–based approach to design and evaluate system solutions to improve patient safety, quality of care, and cost-effectiveness. For more information, see https://www.ssih.org/Interest-Groups/Healthcare-Systems-Modeling-Simulation.

- **Virtual simulations:** Acadicus builds systems that use virtual avatars to engage in healthcare team activities in virtual healthcare systems (https:/acadicus.com). To learn how to use virtual patients and environments for nursing education to explore teamwork, decision-making, and communication, see *Virtual Simulation in Nursing Education,* by Gordon and McGonigle (2018), and "Clinical Virtual Simulation in Nursing Education: Randomized Controlled Trial," in the *Journal of Medical Internet Research,* by Padilha, Machado, Ribeiro, Ramos, & Costa (2019). Gordon & McGonigle (2018) and Padilha et al. (2019) describe the use of virtual patients for education where you can use virtual environments to explore teamwork, decision-making, and communication.

- **Interprofessional simulations:** Chapter 9 of this book fully describes interprofessional simulations and offers examples.

- **Continuum-of-care simulations:** Chapter 2.5 in *Defining Excellence in Simulation Programs* outlines examples of continuum-of-care simulations, including transitions between departments and specialties and using multiple rooms (Navedo & Reidy, 2015). Simulations can also be created to emulate points of a patient's or multiple patients' care. Laerdal provides some continuum-of-care cases on its website (https://www.laerdal.com/us/learn/circle-of-learning/).

- **Electronic health record simulation:** Oregon Health Sciences University has an electronic health record simulation lab (https://www.ohsu.edu/xd/education/simulation-at-ohsu/programs/electronic-health-record-simulation).

Educator Development

It is imperative that those who teach in healthcare environments receive the necessary support to develop and grow their expertise as educators. To ensure that everyone is on the same page, literally and figuratively, training on the fundamentals of learning theories and technology should be provided.

Those in formal leadership roles in academia and service should commit to creating and supporting programs for educators to develop the skills necessary to use technology in their multiple roles. These opportunities can be in many forms. For example, educators can be provided release time from their typical work schedules to attend conferences that are financially supported by educator development funds, or healthcare organizations can bring identified experts into their institutions to provide content that will aid their educators in using the most up-to-date information and educational strategies for their learners.

There should also be mechanisms to reward those who implement best practices in teaching through the use of technology to enhance the educational experience of their learners. This should both highlight their work and encourage others to educate at the highest levels. Educators who have embraced technology can be role models to others by providing workshops and the like to encourage their colleagues in their own use of technology to enhance learner experiences. By becoming formal and informal mentors, educators can form communities of practice that support the use of the latest technologies to enhance teaching.

Ongoing and Focused Professional Practice

The Joint Commission (TJC) has established specific expectations for providers in the acute care setting to engage in continual professional development (TJC, 2008). In 2007, as part of its revision to medical staff standards, TJC introduced the concept of ongoing professional practice evaluation (OPPE) as a mechanism to provide a scorecard of sorts for providers, including physician assistants and nurse practitioners. OPPE is performed on an ongoing basis to provide continuous feedback in an effort to maintain and ideally improve outcomes. In situations in which a provider requests privileges, there is a period of focused professional practice evaluation (FPPE) in which the provider is proctored and monitored during a probationary period. FPPE is also used when there are concerns over a provider's practice pattern and remediation may be in order (Maxworthy & Buczkowski, 2016).

Simulation Support

Healthcare simulation uses experiential learning theory. For many practicing providers, this format is both engaging and relevant to their practice. Simulation can be used for educator development. By allowing educators to participate in simulations, they can identify the best ways to teach specific topics and the tools that would work best within their system. Further, simulation can be used to provide education to and assess performance of providers in the clinical setting.

Educators can use simulation to test and assess education that they themselves develop. Developing simulations can be daunting but with proper training, anxiety can be alleviated (Henricksen, Altenburg, & Reeder, 2017). Piloting new simulation activities can provide necessary feedback to make them more effective. Additionally, the resulting feedback will help these educators become better at their jobs.

With regard to OPPE and FPPE, for those organizations that have invested in simulation and have a mature program, there is a tremendous opportunity to develop scenarios to assess and validate provider competencies. Depending on the particular competency one is assessing, formative or summative evaluation of skills can be provided. If these scenarios are recorded, they can be utilized as part of the providers' ongoing professional practice development.

Those who participate in healthcare simulation activities that are thoughtfully implemented and facilitated by trained educators develop more confidence in their knowledge and skills. Formative learning in such activities can provide the opportunity to learn skills in a safe environment.

Resources

There are multiple resources that can provide the support necessary to be successful. The following are examples of the resources available for educator development in simulation:

- **Professional associations:** SSH, INACSL, and the Association for Standardized Patient Educators (ASPE) develop and share resources to improve the knowledge of those interested in using simulation. Each of these organizations has an annual conference and provides webinars throughout the year for educators to gather additional educational tools.

- **The Stanford Medicine Interactive Learning Initiative** is a centralized resource for Stanford University's medical educators to receive consultation and other services as they consider developing online resources and new in-class sessions for interactive learning programs (http://med.stanford.edu/edtech/portfolio/smili.html).

- **Online teaching pedagogy courses:** The Online Learning Consortium offers programs related to online teaching pedagogy (https://onlinelearningconsortium.org).

- **Educator development courses:** Several organizations offer courses geared toward simulation educator development. Examples include:

  - **National League for Nursing Simulation Innovation Resource Center:** https://sirc.nln.org/

  - **The Center for Medical Simulation:** http://harvardmedsim.org

- **California Simulation Alliance:** https://www.californiasimulationalliance.org
- **The Debriefing Academy:** https://thedebriefingacademy.com
- **HealthySimulation.com:** https://www.healthysimulation.com
- **WISER:** https://www.wiser.pitt.edu/

Realistic Simulations of the Entire System and Healthcare Team

Simulation can be used to accelerate the transformation of health professions education in ways that are affordable and accessible to all learners. There are many options in both the academic and practice setting to assess learners to ascertain their skills and knowledge. It is critical to determine baseline data to truly appreciate the growth of a particular learner over time.

Education should be scaffolded to provide the KSAOs of the teaching points and then built upon to include the realistic complexities in application of those KSAOs, providing new learning points around the system. Education should also be built to include all the component roles to achieve safe care around these cases or topics. Hence, education should be provided in as realistic an environment as possible, including the multiple factors of the system in an interprofessional way.

Simulation Support

One primary advantage of healthcare simulation is the ability to create the same emotional learning as a real event (McGuire & Lorenz, 2018). Neuroscience is increasingly finding the value of creating learning that best triggers the same interpersonal interactions and emotional

responses as real events. This leads to better "imprinting" of learning and windows of enhanced attention where learning can be deepened (Immordino-Yang & Damasio, 2007).

Healthcare simulation can provide a vehicle to assess learners and provide a means by which they can continue to learn in a safe environment. By simulating a particular new procedure or piece of equipment prior to being used with patients, an institution can identify potential issues and mitigate them ahead of time. After an untoward event, simulation can provide a vehicle to re-create the event as part of a root cause analysis, thereby helping to determine what occurred and what needs to be done to prevent the event from occurring again in the future or to mitigate the negative outcomes.

Examples and Resources

Some system simulation examples and resources include:

- **Accreditation standards:** SSH accreditation standards provide the infrastructure needed to ensure that programs run more effectively. For more information, see https://www.ssih.org/credentialing/accreditation/full-accreditation.

- **A model of realism in simulation:** In their article "Which Reality Matters? Questions on the Path to High Engagement in Healthcare Simulation" (2007), Rudolph, Simon, and Raemer provide a model of realism in simulation. This model is based on concepts presented by Dieckmann, Gaba, and Rall (2007) in their article "Deepening the Theoretical Foundations of Patient Simulation as Social Practice." These concepts provide areas to consider when designing simulations.

- **Simulation models:** Kneebone, Weldon, and Bello (2016) provide a number of simulation models blended with realistic social situations in their article "Engaging Patients and Clinicians Through Simulation: Rebalancing the Dynamics of Care." Kneebone, Nestel, and Bello (2017) provide similar information in "Learning in a Simulated Environment," a chapter in *A Practical Guide for Medical Teachers* by Dent, Harden, and Hunt (2017).

Bridging the Education-to-Practice Gap

Technology can provide a means to bridge the education-to-practice gap (National Academies of Sciences, Engineering, and Medicine, 2019). By ensuring that systems are connected, there is greater opportunity for ongoing collaboration. Specific gaps that are frequently mentioned include performance in clinical practice and in the ability to access and effectively use data.

Simulation Support

Healthcare simulation with providers can identify education needs that should be integrated into pre-licensure curriculum. It can also allow for a venue in which students can practice what they learn immediately upon employment and professional practice. Collecting this data can feed into academic settings to integrate the new employee needs, thus closing the education-to-practice gap.

Several healthcare simulation companies have developed their own electronic health record (EHR) software. This software can be made available to educational systems to provide opportunities to learn how to use the EHR for patient information and documentation in multiple clinical sites and departments, with the same information flowing across them all. There are also several education vendors that have created EHRs that can be used to add realism to simulation activities.

Scenario banks have been developed through vendors and institutions to assist with ensuring consistency in content being provided. Templates for various aspects of healthcare simulation activities aid in decreasing variability.

Examples

The following examples show how simulation has bridged the education-to-practice gap:

- **Using simulation in human resources and for resident-matching:** Human resources and resident-matching programs can employ simulation to screen new hires. Seeing employees work under the conditions of the job offers insights into behaviors that are not immediately apparent in a one-to-one verbal interview. For more information, see "Job Simulations: Everything a Hiring Manager Needs to Know—Part I," by Schneider (2017).

- **Using simulation centers:** Simulation centers can provide experiences that otherwise cannot be obtained due to a lack of either clinical placements or specific clinical occurrences during observation experiences. For more information, see "Outcomes of a Simulation-Based Nurse Residency," by Beyea, Slattery, and von Reyn (2010).

- **Simulations for new hires:** Simulation programs can be used to provide both novice and experienced new hires with simulated experiences to gain needed skills in specific patient events that they will encounter in their practice. For more information, see Driscoll's (2018) "The New RN and Emergency Patient Care Scenarios: How Simulation Can Help."

- **Nurse training using a partnership model:** Dudley, Botti, and Hutchinson (2018) found that nursing training in a partnership model buffered the transition for new graduate nurses. For more, see their 2018 presentation, "Does Undertaking Nursing Training in a Partnership Program Buffer Transition Shock in New Graduate Nurses? A Cohort Study," available here: http://knowledgebank.epworth.org.au/epworthjspui/handle/11434/1407.

Collecting and Analyzing Data to Continuously Inform Curriculum Design

The gap between data and curriculum design is one gap in which strengthening communication within the system could powerfully affect education and practice. This gap is visible in many areas, from hospital or needs assessment data that could be useful in prioritizing educational efforts to the reverse—that is, clinical data that show outcomes as a result of education (known as *translational research*). This can also be present in community data that could best inform hospital needs or in population health data that could bridge global efforts to tackle worrisome trends. It may also be new practice research findings that indicate that current practice is ineffective or detrimental to health outcomes. Health informatics can help health systems models best meet the triple (or quadruple) aim of improving population health, reducing costs, and enhancing patient (and provider) experiences.

Innovation must be leveraged to develop better systems to improve our ability to measure and aggregate data that pertain to the performance of individuals, cohorts, and curricula, and the functioning of the institution over time (IOM, 2015). By identifying trends over time, these data can inform how to individualize learner pathways and improve programs.

Simulation Support

The use of simulation can support the collection-analysis-development-implementation cycle at each point within a particular phase of a project. Simulation can be used as a tool to collect data that could inform further design of curricula. Once hospital or systems data are collected, a simulation can be developed to highlight findings from the data, which can provide the information necessary for teams to discuss and potentially come to some critical decisions. There are opportunities to further analyze this simulated experience to shed more light on systems data to better inform decisions in the future.

Simulation can and should be used to test and pilot potential solutions. Once the best solutions are determined, simulation can serve to disseminate this education to identified end users. Finally, simulation can be used to evaluate the impact of the education over time to see if there have been changes made to the desired objective.

Over time, the use of simulation can identify trends in processes. These trends can culminate into a plan on how to best mitigate less-than-optimal outcomes for the short and long term. Simulation can also provide insights into issues and their potential solutions.

Examples

The following simulation activities are examples of how clinical data can inform the curriculum and vice versa:

- **Friday Night at the ER:** This board game simulates the activities of an emergency department and provides an opportunity to better understand systems integration. For more information, see https://fridaynightattheer.com.

- **Systems integration accreditation standards:** SSH has accreditation standards related to systems integration. For more information, see https://www.ssih.org/Credentialing/Accreditation.

- **Rapid Cycle Deliberate Practice (RCDP) simulations:** These allow repeat experiences to solidify KSAOs of specific cases. Hunt et al. (2014) discuss RCDP simulations in more detail in their article "Pediatric Resident Resuscitation Skills Improve After 'Rapid Cycle Deliberate Practice' Training."

- **Translational simulation** (connecting simulation to healthcare services): Brazil (2017) offers examples of continuous data informing curriculum on translational simulation in her article "Translational Simulation, Not 'Where?' but 'Why?' A Functional View of In Situ Simulation."

Sharing Content and the Integration of Data

According to Abraham et al. (2016), the key to the organizational transformation needed to become a CLS is a commitment to providing dedicated resources and ensuring that the individuals involved share, adopt, and ensure that best practices become woven into the fabric of the organization and are sustained over time. Without these commitments, the likelihood of continuous growth is limited.

A *community of practice* is a group of professionals engaged in collective learning within a shared professional domain (Lave & Wenger, 1991). Developing a community of practice can help facilitate the integration of data across systems. Technology can provide the means for movement of data communication across the continuum to ensure that efficiencies can be identified and implemented.

The use of applications by which data can be easily shared among many systems provides an opportunity for interprofessional collaboration, especially when a case is presented to the team with the expectation of a shared solution. Working across entities provides an opportunity to identify cases that have applicability to a multitude of learners at multiple levels and disciplines.

Healthcare in general needs to develop better working relationships with the various accrediting and regulatory agencies to aid with compliance with expected standards so that what is taught in an academic setting has value to those in an acute care setting.

Simulation Support

Simulation can provide a vehicle for organizations to prepare for a visit by an accrediting or regulatory body. Many organizations have used simulation as a means to educate and/or remediate staff after a sentinel event. Organizations also use simulation as a mechanism by which Failure Mode and Effects Analysis can be operationalized and issues mitigated before a piece of equipment or a process is put into general use.

Many simulation programs reinforce closed-loop communication between those involved with the simulation education program and those who focus on patient safety and risk management. To avoid this, consider ensuring that representatives from each sit on the committee of the other—for example, having the Director of Patient Safety and Risk Management sit on the Simulation Program Steering Committee, and having the Simulation Program Director serve as a liaison on Patient Safety and Risk Management Committees.

Examples

The following are examples of how simulation has allowed sharing of content and integration of data:

- **Using simulation to improve patient safety:** Salas, Wilson, Burke, and Priest (2005) have identified ways to use simulation-based training to improve patient safety and noted that the healthcare community can reduce errors by using simulation.

- **Tufts University Sciences Knowledgebase:** This is an open-source curriculum management system from Tufts University (https://tusk.tufts.edu).

Conclusion

Currently, most healthcare simulation efforts exist within departments or within uni-professional curricula, focused on specific practice points. While important, applications of learning and the sustenance of new skills are not well-supported if the context of application is not explored. For example, in a simulation, one can learn ways to manage a case, yet application of these new ways of management are thwarted by other unaccounted-for factors like other professions not having the same education, department-to-

department miscommunications via charting system, etc.

Identifying the critical gaps that exist within a healthcare system can also highlight areas for needed education. Healthcare simulation has the flexibility for educators to develop, as realistically as possible, simulated cases that highlight these gaps and for teams to discover new solutions. It also enables teams to practice solutions and test their realistic applications. Simulation can serve as the mechanism for disseminating new ways of bridging the gaps and can also assist in gathering performance data on these solutions.

Six areas helpful in thinking through how simulation can support a CLS include:

- Integrated learning at all levels

- Educator development

- Realistic simulations of the entire system and healthcare team

- Bridging the education-to-practice gap

- Collecting and analyzing data to continuously inform curriculum design

- Sharing content and integrating data

Simulation provides the opportunity to ensure that integrated learning can occur at all levels of an organization. Educator development can be enhanced through the addition of simulation into their teaching. Providing real-life simulations of day-to-day situations for individuals and systems can give insight into process improvement. Simulation provides a vehicle to bridge the education-to-practice gap. The use of simulations can inform the best ways to make curriculum design changes and identify ways to further refine education over time. Finally, sharing content and integrating data can benefit end users at many levels of an organization.

Acknowledgment

Thank you to the Josiah Macy Jr. Foundation for supporting the use of their work to structure this chapter.

References

Abraham, E., Blanco, C., Castillo Lee, C., Christian, J. B., Kass, N., Larson, E. B., … Lopez, M. H. (2016). Generating knowledge from best care: Advancing the continuously learning health system. *Perspectives*. Discussion Paper. Washington, DC: National Academy of Medicine. doi:10.31478/201609b

Association for Business Simulation and Experiential Learning. (2019, May 15). *Association for Business Simulation and Experiential Learning: About us*. Retrieved from www.ABSEL.org

Berwick, D. M., Nolan, T. W., & Whittington J. (2008). The triple aim: Care, health, and cost. *Health Affairs, 27*(3), 759-769. doi:10.1377/hlthaff.27.3.759

Beyea, S. C., Slattery, M. J., & von Reyn, L. J. (2010). Outcomes of a simulation-based nurse residency. *Clinical Simulation in Nursing, 6*(5), e169–e175. doi: 10.1016/j.ecns.2010.01.005

Bodenheimer, T., & Sinsky, C. (2014). From triple to quadruple aim: Care of the patient requires care of the provider. *Annals of Family Medicine, 12*(6), 573-576. doi:10.1370/afm.1713

Bolton, R. N., McColl-Kennedy, J. R., Cheung, L., Gallan, A., Orsingher, C., Witell, L., & Zaki, M. (2018). Customer experience challenges: Bringing together digital, physical and social realms. *Journal of Service Management, 29*(5), 776–808. doi:10.1108/JOSM-04-2018-0113

Brazil, V. (2017). Translational simulation: Not 'where?' but 'why?' A functional view of in situ simulation. *Advances in Simulation, 2*(20). doi:10.1186/s41077-017-0052-3

Bruynseels, K., Santoni de Sio, F., & van den Hoven, J. (2018). Digital twins in health care: Ethical implications of an emerging engineering paradigm. *Frontiers in Genetics, 9*(31). doi:10.3389/fgene.2018.00031

Dieckmann, P., Gaba, D., & Rall, M. (2007). Deepening the theoretical foundations of patient simulation as social practice. *Simulation in Healthcare, 2*(3), 183–193. doi:10.1097/SIH.0b013e3180f637f5

Driscoll, D. (2018). The new RN and emergency patient care scenarios: How simulation can help. *Open Access Library Journal, 5*, e3904. doi:10.4236/oalib.1103904

Dudley, M., Botti, M., & Hutchinson, A. (2018). *Does undertaking nursing training in a partnership program buffer transition shock in new graduate nurses? A cohort study*. Victoria, Australia. Presented at the Epworth Research Institute. Retrieved from http://knowledgebank.epworth.org.au/epworthjspui/handle/11434/1407

Gordon, R. M., & McGonigle, D. (2018). *Virtual simulation in nursing education*. New York, NY: Springer.

Henricksen, J. W., Altenburg, C., & Reeder, R. W. (2017). Operationalizing healthcare simulation psychological safety: A descriptive analysis of an intervention. *Simulation in Healthcare, 12*(5). 289–297. doi:10.1097/SIH.0000000000000253

Hunt, E. A., Duval-Arnould, J. M., Nelson-McMillan, K. L., Bradshaw, J. H., Diener-West, M., Perretta, J. S., & Shilkofski, N.A. (2014). Pediatric resident resuscitation skills improve after "Rapid Cycle Deliberate Practice" training. *Resuscitation, 85*(7), 945–951. doi:10.1016/j.resuscitation.2014.02.025

Immordino-Yang, M. H., & Damasio, A. (2007). We feel, therefore we learn: The relevance of affective and social neuroscience to education. *Mind, Brain, and Education, 1*(1), 3-10. doi:10.1111/j.1751-228X.2007.00004

Ingle, R. B., Remstad, R. C., Gephart, W. J., & Lampsa, L. V. (1969). Massed versus spaced practice: A classroom investigation. *The Association for Supervision and Curriculum Development, 3*(2), 261-264.

Institute of Medicine. (2007). *The learning healthcare system: Workshop summary*. Washington, DC: The National Academies Press. doi:10.17226/11903

Institute of Medicine. (2015). Measuring the impact of interprofessional education on collaborative practice and patient outcomes. Washington, DC: The National Academies Press. Retrieved from https://www.ncbi.nlm.nih.gov/books/NBK338364/

The Joint Commission. (2008). *Health care at the crossroads: Guiding principles for the development of the hospital of the future*. Retrieved from https://www.jointcommission.org/assets/1/18/Hosptal_Future.pdf

Lave, J., & Wenger, E. (1991). *Situated learning: Legitimate peripheral participation*. Cambridge, UK: Cambridge University Press.

Kneebone, R., Weldon, S. M., & Bello, F. (2016). Engaging patients and clinicians through simulation: Rebalancing the dynamics of care. *Advances in Simulation*. doi:10.1186/s41077-016-0019-9

Kneebone, R. L., Nestel, D., & Bello, F. (2017). Learning in a simulated environment, In J. Dent, R. M. Harden, & D. Hunt (Eds.), *A practical guide for medical teachers* (5th ed.), 92–100. New York, NY: Elsevier.

Maxworthy, J., & Buczkowski, E. (2016). *The complete guide to OPPE and FPPE*. Brentwood, TN: HCPro.

McGuire, K., & Lorenz, R. (2018). Effect of simulation on learner stress as measured by cortisol: An integrative review. *Nurse Educator, 43*(1), 45-49. doi:10.1097/NNE.0000000000000393

Murray, R. E., Ryan, P. B., & Reisinger, S. J. (2011). Design and validation of a data simulation model for longitudinal healthcare data. *AMIA Annual Symposium Proceedings*, 1176–1185.

National Academies of Sciences, Engineering, and Medicine. (2019). *Strengthening the connection between health professions education and practice: Proceedings of a joint workshop*. Washington, DC: The National Academies Press. doi:10.17226/25407

National Academy of Medicine. (2019). *The learning health system series*. Washington, DC: The National Academies Press. Retrieved from https://nam.edu/programs/value-science-driven-health-care/learning-health-system-series/

Navedo, P., & Reidy, P.A. (2015). Continuum of care. In Palaganas, J. C., Maxworthy, J. C., Epps, C. A., & Mancini, M. E. (Eds.), *Defining excellence in simulation programs*. Philadelphia, PA: Wolters Kluwer.

Oregon Health Sciences University. (n.d.). *Electronic health record simulation lab*. Retrieved from https://www.ohsu.edu/xd/education/simulation-at-ohsu/programs/electronic-health-record-simulation/

Padilha, J. M., Machado, P. P., Ribeiro, A., Ramos, J., & Costa P. (2019). Clinical virtual simulation in nursing education: Randomized controlled trial. *Journal of Medical Internet Research, 21*(3), e11529. doi:10.2196.11529

Reed, H. B. (1924). Part and whole methods of learning. *Journal of Educational Psychology, 15*(2), 107-115. doi:10.1037/h0074026

Rudolph, J. W., Simon, R., & Raemer, D. B. (2007). Which reality matters? Questions on the path to high engagement in healthcare simulation. *Simulation in Healthcare, 2*(3), 161–163. doi:10.1097/SIH.0b013e31813d1035

Salas, E., Wilson, K. A., Burke, C. H., & Priest, H. A. (2005). Using simulation-based training to improve patient safety: What does it take? *Joint Commission Journal on Quality and Patient Safety, 31*(7), 363–371. doi:10.1016/S1553-7250(05)31049-X

Schneider, N. W. (2017). Job simulations: Everything a hiring manager needs to know-part 1. Retrieved from https://employmenttechnologies.com/job-simulation-assessment-process-everything-a-hiring-manager-needs-to-know/

Society for Simulation in Healthcare. (2020). Full accreditation. Retrieved from https://www.ssih.org/credentialing/accreditation/full-accreditation

Stroud, J. B., & Ridgeway, C. W. (1932). The relative efficiency of the whole, part and progressive part methods when trials are massed—a minor experiment. *Journal of Educational Psychology, 23*(8), 632-634. doi:10.1037/h0075267

Stuart, G., & Triola, M. (2015). *Enhancing health professions education through technology: Building a continuously learning health system*. Proceedings of a conference sponsored by the Josiah Macy Jr. Foundation in April 2015, New York, NY: Josiah Macy Jr. Foundation. Retrieved from https://macyfoundation.org/assets/reports/publications/macy_foundation_monograph_oct2015_webpdf.pdf

"I hear and I forget. I see and I remember. I do and I understand."

–Confucius

Using Simulation With Specific Learner Populations

8

Carol Noe Cheney, MS, CCC-SLP
Karen Josey, MEd, BSN, RN, CHSE
Linda Tinker, MSN, RN

OBJECTIVES

- Identify basic similarities and differences in simulation with different levels of learners.

- Identify foundational issues that unify all levels of learners.

- Recognize elements of simulation that might affect the learner population and outcomes.

- Understand how simulation can be used to bridge the gap between different types of clinicians from academia to practice.

Simulation foundations and theories largely remain constant while simulation applications are evolving. Simulation has numerous uses in healthcare affecting resilience and reliability, from education and training to process improvement at the individual, team, and system level to improve patient safety, prevent adverse events, and deliver quality and safe patient care (Page, Fairbanks, & Gaba, 2018). Simulation is an educational methodology used to provide learning with patient safety in mind. It is simply no longer necessary to attempt a procedure for the first time on an actual patient when there is a means to practice repeatedly in simulation (Brazil, Purdy, & Bajaj, 2019; Finkelman & Kenner, 2009). Simulation can assure that the learner experiences a specific type of event, whether it is an individual onboarding assessment or an interprofessional simulation of a rare event such as a code or postpartum hemorrhage—without jeopardizing patient safety. In the clinical environment, learners might not often experience rare events; simulation can deliver important and critical standardized learning experiences.

Simulation should be managed and utilized based on the different types and levels of learners. The targeted population of learner, as well as the learning objective, will drive the type of simulation needed. Simulation debriefing methodologies, scenario types, checklists/metrics, and outcomes may vary depending on whether the learner is a novice or experienced or a member of an interprofessional team. Typically, with novice learners, learning occurs in the moment during debriefing. With an experienced team of clinicians, learning is most robust during periods of reflected self-discovery. High, intermediate, or low levels of facilitation may be used in debriefing to guide learners to obtain the best experience (Bauchat & Seropian, 2020; Fanning & Gaba, 2007).

Many simulation activities—regardless of learner type or level—begin with the evaluation or acquisition of motor skills. According to one theory of motor skill acquisition, new learners must think through and perform actions step by step before they can perform in a more rote and fluid fashion, and certainly before adding complexity (Fitts & Posner, 1967). To ensure a new graduate is competent in motor skills, tasks must be repeated over and over, often following a checklist or procedural guideline, like the example shown in Figure 8.1.

For learners who have relevant experience, the simulation team must validate the learner's ability to perform skills independently and competently. Using task trainers is an excellent way to perform this type of assessment. After this occurs for a variety of skills and tasks, these tasks can be superimposed and the learner placed in a more complex environment in which a simulated patient or family receives education while also receiving care or has other complex medical issues. This superimposition of tasks and objectives, using a mannequin to teach and assess, occurs through the scenario-development process.

New Hire Skills Assessment
CVC Care
Onboarding Skills Station

Participant Name: _____ Lawson #: _____ Date: _____

Experience: _____

Instructor: _____

CVC Site Care

Steps	√ = Done X = Not Done
Perform Critical Behaviors: Confirm Order, Verify PT with 2 Identifiers, Explain Procedure, & Hand Hygiene	
1 Removes dressing: demonstrate applying face mask to self and patient, applying clean gloves, removing old dressing and BIOPATCH, removing gloves, and performing hand hygiene	√
2 Cleanses site: demonstrates cleansing site and catheter with 2% chlorhexidine for 30 second friction scrub.	√
3 Secures site: demonstrate applying BIOPATCH then applying skin prep and transparent dressing	√
4 Labels dressing: demonstrate labeling with date and time of dressing change and initials.	√
5 Measures catheter: demonstrate measuring external length of CVC.	√
6 Changes caps: demonstrate changing needleless connectors, cleansing hub with alcohol, and placing disinfectant caps.	√
7 Maintains sterility: demonstrate performing all steps without breaking sterile technique.	√

Quick Comments: _____ 100%

Comments:

FIGURE 8.1   Example of a checklist.

Scenarios can be—and, in the case of scenarios for new graduates, should be—designed to progressively increase in complexity with the addition of distractors (such as noises, interruptions, and so on) found in the natural or live environment. Finally, regardless of the level of learner, factors such as generational differences regarding technology use, vulnerability of the learner in the environment, and group versus individual learning styles must be considered.

All Learners

There are common considerations with all learners in any simulation. These include ensuring all prerequisites have been completed, sending a welcome letter, conducting a pre-briefing and orientation, considering learner vulnerabilities, determining whether the simulation should involve death and dying, and identifying learning objectives.

Prerequisites

All levels of learners should have completed any necessary prerequisites to ensure they have the knowledge and grasp of the content needed to perform in the simulation. For more novice learners who have less experience but more baseline knowledge, study materials may be beneficial. More complex simulations, such as IPE events, entail a different type of preparation due to the different levels of learners involved. On some occasions, prework and a pretest are sent to learners before they participate in simulations.

Welcome Letter

To prepare learners for the simulation and promote a realistic experience, the process may include a welcome letter, which contains information about the content for review. The welcome letter should also include a map, learner expectations, phone numbers, what to wear, and any equipment the learner should bring, such as a stethoscope, pen, etc.

Pre-briefing

The pre-briefing prepares the learner and sets the expectations of the simulation event. Role clarification and orientation to the equipment and environment will lead to a more successful simulation event (Cheng et al., 2016). The pre-briefing also lets learners know whether the event is an assessment of learning needs, a practical learning application, or a high-stakes assessment of performance.

In an assessment of learning needs or practical application, educators and learners should realize that simulation is about learners learning from their mistakes and practicing the events that lead to better patient care. Simulation allows one to practice without harming patients. In a high-stakes simulation, the learner is held accountable for knowing how to perform at a certain level. High-stakes testing is a summative evaluation of a competency that has consequences and is appropriate for more experienced learners. An example of a high-stakes simulation is one that factors into a promotion or advancement—for example, moving from one level to the next in a physician residency training program. A pre-briefing should occur regardless of the type or level of learner or the objective of the simulation experience.

In the pre-briefing, it is important to inform learners that the simulation is to be treated as if they are in actual practice. This "suspension of disbelief" is "the ability of participants to believe the unbelievable and resist judgment of the simulation's authenticity—the cognitive act of accepting an imposter (simulation) as genuine (clinical)" (Muckler, 2017, p. 3). The effectiveness of the simulation depends not only on the high technology of the mannequins or the realistic smells and textures of daily patient care but also on the learner's immersion into the simulation. Whether it's plastic vomit or real vomit, something is occurring with the patient that needs to be addressed. Explaining to learners the importance of assessing, communicating, diagnosing, and treating the patient as they would in the real environment enables the scenario to move forward to meet the intended objectives. Failure to suspend disbelief can halt or make ineffective the scenario or a part of the scenario.

An example of suspended disbelief occurred in our simulation center during a scenario when one of our emergency residents had to perform an emergency C-section on an obstetric mannequin. His hands were shaking as he was cutting as they might if he was cutting on a real patient, yet he was "cutting" a plastic mannequin.

One way to promote the suspension of disbelief is to use a fiction contract (Muckler, 2017; Rudolph, Raemer, & Simon, 2014). A *fiction contract* is an explicit and collaborative agreement proposed by the educator to the learners that transparently acknowledges that the simulation is not real and seeks learner willingness to act as if things are real, participating as fully as possible (Dieckmann et al., 2007). Roh, Ahn, Kim, and Kim (2018) found that pre-briefing strategies for nursing students that included a fiction contract can help improve team psychological safety as well as learning outcomes. They provide an example of a fiction contract in the supplemental materials for their article (https://www.nursingsimulation.org/article/S1876-1399(18)30139-7/addons).

Orientation

Learners should become oriented to the environment, equipment, and mannequin before the simulation. This provides information they need to perform as they would with a typical patient. For example, if the mannequin normally does not have a pulse on one arm and learners are not informed of this, they may make incorrect assumptions, taking away from the real purpose of the experience or impeding learning. Some schools of thought maintain that orientation affects students' ability to suspend their disbelief. To counteract this, some programs embed simulated providers to help learners access the technology being used in a realistic manner, rather than introducing the learners to the mannequin's technical abilities beforehand. For example, the simulated provider will palpate a pulse and say what they feel versus showing learners where to palpate a pulse as part of an orientation.

Vulnerability

Facilitators should account for vulnerability with all learner types. Just as a new graduate or student may feel unsure and uncomfortable being watched while performing alone, experts who are unaccustomed to the simulation environment may hesitate to perform in front of subordinates for fear that their performance might undermine their credibility. Truog and Meyer (2013) speak to the potential for simulation experiences to be "stressful and shameful as well as stimulating and empowering" (p. 3). The authors also discuss building trust and being honest in delivering simulations. This makes simulation an ideal way to teach and assess learners' ability to challenge authority or even question a plan of action to prevent patient harm (Gaba, 2013).

Death and Dying

Whether to allow the simulated patient to die in a simulation is a controversial issue. The level of learner and whether the learner has had experience with death in a real environment are two of several factors in deciding whether to include such a scenario in a simulation (Gaba, 2013).

If death isn't part of the learning objectives, novices who have never experienced death in a real environment may become focused on the death and its emotional aspects, especially if learners are not sure whether actions they took in the scenario led to the patient's passing. This may lead to a traumatic learning experience. On the other hand, learners may benefit from experiencing death for the first time in a simulation environment, with experienced debriefers. Experienced learners may also experience psychological trauma in cases simulating a patient's death, which might affect their impressions of simulation, or they might know their actions did not cause the death and realize that death happens even when appropriate actions are taken. Experienced learners might feel comfortable that they will learn from their mistakes and not repeat them when caring for patients.

Simulations in which dying is not an objective but is a realistic outcome, or the death of a simulated patient in the absence of skilled debriefers, continue to be hot topics in simulation-based education. End-of-life care, communicating about death, and working through feelings about a patient's death have been shown to be valuable simulation experiences. The debriefing process is critical in addressing emotions associated with these events and can enhance learning (Tripathy et al., 2016). According to Corvetto and Taekman (2013), if dealing with death is a planned objective of the scenario and is covered in the pre-briefing, the experience of death can be less stressful and more accepted by learners—especially novice or inexperienced learners.

Learning Objectives

Learning objectives target and prioritize learning to prepare the practitioner for the clinical environment (International Nursing Association for Clinical Simulation and Learning Standards Committee, 2016) and drive the simulation scenario. Staying focused on specific and targeted learning objectives assists in an efficient and positive learning experience. Learners' previous experiences may affect how they perform in future scenarios. An inexperienced learner may be distracted or stray from the intent of the simulation. It is important for facilitators to use the learning objectives to guide the learner to the intended simulation outcome.

Students

A variety of academic programs use simulation to prepare their students for practice in the clinical environment. For example, simulation is widely used in academic environments such as nursing, medicine, dentistry, and social work. It is in an academic setting that many of our newer workforce members experience simulation for the first time.

Simulation experiences in academia often start with basic skills acquisition and practice, such as learning to place an IV line using an arm task trainer with veins. As students master each subsequent skill, the learning progresses to more complex simulated events, such as simulating the collection of a patient history or a head-to-toe assessment. For students, the objectives of a simulation are to learn and master foundational skills. After that, simulations to acquire new skills or principles are introduced sequentially.

Post-simulation debriefing with novice learners such as students may include playing video clips of the simulation prior to discussing the simulation itself to provide visual data for discussion. Debriefing in the moment, during the simulation rather than afterward, might provide a greater benefit to novice learners who may not yet have gained a deep cognitive awareness of what they should or should not do during the simulation and be able to reflect and have an "aha" moment upon watching a recorded playback, as might be expected from an experienced practicing clinician (Fitts & Posner, 1967).

In the academic environment, students learn basic concepts and competencies and have opportunities through simulation and clinical rotations to practice a few firsthand. Mastery of these skills and concepts is not likely to occur, however, as the students might have only performed the skill once and that might have been in a simulation environment rather than with a live patient. There is a difference between practice, demonstration of learning, and competency!

Bridging this gap between academia and the clinical environment has been an ongoing challenge. Simulation offers one way to bridge this gap. It enables learners to experience and practice clinical events before performing them on patients (Hayden, Smiley, Alexander, Kardong-Edgren, & Jeffries, 2014). This helps explain why many state boards of nursing, nursing associations, and academic programs have adopted various "Future of Nursing" recommendations from the Institute of Medicine (IOM)—including the recommendation to use simulation in pre-licensure clinical education (IOM, 2011). In Arizona, for example, this work was led by the Arizona Action Coalition Education-Practice Collaborative (Arizona Action Coalition, n.d.)—a collaboration between education and service originally sponsored by the Arizona Nurses Association. This group worked to bridge the education-service gap for new graduate registered nurses (NGRNs) and

adopted the Massachusetts Nurse of the Future Competency Model (Massachusetts Department of Higher Education [MDHE], 2016). A National Council of State Boards of Nursing landmark study compared competency and knowledge among nurses who received traditional clinical hours pre-licensure to cohorts who had 25% and 50% clinical experience substituted with simulation. The study results showed no statistically significant differences in clinical competency, comprehensive knowledge assessment, NCLEX pass rates, or clinical practice in the first six months of practice among the three groups (Hayden et al., 2014).

Simulation can be used to evaluate common competencies—for example, safety competencies such as those that pertain to infection control, patient identifiers, medication administration, Situation-Background-Assessment-Recommendation (SBAR) communication competencies, therapeutic communication, and hand-offs.

The Quality and Safety Education for Nursing (QSEN) initiative and Massachusetts Nurse of the Future have noted common topics covered in both academic and practice settings delivered through simulation (QSEN, n.d.). Both groups identified these topics (MDHE, 2016; QSEN, n.d.):

- Safety
- Patient-centered care
- Teamwork and collaboration
- Informatics (and technology)
- Quality improvements
- Evidence-based practice

In addition, the Massachusetts Nurse of the Future identified these areas (MDHE, 2016):

- Communication
- Professionalism

- Leadership
- Systems-based practice

Identifying common themes enables collaboration between education and nursing. This type of cooperation is essential to improving NGRN practice readiness to meet the quality and safety needs of patients and families (Arizona Action Coalition, n.d.).

New Graduate Registered Nurses and Other Novice Clinical Staff

NGRNs tend to benefit from well-designed and well-structured training programs that teach not only the concepts and skills they will use routinely but also those they might experience only rarely. Simulation can be a valuable tool to weave together theoretical knowledge, skills, and tasks, as well as insights into communication with patients, caregivers, and colleagues. It also helps integrate clinical reasoning, problem solving, deductive and inductive reasoning, sequencing, pragmatics, and timing into a practice environment. Finally, simulation can reduce precepted time on units and allow unit-based educators and preceptors to focus on the best opportunities and greatest learning needs. That this all happens with zero harm to patients is quite powerful and shows tremendous benefit to the new graduate learner.

Novice learners need opportunities to practice and master what they have learned. Simulation helps identify opportunities for learning and improvement. It provides an opportunity to review what one might have only experienced a few times before or not at all. It also provides a safe environment to remediate and practice for

specific needs, problems, cases, and errors, as well as regulatory requirements.

Physicians graduate from medical school and then go into residency programs to bridge the gap between academia and practice. Physical therapists and pharmacists also have residencies. Paramedic and EMTs have extensive clinical experiences in emergency departments to practice skills they will perform in the field. Such programs are not yet a standard for NGRNs.

Historically, hospital-based nursing programs allowed more time in the clinical setting for learning and practicing nursing skills and for making nursing judgments. Skills were practiced on people first—whether a peer student or a real patient. Over the last 20 years, hospital systems have begun providing NGRN residencies. Today, NGRN residency programs exist, but there is much variation in these programs. They run the gamut from a few weeks' duration to up to a year or more and may be facility-based or a formal standardized program. Guidelines, standards, and accreditations for nurse residency programs, such as the Practice Transition Accreditation Program offered by the American Nurses Credentialing Center (2020) and the Commission on Collegiate Nursing Education (2015), can help build an effective program.

Regardless of the program model used, simulation can play an important part in helping NGRNs translate the knowledge and skills they acquired in their academic studies into a clinical setting. For example, Banner Health uses simulation to onboard NGRNs. First, simulation is used to validate basic practice skills. These skills involve critical actions, which are weighted to assist the validator in the assessment. If the learner does not perform the correct actions, remediation occurs. Next, NGRNs are immersed in one to two full days of patient care simulation scenarios. These scenarios replicate a "typical" day on the unit and target domains such as the following:

- Assessment
- Documentation
- Patient education
- Time management
- Communication with the patient and team
- Procedures
- Critical thinking
- Patient safety

After these simulated scenarios, an individualized report is generated for each learner to rate the learner's opportunities and strengths. This report is sent to the learner's educator or manager, who shares it with the learner's preceptor. Part of the precepting process must include orienting the preceptors to the skills trained in simulation as well as the learning outcomes both intended and achieved by the NGRN. A best practice, then, is to have the preceptors actually experience the simulations firsthand. The preceptor can then adapt the clinical orientation period to focus on areas of opportunity and reinforce strengths. For example, if the learner struggles with communication with physicians but is great with time management, orientation would focus on the communication component. This ensures a more intentional experience for the NGRNs and bridges learning (Deckers & Wilkinson, 2019). Figure 8.2 shows a sample NGRN simulation summary report from Banner Health.

Simulation is an integral part of Banner Health's NGRN residency program. The Banner Health RN residency program includes:

- Clinical orientation
- Electronic medical record (EMR) documentation training
- Specialty academies
- An NGRN forum
- Preceptor training
- Other necessary training such as basic life support, advanced life support, and basic ECG

The specialty academies encompass formative and summative simulations and occur after clinical orientation and EMR training. The purpose of the academies is to help prepare NGRNs and new to service RNs with more advanced knowledge and skills. Figure 8.3 shows the Banner Health RN residency program pathway.

Simulation can be used to reinforce advanced skills and decision-making. However, with NGRNs, it is used more as a development opportunity—that is, as an education, practice, and action-planning strategy to build up to those basic and advanced skills in addition to clinical critical thinking. Simulation can also help new graduates move from didactic concepts and theories to practical application. For new graduate clinicians and healthcare employees, simulation might constitute their introduction to the transference of theory and foundational principles into practice. Less is often more, and the scenarios and skills need not be designed with "intentional" errors, as most NGRNs will make unintentional errors on their own. Note that novices differ from experts in their ability to identify and rectify an error quickly.

New Grad RN Simulation

Report for:	XXXXXXX	Lawson#:	XXXXXX	Attended Day 1 on:	9/17/2018	Attended Day 2 on:	9/18/2018

Newly hired new grad RNs participate in simulation where they are assigned to care for two typical medical surgical patients simultaneously at a Banner Simulation Center as part of the onboarding process. Each session includes a pre-brief, scenarios, and a facilitated debrief which allows for self-reflection, review, and learner-oriented discussion. The scenarios were designed with specific objectives that align with the standards of nursing care and Banner Policies and Procedures. Each of the objectives is categorized into the following Domains: Assessment, Communication, Critical Thinking, Documentation, Impact Patient Experience, Medication Administration, Patient Education, Patient Safety, Procedural, and Timely Interventions. Periodically the scenarios' objectives are evaluated with Risk Management, Patient Safety and simulation remediation data to determine if changes are needed.

This report reflects a baseline assessment of basic skills. The facilitators complete a checklist, while observing the participants, which is used to guide the debriefing and generate this report. Each section will list the objectives, overall percent completed, and a breakdown of missed steps; each participant is remediated on complete basic assessment and any missed steps. The Simulation Specialist may contact the educator or manager if there are significant concerns.

The preceptor, manager, and educator should review this report to become familiar with the learner's strengths and opportunities, share it with the employee to create an individualized orientation, then file the report in the employee's record. The charts and tables below summarize the participant's simulation experience broken out by the different objectives/domains in the scenarios.

Scenario Summary			
SBAR Communication	**91%**	**Measured Domains**	**80%**
Situation	100%	Assessment	81%
Background	100%	Communication	85%
Assessment	60%	Critical Thinking	76%
Recommendation	100%	Documentation	87%
Readback	100%	Impact Patient Experience	50%
Cerner Documentation	**83%**	Medication Administration	86%
Handoff Report	100%	Patient Education	100%
Procedures	50%	Patient Safety	77%
Assessment	50%	Procedural	79%
Physician Notification	100%	Timely Intervention	83%
Vital Signs	100%		
MAR	100%		

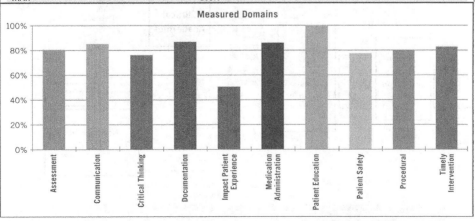

FIGURE 8.2   Sample Banner Health simulation summary report.

continues

New Grad RN Simulation

Report for:	XXXXXXX	Lawson#:	XXXXXX	Attended Day 1 on: 9/17/2018		Attended Day 2 on: 9/18/2018

Tasks observed multiple times *# = Achieved	# Achieved		Observed Opportunities
Hand hygiene	10	of	10
PPE		of	7
Confirms patient identity		of	9
Cluster care		of	7
Pain/Nausea management		of	6
Patient education		of	8
Appropriate use of resource (P&P, Charge RN, CNA)		of	10
Greeting/Opportunity for questions/Anticipating patient needs		of	3
Patient medication education regarding what medication and why		of	8

Comments	Facilitator: 0

Critical thinking/Strengths: Encouraged her post-hypoglycemic pt to eat. Used electronic resources to look up drug compatibilities in MicroMedex; used policies and procedures to look up blood transfusion. Also consulted the pharmacist regarding having both Heparin and Lovenox orders on the same pt. Delegated appropriate tasks to the CNA. Properly administered IV Pepcid diluted and checked labs prior to giving IV Toradol. Started a 2nd IV on her po stop pt. who required a blood transfusion. Used teach back to verify comprehension when instructing on IS use. Left the call light within reach for the pt.

Areas of opportunity: When calling the provider regarding a post-op pt with a low H & H, when the provider inquired about the pt's assessment, she realized she had not completed a focused assessment and could not answer the provider's questions. We discussed the many times we have an opportunity to educate our pts and that it needs to be thorough and occur before we give medications or perform nursing tasks. Continue to use electronic resources and people resources.

FIGURE 8.2   Sample Banner Health simulation summary report. (Cont.)

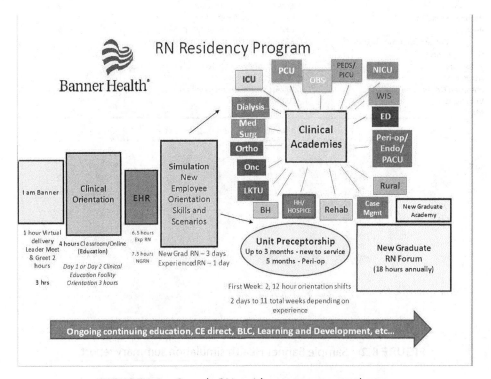

FIGURE 8.3   Sample RN residency program pathway.

Experienced Clinical Staff

As much as NGRNs benefit from progressive structure (e.g., a simulation that progresses in stages of doing), experienced individuals might learn more about themselves and what they have or have not mastered in a more chaotic environment—that is, in large teams, with complex issues, noise, and adrenaline. Sometimes, it is not just the complexity of the simulated event that progresses with experience but also the location in which the simulations occur. Mock codes, for example, address a low-frequency, high-risk event. Most practitioners do not have much experience participating in codes. However, all need to be able to perform at an optimal level when a code occurs. In-situ simulations—simulations that occur in the actual practice environment—such as unit-based mock codes are ideal, in that the team that normally performs together practices together in the actual environment where the event would occur. In-situ simulations, which are complex, high stress, interprofessional events, can identify opportunities for an individual, team, environment, or process.

The expert learner can benefit from a variety of simulations. For example, simulation can be used for:

- Team training
- Exposure to new initiatives
- Skills development and refinement
- Meeting regulatory requirements
- Annual education
- Rollouts that capture a change in process for practice

These experiences refresh expert learners' knowledge and enable them to practice previously learned tasks and previously experienced scenarios. They also assist in ongoing professional development when new clinical practices, equipment, or teams are introduced.

An Example of an Effective In-Situ Simulation

Banner Health's system-wide postpartum hemorrhage process initially was rolled out at every facility throughout seven states using in-situ simulation. These simulations continue as a multidisciplinary effort that includes blood bank employees, transporters, administrative assistants, nurses, physicians, and anyone who would be involved at that facility if an actual event occurred. At almost every facility in which the in-situ simulations were performed, within a day or two, an actual postpartum hemorrhage occurred. The feedback was overwhelmingly positive; because of the simulations, the communication between groups was more efficient, and the process ran more smoothly when it occurred with an actual patient experiencing postpartum hemorrhage. Everyone knew what they had to do to care for the patient and how to respond to a request from another group because they had just practiced it and knew what to expect.

Experienced clinicians benefit from simulation skills practice to retain knowledge or dexterity in situations that may be performed less frequently or that pose a high risk for errors. Examples include:

- Basic airway management
- Chest tube care or insertion
- Lumbar puncture
- Paracentesis
- Thoracentesis

Annual deep sedation training, malignant hyperthermia training (regulatory), and sepsis and pediatric asthma scenarios (initiatives) are other examples of simulation scenarios for experienced practitioners. For an optimum patient experience, clinicians should use simulation to practice effective communication, questioning, and responsiveness. This communication ensures that the patient's concerns, needs, and questions are addressed. Experienced clinicians can use a recorded playback to view their own responses and interactions. If the clinician fails to meet the simulation objectives, remediation should occur, and the scenario should be repeated.

High-stakes testing is another important use of simulation. Normally, simulation is touted as a safe environment in which learners can make errors without retribution. High-stakes testing is an exception as the results may determine whether the learner passes or fails or whether the test-taker can acquire or keep a job or remain in a program. High-stakes testing has been used very extensively to demonstrate knowledge attainment. Simulation can be used in high-stakes testing to demonstrate application of knowledge. A few examples of high-stakes testing in simulation are as follows:

- Emergency residents who must pass emergency-based scenarios to remain or advance in the program
- Critical-care nurses who must demonstrate competence in advanced cardiac life support (ACLS) scenarios to receive ACLS certification and continue in their current positions
- Practitioners who have had complaints about their practice or skills or need to demonstrate competency for credentialing

Community

Simulation is not only used in the medical, aeronautical, or business arenas but also in the community setting. Cardiopulmonary resuscitation (CPR) is a well-known simulated event that has a huge effect on saving lives (Josey et al., 2018). The American Heart Association (AHA) states CPR can double or triple the chance of survival; nonetheless, only 45% of cardiac arrest victims get CPR from a bystander (AHA, n.d.). The motivation and importance for learning and performing bystander CPR is that it is usually performed on someone known to the bystander. Fire departments, community organizations, and medical organizations use simulation to deliver CPR classes to those in the community. Simulation training kits that include a mannequin and video can be obtained from the AHA and used in the community, school, home, or wherever convenient. Simulation has also been successfully used for disaster preparedness drills, which include participants such as local police, fire departments, healthcare organizations, the FBI, Red Cross, and community volunteers.

The community offers many opportunities for simulation, especially in the home care arena, where it can lead to better and safer patient care. Caregivers, including family members, need to know and use simulation to practice skills such as how to give insulin shots, administer tracheotomy care, and manage pediatric asthma. Ideally, individuals in the community could be taught how to deal with worst-case scenarios such as a plugged tracheotomy tube or insulin reaction. Just as nurses need to practice injections, a patient or caregiver can practice to get the feel and confidence to perform in the real setting. Return demonstration ensures learning and safe patient care.

Current simulation centers can be a source of education for other venues that do not have access to simulation support. Banner Health supports physicians who take trauma education and airway management to rural communities Additionally, schoolchildren and high school students can whet their interest in healthcare careers in the safe environment of a local simulation center.

Conclusion

Simulation is a valuable learning modality for all types and levels of learners, with many approaches to simulation-based education. It is important to know which approaches are best used for which groups and levels of learners to maximize learning and meet intended objectives.

Although the foundations of simulation cross all learner levels, the use and complexity of simulation scenarios might differ. For example, novices are typically more focused on acquiring and applying basic skills, such as time management and procedural knowledge.

Advanced learners are typically able to handle much more depth and complexity in simulation scenarios and to have a deeper level of self-reflection. High-stakes simulations can be used to test competencies.

When building simulation scenarios, the learners and the group, as well as the areas of vulnerability of the learners while with the group and during the simulation, are foundational considerations. To ensure an effective learning experience, practical elements such as preparation, pre-briefing, orientation to the simulator, and suspending disbelief should be considered. So should whether the simulated patient should be permitted to die in the scenario.

Using simulation can bridge the gap from academia to practice and can help learners to become ready to practice in a complex, fast-paced environment more quickly, efficiently, and safely than previous apprenticeship models. For both the practitioner and the organization, quick assimilation into the workforce is a desirable outcome.

Simulation allows for the practice, demonstration, and application of learning as well as assessment and validation. All levels of learners can use simulation to safely make errors, learn from mistakes, and avoid patient harm. More research is needed on the transfer of learning in simulation to actual skills, knowledge, and attitudes in the work environment.

References

American Heart Association. (n.d.). *CPR facts and stats.* Retrieved from https://cpr.heart.org/en/resources/cpr-facts-and-stats

American Nurses Credentialing Center. (2020). *Practice Transition Accreditation Program manual.* Retrieved from https://www.nursingworld.org/organizational-programs/accreditation/ptap/

Arizona Action Coalition. (n.d.). *8 recommendations of the future of nursing: Leading change, advancing health.* Retrieved from https://www.aznurse.org/mpage/AzFFN_AzAC

Bauchat, J. R., & Seropian, M. (2020). Essentials of debriefing in simulation-based education. In B. Mahoney, R. Minehart, & M. Pian-Smith (Eds.), *Comprehensive healthcare simulation: Anesthesiology* (pp. 37–46). Cham, Switzerland: Springer.

Brazil, V., Purdy, E. I., & Bajaj, K. (2019). Connecting simulation and quality improvement: How can healthcare simulation really improve patient care? *BMJ Quality & Safety, 28,* 862–865. doi:10.1136/bmjqs-2019-009767

Cheng, A., Morse, K. J., Rudolph, J., Arab, A. A., Runnacles, J., & Eppich, W. (2016). Learner-centered debriefing for health care simulation education: Lessons for faculty development. *Simulation in Healthcare, 11*(1), 32–40. doi:10.1097/SIH.0000000000000136

Commission on Collegiate Nursing Education. (2015). Standards for accreditation of entry-into-practice nurse residency programs. Retrieved from https://www.aacnnursing.org/Portals/42/CCNE/PDF/CCNE-Entry-to-Practice-Residency-Standards-2015.pdf

Corvetto, M. A., & Taekman, J. M. (2013). To die or not to die? A review of simulated death. *Simulation in Healthcare, 8*(1), 8–12. doi:10.1097/SIH.0b013e3182689aff

Deckers, C. M., & Wilkinson, W. J. (2019). Effectively using instructional technologies. In B. Ulrich (Ed.), *Mastering precepting* (2nd ed., pp. 171–196). Indianapolis, IN: Sigma Theta Tau International.

Dieckmann, P., Gaba, D., & Rall, M. (2007). Deepening the theoretical foundations of patient simulation as social practice. *Simulation in Healthcare, 2*(3), 183–193.

Fanning, R. M., & Gaba, D. M. (2007). The role of debriefing in simulation-based learning. *Simulation in Healthcare, 2*(2), 115–125. doi:10.1097/SIH.0b013e3180315539

Finkelman, A., & Kenner, C. (2009). *Teaching IOM: Implications of the Institute of Medicine reports for nursing education.* Silver Spring, MD: American Nurses Association.

Fitts, P. M., & Posner, M. I. (1967). *Human performance.* Belmont, CA: Brooks/Cole Publishing Co.

Gaba, D. M. (2013). Simulations that are challenging to the psyche of participants: How much should we worry and about what? *Simulation in Healthcare, 8*(1), 4–7. doi:10.1097/SIH.0b013e3182845a6f

Hayden, J. K., Smiley, R. A., Alexander, M., Kardong-Edgren, S., & Jeffries, P. R. (2014). The NCSBN national simulation study: A longitudinal, randomized controlled study replacing clinical hours with simulation in prelicensure nursing education. *Journal of Nursing Regulation, 5*(2), S1–S64.

Institute of Medicine. (2011). *The future of nursing: Leading change, advancing health.* Washington, DC: The National Academies Press. Retrieved from http://www.nationalacademies.org/hmd/Reports/2010/The-Future-of-Nursing-Leading-Change-Advancing-Health.aspx

International Nursing Association for Clinical Simulation and Learning Standards Committee. (2016). INACSL standards of best practice: Simulation. Simulation design. *Clinical Simulation in Nursing, 12*(S), S5–S12. doi:10.1016/j.ecns.2016.09.005

Josey, K., Smith, M. L., Kayani, A. S., Young, G., Kasperski, M. D., Farrer, P. … Raschke, R. A. (2018). Hospitals with more-active participation in conducting standardized in-situ mock codes have improved survival after in-hospital cardiopulmonary arrest. *Resuscitation, 133,* 47–52. doi:10.1016/j.resuscitation.2018.09.020

Massachusetts Department of Higher Education. (2016). *Massachusetts nurse of the future nursing core competencies: Registered nurse.* Retrieved from http://www.mass.edu/nahi/documents/NOFRNCompetencies_updated_March2016.pdf

Muckler, V. C. (2017). Exploring suspension of disbelief during simulation-based learning. *Clinical Simulation in Nursing, 13*(1), 3–9.

Page, J. T., Fairbanks, R. J., & Gaba, D.M. (2018). Priorities related to improving healthcare safety through simulation. *Society for Simulation in Healthcare, 13*(3S Suppl. 1), S41–S50. doi:10.1097/SIH.0000000000000295

Quality and Safety Education for Nursing Institute. (n.d.). *QSEN competencies.* Retrieved from http://qsen.org/competencies/pre-licensure-ksas/

Roh, Y. S., Ahn, J., Kim, E., & Kim. J. (2018). Effects of prebriefing on psychological safety and learning outcomes. *Clinical Simulation in Nursing, 25,* 12–19.

Rudolph, J., Raemer, D., & Simon, R. (2014). Establishing a safe container for learning in simulation: The role of the presimulation briefing. *Simulation in Healthcare, 9*(6), 339–349.

Tripathy, S., Miller, K. H., Berkenbosch, J. W., McKinley, T. F., Boland, K. A., Brown, S. A., & Calhoun, A. W. (2016). When the mannequin dies, creation and exploration of a theoretical framework using a mixed methods approach. *Simulation in Healthcare, 11*(3), 149–156. doi:10.1097/SIH.0000000000000138

Truog, R. D., & Meyer, E. C. (2013). Deception and death in medical simulation. *Simulation in Healthcare, 8*(1), 1–3. doi:10.1097/SIH.0b013e3182869fc2

"Coming together is a beginning. Keeping together is progress. Working together is success."

–Henry Ford

Using Simulation for Interprofessional Education and Practice

9

Chad A. Epps, MD, FSSH
Teresa Britt, MSN, RN, CHSE
Janice C. Palaganas, PhD, RN, NP, ANEF, FAAN, FSSH

OBJECTIVES

- Review the evolution of healthcare simulation as a platform for interprofessional education.

- Discuss the benefits and challenges of using simulation for interprofessional education.

- Explore recommendations for the implementation of simulation-enhanced interprofessional education within an organization.

- Provide a framework to achieve successful simulation-enhanced interprofessional education.

With its experiential and boundless features, healthcare simulation is naturally evolving as a platform for interprofessional education (IPE). The need for IPE becomes increasingly evident in patient safety and is recognized by professional, accrediting, and certifying bodies (Aspden, Wolcott, Bootman, & Cronenwett, 2007; Commission on Collegiate Nursing Education [CCNE], 2018; Institute of Medicine [IOM], 2007, 2011; Interprofessional Education and Healthcare Simulation Collaborative [IPEHCS-C], 2012; National League for Nursing Commission for Nursing Education Accreditation [NLN CNEA], 2016; NLN, 2015. (See Figure 9.1.)

Many challenges in the healthcare system support the need for IPE. Over time, separate specialties and professions have been created to focus on specific aspects of patient health and care. As a result, no single profession today can adequately meet all the complex needs of patients. To keep patients safe, healthcare professionals must work together as a team; however, medical error rates, root cause analyses, and patient outcome research reveal that breaches in quality healthcare often result from poor communication within healthcare professional teams (The Joint Commission on Accreditation of Healthcare Organizations [JCAHO], 2005; Parker, Forsythe, & Kohlmorgan, 2018). In assessing situations involving compromised patient care, it has become evident that without effective IPE, professionals have difficulty working together as a team (Fox et al., 2017; Hean, Craddock, & Hammick, 2012).

Teamwork failures stem from a variety of systemic gaps in healthcare processes as well as fundamental human factors. Many systemic gaps have also been revealed in the education of healthcare professionals (Benner, Sutphen,

Leonard, & Day, 2010). One is that students are typically educated in a silo track. After they graduate and go to work in a healthcare setting, they are expected to know how to work with colleagues from other disciplines. Interprofessional practice (IPP) opportunities are not guaranteed in pre-licensure (students) curricula or post-licensure (practicing providers) continuing education. Even when interprofessional conflict does occur, rather than allowing the student or junior clinician to work through the situation and gain the skills needed for effective collaboration, preceptors or experienced clinicians often step in. Another limitation to IPE is that educators tend to teach the way they were taught. They are often hesitant to try other methods, even if they are more effective (Bradshaw & Lowenstein, 2007). This is problematic. Most clinicians learned on the job (e.g., during apprenticeship) and through traditional teaching methods (generally unidirectional education, such as lectures). This style of learning does not match the style of younger, more technologically advanced students (Billings & Halstead, 2008). Fortunately,

accrediting, certifying, and professional bodies have recognized the need for IPE and strongly recommend its implementation. We are currently seeing a trend in IPE adoption within universities and hospitals as a result of awareness from literature, conferences, and media, and through the recommendations of professional bodies.

IPE employs a variety of methods, including simulation. Indeed, healthcare simulation is increasingly recognized as an ideal vehicle for IPE. Simulation activities can occur in an array of settings—for example, simulation centers, in situ, virtual worlds, and so on. These activities also employ a variety of modalities, including mannequin-based simulations, standardized patients, embedded simulated persons, task training, team-based games, and serious games. Not surprisingly, team issues and interactions can be engineered through simulation-enhanced IPE (Sim-IPE), exposing future healthcare providers to relevant encounters that can grow effective teamwork. Examples of the successful use of simulation to teach or improve IPE include the use of peer-led simulation IPE to improve student attitudes, values, and beliefs about IPE as well as increase their understanding of professional roles (Lairamore et al., 2019) and to improve trauma team performance (Harvey et al., 2019).

Although educators and organizational leaders have become fascinated with the benefits of simulation and have even built simulation centers or purchased expensive simulators, many do not have adequate knowledge or resources to use them effectively or to share their knowledge with others. Educators look to the literature to bridge these gaps; however, the existing literature lacks the research evidence needed to guide educators on how to best structure and successfully implement simulation-based IPE (Abualenain, 2018; McGaghie, Issenberg, Petrusa,

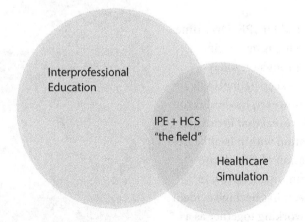

Interprofessional
Education

IPE + HCS
"the field"

Healthcare
Simulation

FIGURE 9.1   The overlapping combined science of the fields of interprofessional education and healthcare simulation.

& Scalese, 2010; Palaganas, Brunette, & Winslow, 2016; Reeves, Abramovich, Rice, & Goldman, 2007; Zhang, Thompson, & Miller, 2011). This chapter seeks to guide educators in understanding healthcare simulation as a platform for IPE by:

- Defining terms of reference to guide educators in Sim-IPE and to suggest a common language when sharing knowledge

- Providing thematic evidence from the research literature

- Providing recommendations from the 2012 Interprofessional Education and Healthcare Simulation Symposium on how to get started in Sim-IPE

- Describing challenges identified in Sim-IPE

- Explaining theoretical frameworks that may serve as a foundation to simulations

- Providing a development, implementation, and practice framework for Sim-IPE that assists in overcoming the challenges in this science

Terms Related to Interprofessional Education

- **Crisis resource management (CRM):** An approach to managing critical situations in a healthcare setting. CRM develops communication skills. Originally conceived in aviation and called crew resource management, CRM emphasizes the role of "human factors"—the effects of fatigue and expected or predictable perceptual errors, as well as different management styles and organizational cultures in high-stress, high-risk environments (Gaba, Howard, Fish, Smith, & Sowb, 2001; Helmreich, Merritt, & Wilhelm, 1999).

- **Interdisciplinary learning:** "Involves integrating the perspective of professionals from two or more professions, by organizing the education around a specific discipline, where each discipline examines the basis of their knowledge" (Howkins & Bray, 2008, p. xviii).

- **Interprofessional education/training (IPE):** "An educational environment where students from two or more professions learn about, from, and with each other to enable effective collaboration and improve health outcomes" (World Health Organization [WHO], 2010, p. 2).

- **Interprofessional learning (IPL):** "Learning arising from interaction between members (or students) of two or more professions. This may be a product of *interprofessional education* or happen spontaneously in the workplace or in education settings (for example, from *serendipitous interprofessional education*)" (Freeth et al., 2005, p. xv).

- **Intraprofessional:** Involves activity between or among individuals within the same profession with similar or different specialties or levels of practice (e.g., surgeon and emergency physician, clinical nurse and nurse practitioner, resident and physician, etc.).

- **Multidisciplinary:** Involves bringing professionals with different perspectives together to provide a wider understanding of a particular problem (Howkins & Bray, 2008).

- **Multiprofessional education (MPE):** "When members (or students) of two or more professions learn alongside one another: in other words, parallel rather than interactive learning. Also referred to as common or shared learning" (Freeth et al., 2005, p. xv).

continues

Terms Related to Interprofessional Education (cont.)

- **Simulation-enhanced interprofessional education (Sim-IPE):** The education of healthcare professionals with different but complementary knowledge and skills in a simulation environment that promotes a collaborative team approach. Sim-IPE occurs when participants and facilitators from two or more professions are engaged in a simulated healthcare experience to achieve shared or linked objectives and outcomes (International Nursing Association for Clinical Simulation and Learning [INACSL] Standards Committee, 2016). It is designed for the individuals involved to "learn about, from and with each other to enable effective collaboration and improve health outcomes" (WHO, 2010, p. 7).

- **Transdisciplinary:** Describes a strategy that crosses many disciplinary boundaries to create a holistic approach to development. A transdisciplinary strategy attempts to overcome the confines of individual disciplines to form a team that crosses and re-crosses disciplinary boundaries and thereby maximizes communication, interaction, and cooperation among team members (Freeth et al., 2005).

- **Uniprofessional education:** When members (or students) of a single profession learn together (Freeth et al., 2005; Howkins & Bray, 2008).

Terms of Reference

Despite defined concepts in interprofessional education and healthcare simulation, terminology often varies across literature, professions, geographical boundaries, and institutions. Acknowledging that a standardized language is essential, these terms of reference are listed in the sidebar on page 153 to create working definitions to facilitate discussions with reduced miscommunications. Most definitions are based on those found in the *Healthcare Simulation Dictionary* (Lioce et al., 2020). Educators and researchers are encouraged to explore and refine these terms through further concept analyses and studies.

The Benefits and Challenges of Simulation-Enhanced IPE (Sim-IPE)

Recognizing the need to assess the community, Wilhaus et al. (2012) surveyed simulation educators who use healthcare simulation for IPE and analyzed the responses. Respondents felt that simulation was an attractive method for IPE because:

- It provides a safe environment by keeping real patients safe.

- Without IPE, there is a lack of opportunities in clinical settings for skill development.

- It provides a realistic experience.

- Learners are more engaged in experiential and active learning.

- It is deliberate practice.

- It provides a standardized experience.

Those who felt that Sim-IPE was more effective than non-simulation IPE at achieving interprofessional learning objectives attributed this perception to the following factors:

- Realism

- Practice

- Debriefing and reflection

- Increased learner engagement

- Relevance of the experience

- Fostered interaction

- Safe environment

- Opportunity for feedback

- Immediacy of feedback

- Immersive experience

- Framework for learning communication

- The emotional experience

Those who felt that Sim-IPE was less effective highlighted the importance of protecting the psychological safety of learners during the simulation—that is, the intrapsychological consequences on an individual from the interpersonal risks or past cognitive connections made during the simulation—and how simulation, if not done "right," may be more detrimental to positive IPL (Palaganas, 2012).

Wilhaus et al. (2012) found that challenges faced during the implementation of simulation-based IPE reflected common challenges found in simulation-based education as well as those found in IPE. Of the common challenges found in simulation, costs and resources were a barrier for Sim-IPE (McGaghie et al., 2010). Of the common challenges found in IPE, scheduling, logistics, and organizing the different programs or professions were large barriers for Sim-IPE (Freeth et al., 2005). Table 9.1 shows simulation-specific challenges during IPE implementation and potential strategies to address these challenges.

Table 9.1   Simulation-Enhanced IPE (Sim-IPE) Challenges and Potential Strategies to Resolve Them

Sim-IPE Challenges	Potential Strategies for Resolution
Problems with audio recording or live streaming	Conduct a dry run of the scenario using audio recording, live streaming, and playback of video.
Scenario development that engages all disciplines and learning levels	Include educators or content experts from all involved disciplines during scenario development.
Scheduling and conflicts	Implement an interprofessional curricula cross-matching committee to bring programmatic curricula and competencies for their programs to the table, to highlight where the curricula or content overlap, and to suggest where courses or labs can be scheduled together.
Mannequin electronic failure	Provide educator development on creative ways to overcome potential mannequin glitches during simulations.
Need for simulator operator training	Schedule in-services with vendor educators or technicians to teach faculty or technicians to use simulators.
	Conduct dry runs with full simulator operation.

continues

Table 9.1   Simulation-Enhanced IPE (Sim-IPE) Challenges and Potential Strategies to Resolve Them   (cont.)

Sim-IPE Challenges	Potential Strategies for Resolution
Lack of faculty expertise in technology, simulation, and debriefing	Send educators to simulation educator development training, or develop an apprenticeship program for faculty.
Interprofessional debriefing	Reflect on personal assumptions. Explore a learner's frame/mental model before opening discussion. Use reflective practice by allowing learners to discover areas of interprofessional practice and improvements.
No technology support	Find educators or students who are technologically inclined. Work with the IT department.
Not having enough time	Prioritize objectives and debriefing points, and limit the simulation or debriefing to critical points.
Lack of pre-briefing	Provide educator development on the importance of pre-briefing and its effect on learning using simulation.
Fidelity/realism/accurate reflection of the phenomenon	Conduct a dry run of the scenario with practicing providers.
Difference in objectives among involved faculty (e.g., one wants team training and the other wants skills training)	Involve educators from each profession in the curriculum and scenario development. Understand each educator's personal objectives for the course and aim for negotiation and consensus of overall course objectives. This maintains educator buy-in and increases the likelihood of the success of the course.
Difficulty assessing team performance	Provide educator development around assessment. Research existing team-performance assessment tools. Contact programs that have performed team assessment.

Themes in Sim-IPE

The IPE literature distinguishes between IPE and multiprofessional education.

- **IPE:** Describes occasions in which two or more professionals learn with, from, and about each other to improve collaboration and the quality of care (WHO, 2010).

- **Multiprofessional education:** Occurs when learners from two or more professions learn alongside one another—in other words, parallel rather than interactive learning (Freeth et al., 2005).

IPE literature offers evidence that learning is better achieved through IPE than multiprofessional education (Canadian Interprofessional Health Collaborative [CIHC], 2010).

This distinction can also be made in healthcare simulation with Sim-IPE and interprofessional simulation (Palaganas, Brunette, & Winslow, 2016; Wilhaus et al., 2012). Interprofessional simulation corresponds with multiprofessional education.

Although both healthcare simulation and IPE have been used for some time, over the last decade, the two fields have merged into an overlapping field called Sim-IPE (Palaganas, Epps, & Raemer,

2014). Sim-IPE refers to a simulation structured according to IPE objectives in which two or more professionals learn with, from, and about each other to improve collaboration and quality of care. It involves learners from two or more professions learning alongside one another in the simulation. In interprofessional simulation, the simulation is structured around a patient condition or situation that requires coordination and demonstration of skills specific to the individual professions.

In a scoping review of simulation and IPE, Lee, Pais, Kelling, & Anderson (2018) found the following themes:

- The most common professions were nursing, medical students, physical therapy, and pharmacy.

- The most common types of simulations were mannequin alone or standardized patient alone.

- Learner size in each simulation was between three to six professions.

They also found common barriers of Sim-IPE to be:

- Recruiting enough learners

- Lack of experience with IPE

- Learners feeling uncomfortable about being observed

- Different knowledge and skill by profession

- Poor learner attitude

- Scheduling

- Cost

- Incorporating learners who are both required and elect to complete the simulation

In a critical review of the literature, Palaganas, Brunette, & Winslow (2016) found the following to be reported attributes that lead to positive Sim-IPE outcomes:

- Realism

- Practice

- Debriefing and reflection

- Increased student engagement

- Relevance of the experience

- Fostered interaction and collaboration

- Safe environment

- Opportunity for feedback

- Immediacy of feedback

- Immersive experience

- Framework for learning communication

- Emotional experience

They also found the following negative issues with Sim-IPE:

- Potentially threatening environment

- Role dissonance

- Unclear objectives

- Lack of formal evaluation and feedback

Given the complexity of the combined science of healthcare simulation and IPE, multiple confounding variables exist from one simulation group and program to another. Single-site studies are one limitation—although given the variability of simulation programs, using multiple sites might contribute a multitude of unnecessary confounding variables. In addition, details of published studies and activities, including potential confounding variables, are limited. This in turn limits the ability to study characteristics that influence positive and negative outcomes.

This limitation also makes generalization and replication extremely difficult.

A review of literature and survey assessment reflects the complexities of healthcare simulation and IPE including:

- The use of multiple teaching methods without comparison

- The lack of valid and reliable measures

- Multiple confounding variables (reported and not reported, with many variables yet to be identified in the field)

- Differences in student learning levels

- Differences in sample sizes of the involved professions (Palaganas, Brunette, & Winslow, 2016).

Palaganas (2012) suggests reporting points—either directly in the publication or as an addendum to the publication—that could enable another site to replicate one's work and provide the ability for future literature synthesis to determine characteristics that influence outcomes. These reporting points (see Table 9.2) could also serve as a development guide for researchers looking to use Sim-IPE (Reeves, Palaganas, & Zierler, 2017).

Table 9.2   Suggested Reporting Points for IPE and Healthcare Simulation Research

Report Sections	Reporting Points
Objectives	Aims and purpose of study (manuscript)
	Objectives of educational activity
	Objectives of simulation activity
Background	Terminology and definitions used by author
	Current existing literature
Learners	Sample sizes (total and per professional group)
	Profession or program
	Grade level
	Team composition in simulation
Educators/researchers	Backgrounds/credentials
	Composition for development of study and educational activity
	Composition for implementation of study and educational activity
Method	Design
	Theoretical framework
	Interventions
Simulation modality	Type, model, and version
	Details of scenario (consider video supplement and scenario appendix)
	Structure of debriefing if incorporated (consider video supplement and appendix if structured or semi-structured)
Measures	Why chosen
	Validity
	Reliability
	Results

Discussion	Simulation factors that may have led to positive outcomes
	Simulation factors that may have led to negative outcomes
	Challenges encountered
	Strengths of study design
	Limitations of study design
	Areas for future study

Source: Palaganas, 2012

The review of literature and survey assessment reflected the complexities of healthcare simulation and IPE, including the use of multiple teaching methods without comparison; the lack of valid and reliable measures; multiple confounding variables (reported and not reported, with many variables yet to be identified in the field); differences in student learning levels; and differences in sample sizes of the involved professions.

Despite the lack of strong findings presented in the literature, literature and survey results as a whole hint that simulation is an excellent platform for IPE. Learners positively perceive simulation as a learning method (McGaghie et al., 2010). The literature has also shown that if an educator did not prepare well enough, was not prepared to deal with an interprofessional group, or did not use a simulation method to reach level-appropriate objectives, then the teaching platform would not be a good fit for learning (Cooper, Carlisle, Gibbs, & Watkins, 2001; Freeth et al., 2005).

Competencies and Recommendations

According to Tekian, McGuire, and McGaghie (1999), expert opinion is the best and most logical source when there is an absence of clear data. The field of IPE and healthcare simulation has advanced through individual simulation programs and the development of professional societies and interest groups. These advancements may be seen through national competencies and recommendations developed by leaders of multiple professional organizations.

To create a coordinated effort across health professions and provide strategies for collaborative learning, an expert panel from the Interprofessional Education Collaborative (IPEC) developed interprofessional competencies in 2010 and revised them in 2016 (IPEC, 2016). Within the interprofessional collaboration domain, four core competencies were identified:

- Values/ethics for interprofessional practice
- Roles/responsibilities
- Interprofessional communication
- Teams and teamwork

Each competency is further divided into sub-competencies. These sub-competencies may be used by educators to set objectives for the Sim-IPE (see Table 9.3).

Table 9.3   Interprofessional Collaborative Sub-Competencies

Values/Ethics Sub-Competencies

VE1	Place interests of patients and populations at the center of interprofessional healthcare delivery and population health programs and policies, with the goal of promoting health and health equity across the life span.
VE2	Respect the dignity and privacy of patients while maintaining confidentiality in the delivery of team-based care.
VE3	Embrace the cultural diversity and individual differences that characterize patients, populations, and the health team.
VE4	Respect the unique cultures, values, roles/responsibilities, and expertise of other health professions and the impact these factors can have on health outcomes.
VE5	Work in cooperation with those who receive care, those who provide care, and others who contribute to or support the delivery of prevention and health services and programs.
VE6	Develop a trusting relationship with patients, families, and other team members (CIHC, 2010).
VE7	Demonstrate high standards of ethical conduct and quality of care in one's contributions to team-based care.
VE8	Manage ethical dilemmas specific to interprofessional patient- or population-centered care situations.
VE9	Act with honesty and integrity in relationships with patients, families, communities, and other team members.
VE10	Maintain competence in one's own profession appropriate to scope of practice

Roles/Responsibilities Sub-Competencies

RR1	Communicate one's roles and responsibilities clearly to patients, families, community members, and other professionals.
RR2	Recognize one's limitations in skills, knowledge, and abilities.
RR3	Engage diverse professionals who complement one's own professional expertise, as well as associated resources, to develop strategies to meet specific health and healthcare needs of patients and populations.
RR4	Explain the roles and responsibilities of other care providers and how the team works together to provide care, promote health, and prevent disease.
RR5	Use the full scope of knowledge, skills, and abilities of professionals from health and other fields to provide care that is safe, timely, efficient, effective, and equitable.
RR6	Communicate with team members to clarify each member's responsibility in executing components of a treatment plan or public health intervention.
RR7	Forge interdependent relationships with other professions within and outside the health system to improve care and advance learning.
RR8	Engage in continuous professional and interprofessional development to enhance team performance and collaboration.
RR9	Use unique and complementary abilities of all members of the team to optimize health and patient care.
RR10	Describe how professionals in health and other fields can collaborate and integrate clinical and public health interventions to optimize population health.

Interprofessional Communication Sub-Competencies

CC1	Choose effective communication tools and techniques, including information systems and communication technologies, to facilitate discussions and interactions that enhance team function.
CC2	Communicate information with patients, families, community members, and health team members in a form that is understandable, avoiding discipline-specific terminology when possible.
CC3	Express one's knowledge and opinions to team members involved in patient care and population health improvement with confidence, clarity, and respect, working to ensure common understanding of information, treatment, care decisions, and population health programs and policies.
CC4	Listen actively and encourage ideas and opinions of other team members.
CC5	Give timely, sensitive, instructive feedback to others about their performance on the team, responding respectfully as a team member to feedback from others.
CC6	Use respectful language appropriate for a given difficult situation, crucial conversation, or interprofessional conflict.
CC7	Recognize how one's own uniqueness—including experience level, expertise, culture, power, and hierarchy within the health team—contributes to effective communication, conflict resolution, and positive interprofessional working relationships
CC8	Communicate consistently the importance of teamwork in patient-centered care and population health programs and policies.

Teams and Teamwork Sub-Competencies

TT1	Describe the process of team development and the roles and practices of effective teams.
TT2	Develop consensus on the ethical principles to guide all aspects of teamwork.
TT3	Engage health and other professionals in shared patient-centered and population-focused problem-solving.
TT4	Integrate the knowledge and experience of health and other professions to inform health and care decisions, while respecting patient and community values and priorities/preferences for care.
TT5	Apply leadership practices that support collaborative practice and team effectiveness.
TT6	Engage self and others to constructively manage disagreements about values, roles, goals, and actions that arise among health and other professionals and with patients, families, and community members.
TT7	Share accountability with other professions, patients, and communities for outcomes relevant to prevention and healthcare.
TT8	Reflect on individual and team performance for individual and team performance improvement.
TT9	Use process-improvement strategies to increase the effectiveness of interprofessional teamwork and team-based services, programs, and policies.
TT10	Use available evidence to inform effective teamwork and team-based practices.
TT11	Perform effectively on teams and in different team roles in a variety of settings.

Source: IPEC, 2016

Another national collaborative met in 2012. The Society for Simulation in Healthcare (SSH) and the National League for Nursing (NLN) Symposium on Interprofessional Education and Healthcare Simulation explored the use of simulation as an instrument for advancing IPE and practice using the competencies developed by an expert panel from IPEC (IPEC, 2011). Commonly reported gaps identified in Sim-IPE knowledge included:

- The lack of substantive and specific accreditation mandates

- Insufficient infrastructure and resources

- A paucity of research support mechanisms that demonstrate the effect of Sim-IPE on quality and safety

- Logistical challenges (e.g., scheduling and coordination)

- Cultural challenges

Symposium attendees developed consensus recommendations for organizations and for individuals. The recommendations for individuals were presented in 10 steps:

1. Examine personal assumptions, knowledge, and skills relative to healthcare simulation, IPE, and Sim-IPE.

2. Identify and engage local spheres of influence and share information about the IPEC competencies.

3. Conduct formal and informal educational offerings.

4. Promote IPE and Sim-IPE through the use of social media.

5. Participate in regional, state, and national conferences to showcase and learn more about Sim-IPE.

6. Submit manuscripts and publications about Sim-IPE.

7. Review and enhance current simulation scenarios to ensure that they align with the IPEC competencies.

8. Use research reports to provide evidence that links Sim-IPE to quality and safe patient outcomes.

9. Employ evaluation tools that focus on IPE.

10. Access and add Sim-IPE resources through the MedEdPortal or iCollaborative.

Educators and organizations can use these steps as a guideline to prepare and implement Sim-IPE.

The Institute of Medicine (IOM, 2015) convened a committee to consider methods necessary to measure the impact of IPE on collaborative practice and patient outcomes. The committee identified four areas that could create a strong foundation for the evaluation of the impact of IPE:

- More closely aligning the education and healthcare delivery systems

- Developing a conceptual framework for measuring the impact of IPE

- Strengthening the evidence base for IPE

- More effectively linking IPE with changes in collaborative behavior

The Health Professions Accreditors Collaborative (HPAC) engaged the support of the National Center for Interprofessional Practice and Education to embark on a multiyear project to develop a consensus guidance document for quality IPE (HPAC & the National Center for Interprofessional Practice and Education, 2019). Although this document is not specific to Sim-IPE, it does provide guidance for institutional administrators and accreditation boards and commissions for developing, implementing, evaluating, and improving IPE programming consistent with HPAC member accreditation expectations. This consensus report provides guidelines that reinforce taking an intentional approach to IPE, which includes:

- A clear rationale for the activity
- Outcome-based goals for the activity
- A deliberate design process
- A plan for the assessment and evaluation of the activity

Characteristics That Influence Outcomes in Sim-IPE

With the technology-integrated lifestyles of today's learners, educators are obligated to change the structured didactic curricula of the past to a more conducive learning platform. The use of simulation in healthcare, in its highly experiential and interactive form, fosters a new culture of learning. For optimal learning using simulation, educators must acknowledge and understand characteristics of Sim-IPE so that educational opportunities can be effectively engineered into the simulation. Examples of foundational characteristics are presented in this section.

The Challenge of Current Literature

Healthcare simulation and IPE continue separately in a discovery phase, attempting to define and redefine their language, taxonomies, characteristics, and the variables that influence outcomes. Limitations are imposed on this combined field in a two-fold fashion, requiring a collaboration of the most artistic, inventive, tolerant, and detail-oriented scientists (Schneider, 2009). Although the literature is deemed "inadequate" with educators frequently "reinventing the wheel," the state of the field is not only appropriate, it is a necessary process. Often it is the social process of working together to understand and find new ways of doing things that generates new capabilities in a healthcare team, rather than the specific techniques or methods that are developed or used. In other words, the "wheel" should not be the focus; instead, the focus should be on the social and relational work that's necessary for replication (e.g., word limits, journal requirements for methods used, etc.). Finding additional venues (such as web addendums to journals) to report details as listed in Table 9.2 is critical to covering gaps in this science.

Case Example: The Challenge of Current Literature

After developing an interest in IPE, Professor Jones has been asked to work with the simulation center to develop IPE for the schools of nursing, pharmacy, and medicine. In search of a model, she has found a journal article that sounds like what she wants to implement and shows significant outcomes in learning teamwork. However, the article only has a paragraph on the simulation scenario. Professor Jones realizes that she needs to fill in details. Taking the advice of this chapter, she assembles a team of faculty from each of the schools to develop the scenario and the objectives of the IPE. The team spends three long meetings coming to agreement on the objectives alone. Although Professor Jones used the model and scenario from the article as a launching-off point, the process of identifying the needs and desires of different faculty and schools, understanding the gaps in the literature, and working together to set objectives generates a sense of teamwork and ownership that is essential to the successful development and implementation of the IPE.

Educator Characteristics

A long-standing variable in education is the expertise, quality, and "likeability" of educators by learners, colleagues, and superiors. Interprofessional education requires additional knowledge in (Hammick, Freeth, Koppel, Reeves, & Barr, 2008; Howkins & Bray, 2008):

- Interprofessional practice as applicable to learner groups

- IPE competencies, as well as the newest research and recommendations for IPE

- IPE planning, design, and implementation, and formulation of design and evaluation teams

- Spheres of influence and change theory

- Translational research

- Assessment of learners in IPE, including existing validated and reliable evaluation instruments

Furthermore, as outlined in the SSH (2019) *Domains for Certified Healthcare Simulation Educators*, educators using simulation require additional knowledge in:

- Experiential teaching and learning theory

- Simulation equipment

- Simulation principles, practice, equipment, and methodology

- Assessment of learners using simulation

- Management of simulation resources and environments

- Engagement in simulation scholarly activities

The level of an educator's knowledge in these areas, along with teaching talent, professional values, and capabilities, can greatly influence a learner group's outcomes.

Preventing Adverse Learning

While creating and implementing Sim-IPE, educators must be mindful that negative perspectives around interprofessional practice may develop. Although adverse learning experiences might occur randomly, the likelihood for positive outcomes may depend on factors of educator knowledge, including substantial planning using an anticipatory design, awareness for and support of possible characteristics that lead to positive outcomes, and recognition and purposeful muting of possible characteristics that lead to negative outcomes. Adverse learning may be minimized by thoughtful adherence to best practices such as the INACSL Standards of Best Practice for Simulation-Enhanced Interprofessional Education (INACSL, 2016).

Case Example: Preventing Adverse Learning

An attending obstetrician who was previously a labor and delivery nurse is leading a debriefing with residents she had mentored previously and new nursing staff. Before the debriefing begins, one of the residents jokes, "At least I wasn't the nurse." The attending chuckles, remembering when she was the nurse, and begins the debriefing.

Throughout the debriefing, the nurses in attendance remain very upset at the resident's joke and do not engage in the debriefing. They also give the IPE low evaluation scores. It is clear that the attending is not aware of her light laughter at the resident's joke, is not transparent in her thought in the moment (her previous nursing experience), and is not aware of the negative effect it caused for the learners.

Modality Matching

All simulators have strengths and limitations. Educators must be aware of the capabilities, strengths, and limitations of available simulation equipment. These capabilities should be matched to the learning objectives set by the educators, the learning level of the learners, and the cues necessary to guide learners toward achieving the learning objectives. This is called modality matching. Although educators involved in healthcare simulation often focus on the realism of the environment and the simulator, there is also a need to focus on the appropriateness of the realism. Highly realistic and complex simulations are not always appropriate (Forneris, 2019). Because Sim-IPE seeks common learning ground, the objectives are often around teamwork, communication, and resource management, and require more focus on making communication opportunities more realistic.

Equal Opportunity for Professions

Educators have ethical obligations that require them to reflect on their individual desires for the education along with their personal assumptions. Often, educators seek participants from other professions to add a more realistic experience to a simulation designed for one profession. This creates a uniprofessional design that may benefit one group of learners more than other professional groups, potentially creating negative learning and proliferating the very stereotypes that IPE strives to alleviate. When designing Sim-IPE activities, there should be participation from all professions involved to ensure equal learning opportunities.

During debriefing, many assumptions arise in conversation—from both learners and educators. In this context, educators are often role models. They should be aware of their own personal assumptions around the professions involved, the value of IPE, and their preferences related to healthcare simulation to prevent modeling views that may be adverse to the intended learning.

Case Example: Modality Matching

The simulation staff receives a scenario developed by the university interprofessional education committee. It involves a traumatic arrest and one objective: for the learners to call the OR team. The simulation staff spends hours moulaging the mannequin and staging the simulated trauma bay, achieving a highly realistic environment. During the simulation, the physicians are so focused on the bleeding mannequin, the nurses are so focused on beeping alarms, and the respiratory therapists are so focused on the mannequin's compromised airway that the learners spend little time speaking and do not access the OR team. This is because the scenario focused mainly on the realism of the environment and did not build in opportunities for communication or prompts to guide learners to meet the objective of the scenario. Instead, it created opportunities for failure to achieve the learning objective. The simulation would have been more effective in reaching the objective if there had been less environmental noise and more social noise—for example, an embedded simulated healthcare provider to facilitate communication with the team.

Case Example: Equal Opportunity for Professions

An attending emergency physician runs a very successful simulation course for emergency resident physicians. Because TJC has encouraged IPE, the attending decides to make the simulation course interprofessional by asking her friend, a school of nursing professor, to bring her senior level BSN students to the simulation. The nursing students participate as learners alongside the residents during the simulation. The attending debriefs the residents as she normally does and then asks the nursing students to share their experience of and perspectives on the simulation. This discussion reveals that although the nursing students were grateful to participate in a simulation with residents, there were no specific objectives developed for the nursing students. The participation of the nursing students, however, helped the residents meet their learning objectives. This simulation might have provided equal opportunity if objectives had been developed for the nursing students to meet their specific learning needs, and the residents helped them meet those learning objectives.

Debriefing Facilitation Skills

Whether learning really occurs primarily during the simulation (by working together) or during the debriefing (reflecting on team skills using a common experience) is unclear. Fanning and Gaba (2007) posit that debriefing, more than the active simulation, is where learning takes place. The idea is that guided reflection or facilitator-led discussions create prolonged learning through reconstruction of the events, self-reflection, and cognitive assimilations. In debriefing, students also learn how to provide peer-to-peer and profession-to-profession feedback and, in this process, learn how to communicate their thoughts to a team of other professions. This skill is relevant to clinical practice and often lacking in the clinical setting, contributing to compromises in patient care. A focus on developing this skill of feedback and communication may be key in teaching healthcare providers how to work together.

Debriefing interprofessional groups can present unique challenges. Validated interprofessional debriefing tools (Poore, Dawson, Dunbar, & Parrish, 2019) may be helpful. Co-debriefers from differing professions are preferred, but a single debriefing may equate to co-debriefing for Sim-IPE (Brown, Wong, & Ahmed, 2018).

The hard part of IPE debriefing is getting learners into their comfort zone so they become willing to share their thoughts about each other and each other's professions. However, debriefings after in-situ Sim-IPE are often held in less private areas such as a staff break room or at the bedside of the mannequin. And, they typically last only 15 minutes or so. A less private area and limited time become significant barriers to creating this comfort and opportunity for deep reflection and feedback. Hence, the debriefer must possess effective facilitation skills that can either overcome these barriers or be effective within the limitations presented.

Learner Characteristics

In IPE, participants are learning with, from, and about each other. Each participant brings unique knowledge, previous experiences, energy, attitudes and perspectives, personality, mental frames, and communication skills. The combination of these unique factors affects the co-creation of knowledge and can greatly influence interprofessional learning. Therefore, depending on characteristics of the participants who compose a group (e.g., their ages, ethnicities, genders, and clinical experiences), the learning will differ from group to group.

Group Familiarity

Familiarity with one or more group members influences learning outcomes. In groups that have more than one member from a profession (e.g., three nursing students and one medical student), the within-profession learners are typically familiar with each other. Knowing how team members work together might increase team comfort or, to the contrary, create subgroup fragmentation if there are only a few members who are familiar with each other. Whether the interprofessional learning is more efficient in working teams than ad hoc teams has not yet been studied in Sim-IPE, but it might be a significant group characteristic affecting outcomes.

Observers Versus Active Participants

Due to larger group sizes and limitations on simulation resources, simulation often involves observers and active participants. Observers of a simulation in which active participants are in a clinical environment often actively engage in reflection using team-structured debriefings. Observers may also be "activated" by using structured observational tools. Whether observation through video projection and one-way mirrors serves as a concrete experience or not is unclear. It is also unclear whether debriefing serves as a concrete experience.

Some Sim-IPE have members of one profession participate in simulations as members of another profession to gain a sense of role differences and similarities. Although this may be a valuable experience, it should be used only for activities that pertain to objectives around role clarity or other appropriate objectives. If the objectives are around communication and a nurse is participating as a physician, the realism of the simulation is compromised because the nurse might not communicate the way a physician would, but rather the way the nurse believes a physician communicates, and vice versa. This dilemma is also present with cross-profession evaluations or observations. Healthcare professions are beginning to realize that each profession has a specialized language and culture that another profession might not understand; therefore, if one profession is evaluating another, gaps in the observation might occur.

Psychological Safety

A fundamental characteristic for the use of simulation is the establishment of psychological safety (SSH Council for the Accreditation of Healthcare Simulation Programs, 2018). For learners to fully engage in a simulation, their fears or potential fears should be addressed and their insecurities resolved (Rudolph, Raemer, & Simon, 2014). For example, students might be worried about whether their grading professor is behind the mirror or will be reviewing the video (if used). Ensuring confidentiality may positively affect their behavior during the simulation and the resulting learning outcomes.

Although scenarios are typically developed to fit curricular needs, a particular scenario may elicit memories in participants that could affect the learning of the group. These memories may be personal, traumatic, or sad. Educators must be able to address such a breach in psychological safety should it arise.

Psychological safety is particularly important to clinical-based learner groups or learners who work together on a day-to-day basis. If mistakes are made during the scenario, then fear, embarrassment, and judgments may carry over to the day-to-day setting. This can create discomfort and mistrust among the clinical team, which may contribute to ineffective patient care. Thus, educators must establish safety to address team issues and hold these as priorities during the debriefing.

Case Example: Psychological Safety

The nurse educator of a unit is asked to be an embedded simulated provider in a simulation involving nurses and physicians on the unit. In the simulation, the nurse educator plays the role of a clinical staff nurse who makes a medical error. The day after the simulation course, the nurse educator works on the unit. She is paranoid that the physician she is working with during the shift might think that she is likely to make medical errors.

Sim-IPE often requires the use of an embedded simulated provider, often played by a clinician familiar to the learners. If this embedded simulated provider is a clinician who interacts with the learners frequently, that person's role in the scenario must be made clear to learners. This is to break the link in learners' minds between the clinician and his or her actions during the scenario—in other words, to ensure the learners don't associate those actions with the clinician after the simulation.

Simulation and Evaluation Design

Characteristics identified in Sim-IPE frequently concern the logistical design of the simulation. Questions regarding simulation design still in need of study include:

- What effect is there on interprofessional learning if the Sim-IPE course is a required course versus an elective course?

- What is the most effective number of members and disciplines composing a team for Sim-IPE?

- With pre-licensure students, is it more effective for students to engage in Sim-IPE in their current role as students or in their post-licensure role?

- What effect does clinical experience have on an individual and team involved in IPE?

Overcoming Challenges

There are many challenges in Sim-IPE. Having a solid grasp of theoretical frameworks can provide options and solutions. Chapter 1 contains a detailed discussion of theoretical frameworks. In addition, a framework specific to establishing content validity, reliability, and assessment in Sim-IPE is suggested in this section. This framework may be helpful in the development of quality simulations.

Theoretical Frameworks

Discovering undeveloped areas of the IPE field, educators have turned to theoretical frameworks to guide the development of a learning program and to guide the facilitation of learning. Traditionally, *theory* has been defined as "an abstract generalization that offers a systematic explanation about how phenomena are interrelated" (Polit & Beck, 2012, p. 126). Generally, theory connotes an abstraction (Polit & Beck, 2012). Hence, IPE or healthcare simulation educators are basing their methods on varied theories (from opinions, suggestions, and recommendations). Educational theories such as those shown in Table 9.4 provide structure and guidance to instructional strategies and learning activities in Sim-IPE.

Table 9.4 Educational Theories	
Theory	**Description**
Adult learning (Knowles, 1980)	Andragogy is the study of adult learning. Malcolm Knowles states six assumptions that motivates adults to learn. These assumptions include: 1) adults need to know the reason why they are learning what they are learning, 2) adults need to be involved in their plan and decisions around education (be self-directing), 3) adults bring vast experiences to the discussion, 4) adults are most interested in material that is relevant to their lives, 5) adults learn best when the activity is problem-centered, and 6) adults are internally driven.
Experiential learning (Kolb & Fry, 1975)	David Kolb and Roger Fry developed a model of learning that conceptualizes learning as a process through the transformation of experience from the work of Dewey, Lewin, and Piaget. The model posits four cycles: experience (e.g., work, "real-world" experience, simulations), reflection (e.g., reflecting on a specific action), conceptualization (e.g., analyzing and understanding what drove the action and effect), and experimentation (e.g., planning and executing a course of action).
Situated learning (Lave & Wenger, 1991)	Lave & Wenger describe a social process where knowledge is co-created within the context of how that skill or knowledge is applied. Situated learning theory also embraces a concrete experience (i.e., simulation) and reflective observation on the experience (i.e. debriefing). Learning is constructed in a way where knowledge is contextualized. This deep understanding of the context becomes the means for understanding that situation and the meaning made by the learner. This dynamic perspective adds a larger context to debriefing and suggests that learning is supported and altered through the exchange and interaction of individuals. Lave & Wenger complement situated learning with the concept of a "community of practice." The learning in IPE should include the same members with their perspectives and contribution of the event explored.
Reflective practice (Schön, 1983)	Donald Schön's work describes how we create new meaning through the analysis and understanding of actions and values. There are two types of reflection: reflection-in-action (i.e., during the simulation) and reflection-on-action (i.e., after the simulation) during debriefing. Debriefing should also allow for a third type of reflective practice identified by Thompson and Pascal reflection-for-action (i.e., how to apply new meaning for new action in practice or for the next simulation).
Deliberate practice (Ericsson, 2004)	K. Anders Ericsson outlines essential components of deliberate practice that optimizes learning and performance, including internal motivation to engage in a task to improve; building upon previous experience, skill, and knowledge; immediate feedback on the performance; and repetition of the task. Ericsson underscores the point that healthcare students need representations that can support planning and practice of the actual performance to allow for adjustments toward mastery and there is a need where feedback can be immediate. With careful planning and skilled facilitation, simulation with debriefing helps to fill this need.
Psychodynamic theory (Bion, 1961)	Bion brings to light psychodynamic perspectives where learning depends on cultivating critical awareness of behavior in, as, and between groups.
Contact hypothesis /theory (Allport, 1954)	Allport posits that contact modifies prejudice and stereotypes between professions and, therefore, modifies relationships between professional groups.

continues

Table 9.4 Educational Theories (cont.)	
Theory	**Description**
Identity theories (Brown, Condor, Mathews, Wade, and Williams; Tajfel & Turner, 1986; Turner, 1999)	In social identity theory, Tajfel and Turner describe how our identity comes from our membership of social groups in which we perceive our group more positively than others. Turner explores self-categorization theory as an expansion of social identity theory in the context of one's organization. Brown, Condor, Mathews, Wade, and Williams focus on group objectives in realistic conflict theory, where the objectives in each group surface through attitude and behavior.
Practice theory (Bourdieu, 1977)	Bourdieu describes how professional identity is acquired through one's culture and how each profession has its own "cultural capital." Under this theory, IPE should be a common, long, and consistent experience.
Self-determination theory (Deci, 1971)	SDT seeks to understand motivation, contrasting intrinsic and extrinsic motivators. In online engagement, there are multiple factors from the individual and from the environment. SDT highlights what people have in common, and this was important to us since it seemed that each response and interview revealed many differences in values and interests. It was helpful to view the data as common themes and common areas of difference.
Psychological safety (Edmondson & Lei,, 2014)	Edmondson and Lei describe how the feeling of safety for interpersonal risk-taking is a mediator of relationships and critical to teaching and learning.
General systems theory (von Bertalanffy, 2015)	Von Bertalanffy views the whole individual-community-environment as beyond professional and political bounds typically of focus, taking into account each profession's complexity. Cause and effect are interdependent, and this theory seeks to unify how each profession relates its work to the needs of all involved components.
Organizational theory (Senge, 1990)	Senge describes conditions that nurture learning, creating "a culture of enquiry." An environment capable of respectful, proactive, and innovative continuous and iterative process of change and reframing allows this culture of inquiry.
Activity theory (Engeström, 2001)	Engestrom focuses on understanding and intervening in interactions to effect change in relations at the micro (individual) and macro (community rules) levels. This requires a joint activity.
Complexity theory (Fraser & Greenhalgh, 2001)	Fraser & Greenhalgh account for the unpredictable complex adaptive systems in organizations, professions, and learners. Learning takes place between familiar and unfamiliar tasks and environments. To address each complexity, multiple remedies are more effective.
Transformative learning theory (Mezirow, 1978)	Transformational learning is a branch of Adult Learning. Mezirow describes a 10-step process for transformative learning to offer a guideline in developing the skills needed for optimal team performance in a complex environment.

SimBIE Reliability-Validity-Assessment Framework

When used for IPE, simulation is most often a tool to achieve interprofessional learning. Just like any educational tool, quality education results from validation and reliability testing. Based on findings from a study by Palaganas (2012), the Simulation-Based Interprofessional Education Reliability-Validity-Assessment (SimBIE RVA) framework shown in Figure 9.2 is offered to educators and researchers in the field.

The SimBIE RVA framework might fill gaps identified in this chapter and reinforce the endeavors of the field (Palaganas, 2012). It can also serve as a resource for educators,

researchers, and simulation programs intent upon building interprofessional learning through Sim-IPE. Finally, as noted in this chapter, establishing reliability, validity, and accurate assessment is difficult due to the complexity of and uncertainties within the IPE field. The SimBIE RVA framework can help educators and researchers further understand their simulation and IPE practice, clarify complex areas already studied, and build their own curriculum for interprofessional learning using existing evidence and findings as a foundation. Many educators or organizations have already developed a similar Sim-IPE. Seeking these resources may provide roadmaps that can help to develop new programs or improve existing programs.

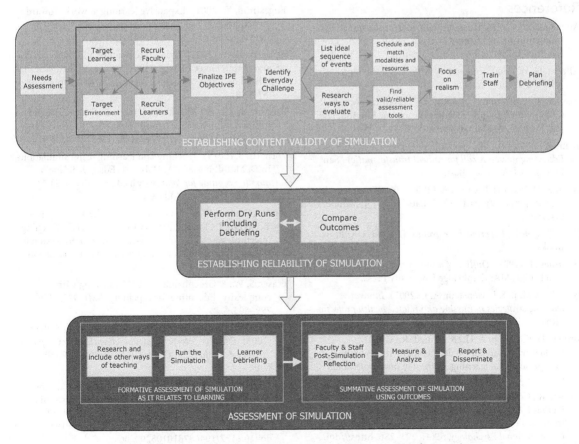

FIGURE 9.2 The SimBIE RVA framework (©Janice C. Palaganas).

Conclusion

Because the fields of healthcare simulation and IPE have entered a discovery and exploratory stage, thoughtful reporting will be crucial to future developments. This chapter has provided information on healthcare simulation and IPE from the literature, national discussions and efforts, and considerable reflection of terminology and characteristics. It contributes to the growing findings around factors in IPE methods that influence positive and negative outcomes and also reveals many questions that are foundational for this science. Use of the information and tools presented in this chapter can assist in thoughtful planning for future Sim-IPE and research.

References

Abualenain, J. (2018). Hospital-wide interprofessional simulation-based training in crisis resource management. *Eurasian Journal of Emergency Medicine, 17*(3), 93–96.

Allport, G. W. (1954). *The nature of prejudice*. Oxford, UK: Addison-Wesley.

Aspden, P., Wolcott, J. A., Bootman, J., & Cronenwett, L. R. (2007). Preventing medication errors. Washington, DC: The National Academies Press.

Benner, P., Sutphen, M., Leonard, V., & Day, L. (2010). *Educating nurses: A call for radical transformation*. San Francisco, CA: Jossey-Bass.

Billings, D. M., & Halstead, J. A. (2008). *Teaching in nursing: A guide for faculty* (3rd ed.). Philadelphia, PA: Saunders Elsevier.

Bion, W. (1961). *Experiences in groups*. London, UK: Basic Books.

Bourdieu, P. (1977). *Outline of a theory of practice*. Cambridge, MA: Cambridge University Press.

Bradshaw, M. J., & Lowenstein, A. J. (2007). *Innovative teaching strategies in nursing and related health professions* (4th ed.). Burlington, MA: Jones & Bartlett Learning.

Brown, D. K., Wong, A. H., & Ahmed, R. A. (2018). Evaluation of simulation debriefing methods with interprofessional learning. *Journal of Interprofessional Care, 19*, 1–3. doi:10.1080/13561820.2018.1500451

Brown, R., Condor, S., Mathews, A., Wade, G., & Williams, J. (1986). Explaining intergroup differentiation in an industrial organization. *Journal of Occupational and Organizational Psychology, 59*(4), 273–286. https://doi.org/10.1111/j.2044-8325.1986.tb00230.x

Canadian Interprofessional Health Collaborative. (n.d.). A national interprofessional competency framework. Retrieved from https://www.mcgill.ca/ipeoffice/ipe-curriculum/cihc-framework

Commission on Collegiate Nursing Education. (2018). *Standards for accreditation of baccalaureate and graduate degree nursing programs*. Washington, DC: Commission on Collegiate Nursing Education. Retrieved from https://www.aacnnursing.org/Portals/42/CCNE/PDF/Standards-Final-2018.pdf

Cooper, H., Carlisle, C., Gibbs, T., & Watkins, C. (2001). Developing an evidence base for interdisciplinary learning: A systematic review. *Journal of Advanced Nursing, 35*(2), 228–237.

Deci, E. L. (1971). Effects of externally mediated rewards on intrinsic motivation. *Journal of Personality and Social Psychology, 18*, 105–115.

Edmondson, A. C., & Lei, Z. (2014). Psychological safety: The history, renaissance, and future of an interpersonal construct. *The Annual Review of Organizational Psychology and Organizational Behavior, 1*, 23–43. doi:10.1146/annurev-orgpsych-031413-091305

Engeström, Y. (2001). Expansive learning at work: Toward an activity theoretical reconceptualization. *Journal of Education and Work, 14*(1), 133–156.

Ericsson, K. A. (2004). Deliberate practice and the acquisition and maintenance of expert performance in medicine and related domains. *Academic Medicine, 79*(10 Suppl.), S70–S81.

Fanning, R. M., & Gaba, D. M. (2007). The role of debriefing in simulation-based learning. *Simulation in Healthcare, 2*(2), 115–125. doi:10.1097/SIH.0b013e3180315539

Forneris, S. (2019). Teaching and learning using simulations. In D. M. Billings & J. A. Halstead (Eds.), *Teaching in nursing: A guide for faculty* (6th ed., pp. 353–372). St. Louis, MO: Saunders Elsevier.

Fox, L., Onders, R., Hermansen-Kobulnicky, C. J., Nguyen, T., Myran, L., Linn, B., & J. Hornecker. (2017). Teaching interprofessional teamwork skills to health professional students: A scoping review. *Journal of Interprofessional Care, 32*(2), 127–135.

Fraser, S. W., & Greenhalgh, T. (2001). Coping with complexity: Educating for capability. *BMJ, 323*(7316), 799–803.

Freeth, D. S., Hammick, M., Reeves, S., Koppel, I., & Barr, H. (2005). *Effective interprofessional education: Development, delivery & evaluation*. Oxford, UK: Blackwell Publishing Ltd.

Gaba, D. M., Howard, S. K., Fish, K. J., Smith, B. E., & Sowb, Y. A. (2001). Simulation-based training in anesthesia crisis resource management (ACRM): A decade of experience. *Simulation & Gaming, 32*(2), 175–193. doi:10.1177/104687810103200206

Hammick, M., Freeth, D., Koppel, I., Reeves, S., & Barr, H. (2008). A best evidence systematic review of interprofessional education: BEME guide no. 9. *Medical Teacher, 29*(8), 735-751. doi:10.1080/01421590701682576

Harvey, E. M., Freeman, D., Wright, A., Bath, J., Peters, V. K., Mwadows, G., ... Collier, B. R. (2019). Impact of advanced nurse teamwork training on trauma team performance. *Clinical Simulation in Nursing, 30*, 7–15.

Health Professions Accreditors Collaborative & the National Center for Interprofessional Practice and Education. (2019). *Guidance on developing quality interprofessional education for the health professions.* Retrieved from https://healthprofessionsaccreditors.org/wp-content/uploads/2019/02/HPACGuidance02-01-19.pdf

Hean, S., Craddock, D., & Hammick, M. (2012). Theoretical insights into interprofessional education: AMEE guide No. 62. *Medical Teacher, 34*(2), 78-101. doi:10.3109/0142159X.2012.650740

Helmreich, R. L., Merritt, A. C., & Wilhelm, J. A. (1999). The evolution of Crew Resource Management training in commercial aviation. *International Journal of Aviation Psychology, 9*(1), 19-32.

Howkins, E., & Bray, J. (2008). *Preparing for interprofessional teaching: Theory and practice.* London, UK: Radcliffe Publishing Ltd.

Institute of Medicine. (2007). *The learning healthcare system: Workshop summary.* Washington, DC: National Academies Press. doi:10.17226/11903

Institute of Medicine. (2015). *Measuring the impact of interprofessional education on collaborative practice and patient outcomes.* Washington, DC: The National Academies Press. Retrieved from https://www.ncbi.nlm.nih.gov/books/NBK338360/

International Nursing Association for Clinical Simulation and Learning Standards Committee. (2016). INACSL standards of best practice: Simulation. Simulation-enhanced interprofessional education (Sim-IPE). *Clinical Simulation in Nursing, 12*(S), S34-S38. doi:10.1016/j.ecns.2016.09.011

Interprofessional Education and Healthcare Simulation Collaborative. (2012). *A consensus report from the 2012 interprofessional education and healthcare simulation collaborative.* Washington, DC: Society for Simulation in Healthcare.

Interprofessional Education Collaborative. (2011). *Core competencies for interprofessional collaborative practice: Report of an expert panel.* Retrieved from https://www.ipecollaborative.org/resources.html

Interprofessional Education Collaborative. (2016). *Core competencies for interprofessional collaborative practice: 2016 update.* Retrieved from https://nebula.wsimg.com/2f68a39520b03336b41038c370497473?AccessKeyId=DC06780E69ED19E2B3A5&disposition=0&alloworigin=1

The Joint Commission on Accreditation of Healthcare Organizations. (2005). *Health care at the crossroads: Strategies for improving the medical liability system and preventing patient injury.* Retrieved from https://www.jointcommission.org/assets/1/18/Medical_Liability.pdf

Knowles, M. S. (1975). *The modern practice of adult education: From pedagogy to andragogy.* Wilton, CT: Association Press.

Kolb, D., & Fry, R. (1975). Towards an applied theory of experiential learning. In C. L. Copper (Ed.), *Theories of group processes* (pp. 33–58). London, UK: John Wiley.

Lairamore, C., Reed, C. C., Damon, Z., Rowe, V., Baker, J., Griffith, K., & VanHoose, L. (2019). A peer-led interprofessional simulation experience improves perceptions of teamwork. *Clinical Simulation in Nursing, 34*, 22–29.

Lave, J., & Wenger, E. (1991). *Situated learning: Legitimate peripheral participation.* Cambridge, UK: Cambridge University Press.

Lee, C. A., Pais, K., Kelling, S., & O. S. Anderson. (2018). A scoping review to understand simulation used in interprofessional education. *Journal of Interprofessional Education & Practice, 13*, 15–23.

Lioce, L., Lopreiato, J., Downing, D., Chang, T. P., Robertson, J. M., Anderson, M., ... the Terminology and Concepts Working Group. (2020). *Healthcare simulation dictionary* (2nd ed.). Rockville, MD: Agency for Healthcare Research and Quality. AHRQ Publication No. 20-0019. doi:https://doi.org/10.23970/simulationv2

McGaghie, W. C., Issenberg, S. B., Petrusa, E. R., & Scalese, R. J. (2010). A critical review of simulation-based medical education research: 2003–2009. *Medical Education, 44*(1), 50–63. doi:10.1111/j.1365-2923.2009.03547.x

Mezirow, J. (1978). Perspective transformation. *Adult education, 28*(2), 100-110.

National League for Nursing. (2015). *Guide to effective interprofessional education experiences in nursing education.* Retrieved from http://www.nln.org/docs/default-source/default-document-library/ipe-toolkit-krk-012716.pdf?sfvrsn=6

National League for Nursing Commission for Nursing Education Accreditation. (2016). Accreditation standards for nursing education programs. Retrieved from http://www.nln.org/docs/default-source/accreditation-services/cnea-standards-final-february-201613f2bf5c78366c709642ff00005f0421.pdf?sfvrsn=12

Palaganas, J. C. (2012). *Exploring healthcare simulation as a platform for interprofessional education* (Doctoral dissertation). Available from ProQuest Dissertations and Theses database.

Palaganas, J. C., Brunette, V., & Winslow, B. (2016). Prelicensure simulation-enhanced interprofessional education. *Simulation in Healthcare, 11*(6), 404–418. doi:10.1097/SIH.0000000000000175

Palaganas, J. C., Epps, C., & Raemer, D. B. (2014). A history of simulation-enhanced interprofessional education. *Journal of Interprofessional Care, 28*(2), 110–115. doi:10.3109/1356 1820.2013.869198

Palaganas, J. C., Scott, E., Mancini, M. B., & Stryjewski, G. (2016). Simulation-enhanced interprofessional education. In V. Grant & A. Cheng (Eds.), *Comprehensive healthcare simulation: Pediatrics* (1st ed.). New York, NUY: Springer.

Parker, A. L., Forsythe, L. L., & Kohlmorgan, I. K. (2018). TeamSTEPPS: An evidence-based approach to reduce clinical errors threatening safety in outpatient settings: An integrative review. *Journal of Healthcare Risk Management, 38*(4), 19–31.

Polit, D. F., & Beck, C. T. (2012). *Nursing research: Generating and assessing evidence for nursing practice* (9th ed.). Philadelphia, PA: Lippincott Williams & Wilkins.

Poore, J. A., Dawson, J. C., Dunbar, D. M., & Parrish K. (2019). Debriefing interprofessionally: A tool for recognition and reflection. *Nurse Educator, 44*(1), 25–28. doi:10.1097/NNE.0000000000000518

Reeves, S., Abramovich, I., Rice, K., & Goldman, J. (2007). *An environmental scan and literature review on interprofessional collaborative practice settings: Final report for Health Canada.* Li Ka Shing Knowledge Institute of St Michael's Hospital: University of Toronto.

Reeves, S., Palaganas, J., & Zierler, B. (2017). An updated synthesis of review evidence of interprofessional education. *Journal of Allied Health, 46*(1), 56–61.

Rudolph, J. W., Raemer, D. B., & Simon, R. (2014). Establishing a safe container for learning in simulation: The role of the presimulation briefing. *Simulation in Healthcare, 9*(6), 339–349. doi:10.1097/SIH.0000000000000047

Schneider, A. M. (2009). Four stages of a scientific discipline; four types of scientist. *Trends in Biochemical Sciences, 34*(5), 217–223. doi:10.1016/j.tibs.2009.02.002

Schön, D. (1983). *The reflective practitioner: How professionals think in action.* New York, NY: Basic Books.

Senge, P. M. (1990). *The fifth discipline: The art and practice of the learning organization.* New York, NY: Doubleday/Currency.

Society for Simulation in Healthcare Council for Certification. (2019). *SSH certified healthcare simulation educator handbook.* Retrieved from https://www.ssih.org/Portals/48/Certification/CHSE_Docs/CHSE%20Handbook.pdf

Tajfel, H., & Turner, J. C. (1986). *The social identity theory of intergroup behavior.* Chicago, IL: Nelson Hall.

Tekian, A., McGuire, C. H., & McGaghie, W. C. (1999). *Innovative simulations for assessing professional competence: From paper-and-pencil to virtual reality.* Chicago, IL: University of Illinois at Chicago, Department of Medical Education.

Turner, J. C. (1999). Some current issues in research on social identity and self-categorization theories. *Social identity: Context, commitment, content, 3*(1), 6–34.

von Bertalanffy, L. (2015). *General systems theory. Foundations, development, applications.* New York, NY: George Braziller Inc.

Wilhaus, J., Palaganas, J., Manos, J., Anderson, J., Cooper, A., Jeffries, P., ... Mancini, M. E. (2012). *Interprofessional education and healthcare simulation symposium.* National League for Nursing. Retrieved from http://www.nln.org/docs/default-source/professional-development-programs/white-paper-symposium-ipe-in-healthcare-simulation-2013-(pdf).pdf?sfvrsn=0

World Health Organization. (2010). *Framework for action on interprofessional education & collaborative practice.* Retrieved from https://apps.who.int/iris/bitstream/handle/10665/70185/WHO_HRH_HPN_10.3_eng.pdf;jsessionid=430EAAE58D8EE194396BA68B4E59FE50?sequence=1

Zhang, C., Thompson, S., & Miller, C. (2011). A review of simulation-based interprofessional education. *Clinical Simulation in Nursing, 7*(4), e117–e126. doi:10.1016/j.ecns.2010.02.008

"Learning is the process whereby knowledge is created through the transformation of experience."

–David Kolb

Using Simulation in Academic Environments to Improve Learner Performance

Deborah Becker, PhD, RN, ACNP, BC, CHSE, FAAN

10

OBJECTIVES

- Relate simulations and simulated learning strategies to educational theories.

- Identify a variety of ways simulation can be used for content delivery and the development of psychomotor skills.

- Describe approaches to teach early recognition and rescue situations.

- Discuss the importance of aligning technology with simulation objectives.

- Compare and contrast the benefits of using various types of simulation approaches.

- Explain how simulation can be used for instruction and evaluation.

Providing education for health professionals in the academic setting has changed significantly since the days of training with the mantra "See one. Do one. Teach one." Today, in addition to developing competent and confident healthcare professionals, educators are concerned with the ethics of training with actual patients. They must also ensure consistent access to specific clinical experiences to prepare increasing numbers of clinically competent providers who are confident in simple to highly technical skills and complex reasoning (Ziv, Wolpe, Small, & Glick, 2003).

Simulation is uniquely suited to help meet the challenges of educating healthcare students in the academic environment. As a teaching strategy, simulation has been demonstrated to provide a safe and effective approach to learning skills, developing clinical thinking, and making critical decisions without placing patients at risk for harm (Institute of Medicine, 2011). Simulations can be constructed to deliver content in place of traditional lectures and to teach students how to perform specific skills as well as how to critically think through a clinical situation. Simulations also can be designed to provide learners with a series of experiences that cannot be guaranteed to occur during their clinical practice time as well as encourage teamwork, leadership, interprofessional practice, and communication. Learner acquisition of knowledge, skills, and abilities can be evaluated using simulation. These evaluations can be formative or summative. When properly designed, simulations can ensure consistency in evaluative approach and can be used in high-stakes testing such as determining progression to the next level within a program or to graduation.

Educational Theory and Simulation

The concept of learning as a function of activity, context, and culture is based on the theory of contextual or situated learning. *Active learning*—in which participants are physically, mentally, and emotionally involved in the learning, usually within context and situation—is a profoundly more effective teaching strategy than more passive methods. Learners and their learning needs are at the center of active learning. Any number of teaching strategies can be employed to actively engage students in the learning process, including group discussions, problem-solving, case studies, role-play, journal writing, and structured learning groups. The benefits to using such activities are many, including improved critical-thinking skills, increased retention and transfer of new information, increased motivation, and improved interpersonal skills.

Simulation puts the learner into action, providing a contextually realistic environment in which the student is expected to demonstrate techniques, make clinically sound judgments, and respond dynamically to the situation (Lateef, 2010). Simulation supports the educational theory of constructivism. *Constructivism* posits that people construct their own understanding and knowledge of the world by experiencing things and then reflecting on those experiences (McGaghie & Harris, 2018; Thomas, Menon, Boruff, Rodriguez, & Ahmed, 2014). When people encounter something new, they have to reconcile it with their previous ideas and experiences—maybe changing what they believed or maybe discarding the new information as irrelevant. In any case, learners are active creators of their own knowledge. Constructivism modifies the role of the educator to one that helps students construct knowledge rather than recall facts. The educator provides

tools such as problem-solving and inquiry-based learning activities to provide students with opportunities to apply their existing knowledge and real-world experience, learn to hypothesize and test their theories, and, ultimately, draw conclusions from their findings (Kolb, 1984). By actively participating in simulations, learners use previously gained knowledge along with newly acquired abilities to work through new experiences. Afterward, learners participate in a debriefing session in which they are asked to reflect on their performance and decision-making during the simulation. This allows them to construct their own understanding, making changes to what they believe and either keeping or discarding the information as relevant or irrelevant.

Adult learning principles are often employed when educating health professionals. These principles form a model of assumptions about the characteristics of adult learners that are different from the traditional pedagogical assumptions made about children. Adult learning theory suggests that adults have a need to know why they should learn something; they need to be self-directed; and, because they have more experiences than youths, they become ready to learn when they experience situations in which they determine a need to know or a need to be able to perform something to be more effective (Clapper, 2010; Knowles, 1996). Simulation provides opportunities for educators to develop reality-based situations in which these principles can be applied and tested in practice almost immediately.

Achieving Objectives Through Simulation

Simulation supports the achievement of an array of objectives. Students can learn skills ranging from basic to complex through the use of task trainers when the psychomotor components of the skill are deliberately practiced. In addition, clinically based scenarios can be developed in which participants determine whether the patient's status warrants performance of the skill. If the learner's judgment is to proceed with the skill, then the learner must prepare the patient, perform the skill, and evaluate the patient's response to the intervention. This leads to greater mastery of the skill while also providing the opportunity to demonstrate the knowledge and abilities necessary to work through a dynamic situation. It also allows the learner to develop and exhibit critical thinking and clinical judgment.

Academic institutions might have access to elaborate simulation centers with a number of rooms that simulate a variety of practice settings, or they might have access only to a multipurpose space. Simulation centers typically provide contextual realism that can be important for specific educational objectives and often are equipped with technologies such as a video-recording system. But just because these centers exist does not mean that all simulations have to occur in them. Sometimes bringing the simulation into the classroom is appropriate, particularly when the objective is to demonstrate how to apply newly acquired information. Novices need opportunities to observe experts applying information and making clinical judgments. Bringing a simulation into the classroom can help solidify knowledge acquisition. It also demonstrates how new information and concepts are applied to situations or how this information is used to set priorities and make clinical decisions.

Content Delivery

Simulation can be an effective way to teach students in health professions programs about concepts and processes while also fostering an interesting and engaging experience. Bringing a mannequin into a classroom setting and demonstrating the steps of assessment (or asking for volunteers and walking students through the steps) is an effective way of not only delivering material but also placing it in context by showing how it is done. Educators can set up a mannequin so that the signs and symptoms of a particular disease are manifested, and students can apply their newly obtained knowledge to simulated patient situations. In this way, core content is delivered along with expert modeling by the instructor. This enables students to develop a better understanding of their roles as care providers. When delivering content in this way, educators can allow the simulation to be interrupted and can give clarification at key points. Students can ask questions about approaches demonstrated, allowing for discussions around the nuances of care provision.

Simulation can be used as a means for students to demonstrate their understanding of classroom material. Educators can offer scenarios that purposely omit relevant data and include irrelevant or incomplete data that can be presented so students can engage in identifying cues and generating inferences (Su & Juestel, 2010). Educators creating the scenario must consider the background knowledge that students have on the content. By doing so, educators have the opportunity to consider where the student might get stuck and develop prompts that can redirect the student. It also provides an opportunity for the educator to consider alternative paths that students might take and determine if this will be permitted or deterred in some way. This allows educators to determine the type of pre-scenario preparation the students require and provide assignments that meet this need (Su & Juestel, 2010).

Participation in simulations provides the chance for students to show their mastery of content and their ability to apply their newly acquired knowledge to a variety of clinical situations. The idea of using simulation to replace clinical experiences is currently receiving much attention. Educators can use simulation as preparation for clinical experiences by having scenarios set up around normal findings as a way to prepare students for their assigned clinical placements (Bantz, Dancer, Hodson-Carlton, & Van Hove, 2007). Or, scenarios demonstrating commonly encountered but abnormal findings can be used to prepare students to recognize and respond in an environment that is safe and that allows for mistakes and corrections without doing harm.

When providing simulation experiences focused on replacing or enhancing hours traditionally spent in direct clinical experiences, the educator must consider the level of the learner, the number of students, the allotted time and space, and the desired clinical objectives for the experience. After the educator has determined these characteristics, scenarios can be constructed to provide the students a consistent set of experiences that requires the type of clinical thinking and decision-making that occurs in clinical settings. As students' knowledge and decision-making capacity grows, the need for more complex and realistic scenarios grows. One way to accomplish this objective is to use a full-sized, highly automated mannequin that exhibits vital signs; emits heart, lung, and bowel sounds; has palpable pulses; perspires; vomits; cries; and speaks, among a host of other features. These mannequins can be programmed to display realistic physiologic responses to actions taken by a student or progress through a series of clinical presentations reflecting a preestablished clinical condition.

Another way to create more realistic scenarios is to use a standardized patient. A *standardized patient* is a person who might or might not have formal acting experience, but who has been trained to act like a patient with a particular disease or disorder. Standardized patients are taught how to answer questions or are provided a script from which they cannot deviate. They are instructed to interact in a specific way with the provider. Their responses, reactions, and behaviors are maintained in a narrow range to provide consistency in the scenario, especially if the scenario will be offered to several students sequentially. In most educational programs, this type of simulation is ideal. However, it has limitations. First, the realism of the scenario depends on the standardized patient's ability to act, maintain character, and provide consistency in the scenario. Second, if the scenario requires the patient to exhibit certain physical findings, this might be difficult unless the actor actually has the condition.

Hybrid simulations use a standardized patient for the interactive segments of the scenario, and when physical findings—such as being in labor or having a murmur—cannot be simulated, a partial simulator (for example, birthing simulator or an auscultative model) is used to exhibit the required physical condition or symptoms. Hybrid simulations provide opportunities for the student to assess the patient, including asking questions and receiving responses from a "real" patient. If the student decides that the patient's condition requires the performance of a particular skill, this skill can be performed on the manufactured body part attached to or in the vicinity of the standardized patient.

Standardized patient programs can be costly if professional actors are used. A way to reduce costs is to use volunteers such as students, staff members, retired healthcare providers, or retired members of the community. It is amazing how many people are willing to help teach students in health professions programs for free or very little money. However, a shortcoming to using volunteers can be varying levels of commitment.

Mannequin-based or standardized patient simulations are not the only types of simulations that can be used to deliver content. Screen-based simulations—such as those that demonstrate anatomy and physiology and physical assessment techniques for evaluating function and structure—make excellent learning tools. These include numerous online games and tutorials, which provide information in an engaging and interactive manner.

There are also simpler games for use in health professions education. One such game is Six Second ECG. Six Second ECG teaches learners to identify different cardiac rhythms (Skillstat Inc., 2013). During the game, a series of rhythm strips appear. The object is for the player to identify as many as possible. The game then calculates the ratio of correct to incorrect answers and provides direct feedback that ranges from "mastery of content" to "more preparation is needed." Case-based simulations that include video, audio, and imagery—referred to as *adaptive educational technologies*—create an immersive environment in which learners interact with a computer-generated image of a patient and make decisions relevant to the patient scenario presented. The scenario progresses based on individualized learner decisions, and the case adaptively progresses based on those decisions. This allows students to experience the consequences of their decisions and provides an opportunity for learners to continue as the case unfolds. Learners

gain insight into their decision-making; coaching specific to learner decision-making can be solicited upon request (Lineberry, Dev, Lane, & Talbot, 2018).

Other screen-based simulation modalities that can be used effectively in the academic setting are computer screen-based simulations (with and without haptic technology devices that provide tactile feedback to the learner; see Figure 10.1) and virtual-reality simulations (computer-simulated environments that simulate the learner's presence in real-world situations). Virtual phlebotomy simulators are an example of a screen-based simulation that integrates haptic technology to provide content and psychomotor skill training. These comprehensive, interactive, self-directed learning systems can be used in academic settings to teach both cognitive and psychomotor skills.

The learning management system embedded in this type of simulation product typically allows for use in teaching and testing modes and thus can serve multiple purposes in the academic setting. In the case of a program focused on the knowledge and skills associated with establishing intravenous (IV) access, instruction on how to insert a catheter and the issues that should be considered before, during, and after performing the skill are provided via a screen-based computer program. When ready, the learner can move on to practicing actual psychomotor skills of catheter insertion using the haptic device that provides tactile and resistance feedback, with the screen showing the learner's actions. When the learner feels confident, the program provides a scored checklist and a detailed debriefing on performance. A variety of patient situations requiring catheter insertion are provided.

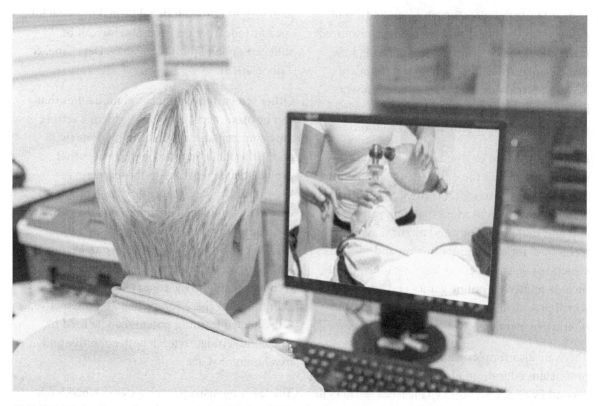

FIGURE 10.1 Example of a screen-based simulation that integrates haptic technology to provide content and psychomotor skill training.

Virtual reality is a computer-simulated environment that replicates the learner's presence in a real-world situation. The use of virtual-reality simulations is becoming increasingly popular in academic settings. Virtual reality allows learners to explore and manipulate computer-generated or three-dimensional (3D) environments in real time (Kyaw et al., 2019). The immersive nature of this technology promotes the learner's suspension of disbelief and allows learners to believe they are in the environment. Active learning occurs because learners are able to interact with or manipulate objects in the virtual environment. Hence, virtual reality is highly conducive to clinical and surgical procedures–focused training.

There are several commercially and faculty-developed virtual-reality programs available that provide educators with interactive and highly engaging platforms to develop learning encounters that can accommodate numerous students at one time. Examples include:

- **Second Life (https://www.secondlife.com):** An online world that allows interaction between individuals in various settings.

- **Nightingale Isle (http://nightingaleisle. blogspot.com):** A virtual space created to foster collaboration, research, and education for nursing students, educators, and health professionals.

- **Xtranormal (http://www.xtranormal.com):** A website that allows individuals to create animated videos.

Virtual worlds that can engage numerous students at one time are called multiuser virtual worlds (MUVWs). Although a variety of healthcare settings exist in these virtual worlds, some educators might want to create their own hospitals, clinics, or community centers and customize their appearance. The same activities that can be conducted in an actual or simulated situation can be created in these virtual worlds. Faculty and students can interact in these settings in a number of ways. They can create avatars (computer-generated representations of themselves) and participate in activities that provide new content or require them to apply newly gained knowledge to patient-care scenarios (Creutzfeld, Hedman, & Felländer-Tsai, 2016).

The level of complexity in virtual-reality settings typically can be manipulated in much the same way face-to-face simulations can be adjusted based on the objectives of the activity. Although there is limited research on the effect of these programs on actual educational outcomes (Graafland, Schraagen, & Schijven, 2012; Kyaw et al., 2019; Moro, Štromberga, Raikos, & Stirling, 2017), students—especially those of the millennial generation who have much computer and gaming experience—quickly accept this format and enjoy participating in these simulations (Tan et al., 2017; Weiss, Bongartz, Boll, & Heuten, 2018).

The most recent development in virtual worlds is *mixed reality*, or hybrid reality—the merging of real and virtual worlds to produce new environments and visualizations in which physical and digital objects co-exist and interact in real time (Condino et al., 2018; Pfandler, Lazarovici, Stefan, Wucherer, & Weigl, 2017). For example, for lumbar laminectomy training, a digital virtual world could show the immersive operating room (OR) and the patient set up for the learner to perform the laminectomy. After the learner

ensures the right patient has moved to the OR, the patient is properly positioned, and anesthesia is being administered, the learner can move over to the physical laminectomy simulator, which uses augmented reality to digitally enhance a real environment that includes the simulator, and begin the surgery. The learner incises the skin, dissects the layers of tissue, performs the laminectomy, places the pedicle screw, and performs the lumbar stenosis decompression surgery (Coelho & Defino, 2018; Pfandler et al., 2017). Through mixed reality, the learner visualizes the incision made and the layers of tissue, selects the site, and performs the screw placement while in the digital environment. The learner practices the technique and receives feedback on the consistency of his or her technique.

Serious gaming—the use of a game designed with a purpose other than entertainment— is another form of simulation that is being integrated into the academic setting. In healthcare education, games are being developed to teach specific content, technical skills, and teamwork. Similar to computer screen–based simulations, serious games are a more sophisticated form of simulation that allows learners to make clinical decisions and respond to the patient or team reactions (Chang, Poh, Wong, Yap, & Yap, 2015; Ijaz, Khan, Ali, Qadir, & Kamel Boulos, 2019; Tan et al., 2017). The environment is typically more visually enhanced and realistic, often with avatars. Individual learners and teams can work together on a common objective. Points can be accrued, and "leveling up" can be achieved by demonstrating greater content mastery.

Although games developed for educational purposes should be validated before being integrated into the curricula of academic programs, faculty should consider how this type of simulation might be used to achieve course objectives and acquire competencies. The University of Wisconsin keeps an updated list of online games and simulations for healthcare (http://healthcaregames.wisc.edu/index.php).

Acquisition and Mastery of Psychomotor Skills

When the ethics of learning skills on real patients began to be questioned, educators knew they had to find a better way, which led to the adoption of simulation. Effective practice includes both technical and cognitive components (Shinnick, Woo, & Mentes, 2011; Smiley, 2019). Simulation presents the unique opportunity for deliberate practice in the quest to obtain mastery of psychomotor skills (Clapper & Kardong-Edgren, 2012).

Educators can use several approaches to help students to develop their psychomotor skills. The skill can be deconstructed into parts, providing students with smaller tasks that might be more manageable in the beginning. After students can perform the smaller tasks, the skill is reconstructed into the whole. An alternative is to have students watch someone perform the skill and then demonstrate the skill themselves. The educator can walk students through the skill the first time and then have students try to perform the skill without any guidance. It is imperative that learners practice performing the skill correctly. If students have a question or need guidance and an educator is not available, they can use a video that demonstrates the procedure as the guide.

After students have been shown how to perform a skill, the road to mastery is practice. Students must identify the need to perfect their performance. Self-regulated learning is essential in developing and maintaining competence (Artino et al., 2012). Practicing healthcare providers have an obligation to self-regulate and

seek opportunities to practice to maintain a level of proficiency. Promoting this accountability should begin during initial academic preparation for the role of a healthcare provider. For self-regulated learning to be successful, the deliberate practice process must be taught. Critical reflection causes learners to actively seek new learning experiences fueled by the thought that they do not know how to do a skill well enough (Clapper & Kardong-Edgren, 2012).

Deliberate practice is designed for learners to practice skills. It is good to consider selecting skills for deliberate practice that learners fear or dislike practicing because those skills are the ones that often lead to failure or error (Cloud, 2008; Ericsson, 2006). Deliberate practice can result in learners increasing the speed at which the task is performed, but that is not the goal. The goal is for learners to master skill performance and to gain the cognitive knowledge and attitudes needed to anticipate potential problems and the next steps to take if these problems arise (Ericsson, 2006).

It is essential, therefore, to provide students with adequate opportunities to practice performing skills in a safe environment. Ericsson (2008; Ericsson & Harwell, 2019) proposes that the best training situations for developing mastery are most often those that include immediate feedback, reflection, and correction, followed by opportunities to practice the task again until it can be completed with consistent success. A meta-analysis of literature addressing simulation-based medical education (SBME) with deliberate practice compared to results from traditional clinical education found that SBME is superior for acquiring a range of medical skills (Fraser et al., 2009; McGaghie, Issenberg, Cohen, Barsuk, & Wayne, 2011; Nestel, Groom, Eikeland-Husebø, & O'Donnell, 2011). However, concerns remain about students' ability to transfer knowledge and skills from the learning laboratory to actual patient care areas (Ross, 2012). Learning a skill in isolation without the complexities of real clinical practice is not necessarily sufficient. Educators can create integrated simulated scenarios that provide a contextual learning environment along with clinical scenarios that are either commonly encountered or occur infrequently but require application of cognitive knowledge. These simulations should challenge students to think about individual patient characteristics or clinical nuances that might affect the decision to continue on to skill performance or to determine another course of action.

A novel approach to SBME that is receiving increasing attention is rapid cycle deliberate practice (RCDP). *RCDP* combines deliberate practice and customized directive feedback. In this approach, learners are interrupted when an error in skill performance, decision-making, or other area of interest occurs. Facilitators provide targeted feedback on what was done incorrectly, and learners can ask questions. The simulation is then "rewound" to an earlier point, and the scenario restarts. Progress continues until the next time an error is made, at which point the scenario is halted again, directed feedback is provided, and the scenario is restarted at a point before the most recent error occurred. This cycle continues with the goal of mastery learning.

Preparing Students for Clinical Practice

The Agency for Healthcare Research and Quality (AHRQ) has identified failure to identify early signs of deteriorating patient conditions, as well as failure to rescue patients in a timely fashion after a complication has occurred, as a quality and efficiency issue (AHRQ, 2017). For almost two decades, failure to rescue has been recognized as a preventable patient complication (Coates et al., 2017; Ghaferi & Dimick, 2015). Level of

education, human error, lack of knowledge, and poor performance contribute to the lack of safety.

Simulation is a method to address failure-to-rescue events (Blackburn, Harkless, & Garvey, 2014; Schubert, 2012; Sheetz, Dimick, & Ghaferi, 2016). Exposure to these sorts of situations in a simulated environment enables students to work through potential emergent or infrequent situations that occur in clinical practice, so they become proficient in responding. Preparing students to care for patients in these dynamic situations is the goal of all healthcare educators, and simulation is a powerful tool to achieve this goal. Simulation activities focused on developing cue recognition, clinical judgment, diagnostic reasoning, and managing responses to quickly changing situations can be interspersed throughout the academic program. Situations encountered in clinical practice are often unpredictable. As such, behaviors taught to students cannot be so rigid that clinical reasoning is not expected or permitted. In fact, clinical judgments based on the information known and a reasonable understanding of similar situations must be cultivated in students.

In actual clinical settings, patient information is often missing or incomplete, but decisions must still be made. Using unfolding case studies is a popular way to promote clinical reasoning and provide students with opportunities to make decisions about patient needs. In unfolding cases, a staged scenario approach is used to incorporate the fluid nature of clinical reasoning. This approach enables students to experience changes in a client's condition based on the planned scenario and the decisions and actions taken by the learner within that scenario (Baldwin, 2007; Bowman, 2017; Zook, Hulton, Dudding, Stewart, & Graham, 2018). A series of scenarios related to the initial case, set in consecutive time frames, provides an opportunity to react to various situations at each point along a timeline. After the series of cases is complete, learners are required to reflect on the decisions they made. These exercises provide opportunities to think in ways similar to that required in actual clinical practice.

Regardless of the specific simulation method used, simulation provides effective ways to prepare students for clinical practice. Establishing scenarios in which students encounter commonly occurring abnormal findings prepares students to more quickly recognize subtle variations in physiologic and physical data and prepare them to respond appropriately. Designing scenarios around low-frequency, high-risk situations can prepare students to recognize the signs and symptoms of situations that often result in poor outcomes. Simulation has also been found to be an effective method to develop students' ethical decision-making skills (Basak & Cerit, 2019), provide culturally competent care (Levett-Jones, Everson, & Lapkin, 2019), develop prioritization skills (Harder, Stevenson, & Turner (2019), and improve knowledge and attitudes of end-of-life care (Campbell, Trojanowski, & Smith, 2020).

When educators are sure that students' confidence is strong, they can include greater complexity, more complicated patients, greater numbers of patients, and misinformation or misleading information. Deliberately misleading students so they make mistakes might seem to be unethical, but it provides students with opportunities to make mistakes and manage the consequences.

The number of training programs for nurses, occupational therapists, and other healthcare professionals continues to increase, resulting in greater competition for quality clinical placement sites. At the same time, quality initiatives within acute care settings have reduced the number of healthcare providers-in-training permitted to be on a medical unit at one time. Until recently, there were no alternatives to clinical fieldwork.

With the adoption of high-fidelity simulation, and educators' increasing familiarity with simulation technologies, their application to patient care, and improved debriefing techniques, the question of whether simulation can be used as an alternative to traditional clinical training has arisen. The National Council of State Boards of Nursing (NCSBN) designed a longitudinal, randomized, controlled, multisite trial using nursing programs from across the United States to examine if time and the activities in a simulation laboratory could effectively substitute for traditional clinical hours in the pre-licensure nursing curriculum. Results indicate that up to 50% of traditional clinical experience in all pre-licensure core nursing courses can effectively be replaced by simulation with trained simulationists under conditions comparable to those described in the study (NCSBN, 2014). A recent meta-narrative review by Roberts, Kaak, and Rolley (2019) found support for these results. There is, however, great variability in the United States in how State Boards of Nursing are defining and regulating the use of simulation in prelicensure nursing programs (Bradley et al., 2019). Comparable studies in other healthcare areas may show similar results and provide alternatives to clinical placements.

Developing Team-Based and Interprofessional Practice Competencies

Developing the competencies associated with interprofessional practice, including effective communication and teamwork, is recognized as essential to maximizing patient outcomes and improving patient safety (Interprofessional Education Collaborative [IPEC] Expert Panel,

2011). Because communication and teamwork are such important issues, interprofessional collaborative simulations in academic programs typically focus on closed-loop communication, role identity, and leadership. Interprofessional education (IPE) addressing these core concepts, followed by a series of simulations involving commonly encountered clinical situations, can result in greater understanding of team member roles, knowledge base, perspective, and contributions to clinical issues (Robertson et al., 2010). With these improvements, interprofessional collaboration is enhanced, resulting in the provision of safe and quality care, improved systems, and cost reduction. Participation in simulations with students from other healthcare disciplines in which effective approaches to interprofessional collaboration are explored is expected to become a core content area for health professions education (IPEC Expert Panel, 2011).

Numerous challenges exist when attempting to conduct IPE in academic settings. The most significant challenge is that education in healthcare programs typically occurs in silos. Course and clinical schedules are often so diverse that it is exceedingly difficult to find a mutually agreeable time to bring students together for IPE (IPEC Expert Panel, 2011; Robertson et al., 2010). Another challenge can be a lack of administrative leadership support to provide resources for IPE. Many health professions schools are not on academic health science campuses. Thus, the students from one school have no students representing other healthcare disciplines with whom they can conveniently interact. Regardless of whether the various schools for the different healthcare professions are located on the same or different campuses, faculty from the schools involved in IPE need to be knowledgeable about

the interprofessional competencies as well as the techniques of IPE.

Historically, there has been a lack of recognition by accreditors of health professions schools of the vital need to provide substantive opportunities for their students to acquire the competencies for effective interprofessional practice. However, these bodies are increasingly mandating the inclusion of IPE in schools that prepare health professionals. Simulation is an effective way to meet this requirement. In 2012, the Society for Simulation in Healthcare (SSH), in partnership with the National League for Nursing (NLN & Laerdal Medical, 2010), produced a white paper describing the advantages of simulation-enhanced IPE and providing a roadmap to its integration into both academic and clinical settings (Wilhaus et al., 2012). The work of Gannon et al. (2020) provides an example of using simulation to teach students IPE. They used multistation simulations to reinforce interprofessional communication and huddle behaviors to nursing, pharmacy, and medical students. Communication improved, and there were fewer care delays and less harm when huddle time increased.

An important aspect of learning with simulation is the debriefing that occurs after the scenario is over (see Chapter 5). Debriefing an IPE experience has some unique challenges. During debriefing, discussion and reflection help move learners to new perspectives, understanding, and skills. In simulation scenarios designed to acquire competencies associated with interprofessional practice, facilitators in the debriefing need to be sure to focus on the knowledge, behaviors, skills, and attitudes associated with interprofessional practice—not necessarily the clinical situation itself. It is also important for facilitators to discuss in advance how role-specific questions and reflections will be handled. For example, will there be representation from the faculty from each school present during the debriefing? See Chapter 9 for tips on how to develop interprofessional simulations. Some simulations associated with team training require little technology to be successful. Role-playing activities involving students, educators, or actors do not need to be held in a simulation center. They can be held in the classroom. Simulations used to teach or evaluate communication skills require only one other person acting in a particular way for the student to learn how to employ effective communication skills. If faculty members role-play first, students can observe how they communicate effectively in challenging situations. Students then can be asked to participate in subsequent scenarios. Communication scenarios for students in the health professions typically focus on patient encounters, interprofessional communication challenges, and topics such as breaking bad news. Communication approaches such as active listening skills and the use of nonverbal/body language can be areas explored in simulations. Debriefing after these simulations can concentrate on challenges encountered and alternative approaches that could be used.

Likewise, scenarios exploring leadership skills can be conducted with little use of technology. Role-playing conducted around a conference table can be used to explore students' abilities to negotiate, bargain, and build consensus. Scenarios can be conducted using a few students at a time. If the capability exists, additional students in an adjacent room can observe through a one-way window. If video recording is available, simulations can be taped and viewed in class at a later time or broadcast synchronously to a classroom where students are observing. This provides an opportunity for all students of different professions to participate in the scenario by asking student observers to critique approaches and explore various alternatives.

Aligning Technology With Objectives

For the purpose of educating new healthcare professionals, beyond the ethics, the use of simulators has several significant advantages over the use of actual patients:

- Simulators enable educators to create the "deliberate practice" training conditions that expedite skills development (AHRQ, 2013; Marcus, Vakharia, Kirkman, Murphy, & Nandi, 2013).

- Simulators make it possible for educators and learners, rather than patient availability, to set the learning agenda.

- Simulators give learners permission to fail and to see the natural consequences of making an error without patients suffering adverse clinical consequences (Gordon, Wilkerson, Shaffer, & Armstrong, 2001; Lame & Dixon-Woods, 2018).

- Simulators provide greater opportunity for practice (Kneebone, 2003; Mahoney & Saloum, 2020).

Using the vast array of available simulators for these purposes requires an educator who is highly familiar with the capabilities of the simulators to achieve the desired educational outcomes.

To create a successful simulation, educators must first have clear learning objectives. With these in mind, it is essential to select a methodology and technology (simulator) with capabilities that are aligned with the objectives. For example, if the objective is to teach students how to record a 12-lead electrocardiogram (ECG), choosing a technology that requires the student to attach leads to a patient's chest is essential. Whether a full-sized, lifelike mannequin or a static torso should be used depends on the objectives to be achieved. If the objective is to have the student demonstrate appropriate lead placement, then either type of mannequin will work. A few online programs—some available free of charge and others accessible for a small fee—require students to place the leads appropriately before permitting them to progress to the next step. However, if the learner is expected to determine whether the ECG tracing obtained from the machine is appropriate, then a simulator that provides a 12-lead ECG tracing must be used. This can be done with a full-sized mannequin or with actors who have the ECG actually performed on them. This example illustrates why determining the objectives before choosing the simulator is so important.

Another example of aligning technology with objectives is teaching skill acquisition. Task trainers are designed to replicate a part of a system (e.g., the human body) or process. The learning objectives associated with these simulators are often task specific. Examples include intubation mannequins, IV arms, and surgical device or procedure simulators. The advantages of these devices include standardization, portability, and skill specificity. The disadvantages include a lowered ability to suspend disbelief due to the single task purpose of the trainer. When used in conjunction with integrated simulators or higher technology simulators, however, this disadvantage can largely be overcome (Beaubien & Baker, 2004).

Some simulators not only teach skill acquisition but also evaluate diagnostic abilities. An example is OtoSim. OtoSim is a simulator that provides the learner with the opportunity to hold and use an otoscope, manipulate the auricle of the ear, and diagnose a variety of internal ear canal or tympanic membrane disorders. Verifying accuracy of the learner's diagnosis of the ear malady requires re-instrumentation of the ear and

may cause discomfort. However, using a simulator such as OtoSim provides an alternative to learning on a real patient. This technology has multiple examples of ear disorders; with the attached laptop, the instructor can display a particular disorder and require the learner to correctly diagnose it and describe where in the simulated ear canal it is found.

When learners need to be able to perceive tactile or other stimuli, educators can use haptic systems. This virtual-reality technology offers an opportunity for learners to practice skills, including surgical techniques, bronchoscopy, and intravenous and central line catheterization. Sensors can be placed within a task trainer to detect pressure and presence during learner activities such as those associated with learning pelvic exams and surgical procedures (Durham & Alden, 2008). These high-technology simulators lend an added high-fidelity dimension to simulations (Decker, Sportsman, Puetz, & Billings, 2008), but can also increase the overall cost of the simulation experience. Starting with the educational objective in mind helps educators make cost-effective decisions.

When a high degree of realism is needed for the simulation scenario, full-body simulators of an adult, child, or infant that are capable of responding to certain medications, chest compressions, needle decompression, chest tube placement, and other physiologic interventions and subsequent responses are desirable (Galloway, 2009). Full-body simulators help suspend disbelief during a simulation. This is due to computer technology housed in the mannequin that enables it to respond in real time to specific care interventions and treatments.

Role-play can be an effective and efficient simulation method, especially in the realms of team training or changing attitudes (Aldrich,

2005). Role-play, using students, educators, or staff to act out a particular role, can be an effective way to simulate a situation. Although it is helpful to role-play in a contextually relevant setting (e.g., home, hospital, or office), it is not essential to do that for the simulation to be effective.

For objectives such as learning how to conduct a physical assessment, take a patient history, communicate bad news, practice a psychiatric intervention, or even perform a pelvic or prostate examination, standardized patients or actors can be the simulation technology of choice. The use of standardized patients has been found to help students gain self-awareness of their communication and clinical strengths and weaknesses, their reactions to stressful situations, and their biases (Shemanko & Jones, 2008). A well-trained standardized patient with a good script is very effective at suspending disbelief in the scenario and creating a valuable learning experience.

Using Simulation for Instruction or Evaluation

Simulation can be used for instructional or evaluative purposes. Designing an effective and efficient simulation requires clarity of purpose. Is the session being designed as a formative learning experience (to monitor the student's learning and provide feedback) in which learners are allowed to make mistakes and the educator can suspend time, provide needed instruction, and then restart the scenario? Or, is the simulation being used as a summative experience (to evaluate learning by comparing to a benchmark or standard of performance) in which the participant is expected to make clinical decisions and provide safe and competent care with little or no interference from the educator? Having clarified the purpose of the simulation, educators are better able to decide on

the most appropriate technology and approach to use to achieve the educational objectives and purpose.

The decision to interrupt the flow of the simulation to provide instruction to learners or to enable learners to work through the entire scenario without direction or interference from the instructor or facilitator dictates how the scenario will be built. This is an important decision that affects the performance and confidence of participants and the perceived success of the simulation. Educators should consider two issues before finalizing this decision:

- **The level of students participating in the simulation:** Will the simulation involve first-semester students learning basic tasks or senior students with the knowledge, skills, and abilities to successfully participate without assistance or direction? If the students are at the beginning level of knowledge development, then educators should be prepared to interrupt the flow of the scenario to clarify concepts or to redirect the scenario and should allot time for the interruptions.

- **The educators' ability to respond to all possible responses learners might have to the clinical situation presented:** This takes much planning with novice learners because the likelihood of them straying from expected approaches is high. However, as the level of learner knowledge and sophistication increases, the alternatives are more easily anticipated, and the scenario can be permitted to progress with little to no interruption.

An example of a simulation that can be interrupted so feedback and instruction can be provided is a scenario in which nursing students are learning safe medication administration. In this example, students have had several opportunities to practice the five rights of medication administration, so they are aware they should perform three medication checks before dispensing the medication. In this simulation, the students are to enter a patient's room in the simulation center. After washing their hands, they are to introduce themselves to the patient, confirm that the patient in the bed is indeed the right patient, and administer the medication. But the students don't do that. Instead, they introduce themselves and tell the patient they are going to prepare the medications. They don't check the patient's armband, check the patient's name, or ask the patient for his or her date of birth. Instead, the students move directly to getting the medications from the drawer. Should the simulation be stopped, and the students told what has happened, or should the simulation be allowed to progress? If the objective of this simulation experience is learning as opposed to evaluation, stopping the simulation and discussing what has happened is appropriate. Before moving forward, the students can be refocused on the correct process and reflect on what they need to know and how they might do things differently. When this is complete, the scenario can be restarted, or the group can be moved to a more intensive debriefing session for further exploration.

Although it is easy to see why one would design uninterrupted simulations for evaluation purposes, simulations designed for learning also can be developed to run uninterrupted. These types of simulations are often used in academic environments to allow learners the opportunity to apply knowledge they have gained, work with others, respond to available data, and experience the natural outcomes of their decisions. When the scenario is completed, a debriefing session is conducted to allow for reflection and to review

perceptions of what actually occurred. In the debriefing, facilitators cover the cause and effect of decisions made and actions taken. In addition, facilitators should ensure that any problems encountered are explored.

An example of a learning simulation that would be permitted to go to its conclusion is one in which a nurse calls the rapid response team to evaluate a patient who has become progressively more dyspneic, tachycardic, and hypoxic, with a pulse oximetry reading of 86%. To determine whether students have developed the skills to quickly gather data, assess the patient, and decide whether the patient requires intubation, this scenario is allowed to unfold naturally without interruption. The students recognize the need to increase the patient's oxygen supply. And after placing a 100% non-rebreather mask on the patient and not achieving a response, the students decide to call anesthesia to intubate the patient. The students support the patient until intubated. The scenario ends. Afterward, a debriefing session provides participants the opportunity to react to the scenario, reflect on their actions and interactions with the patient and team, and discuss whether alternative approaches to care should have been considered. After all points are reviewed, the facilitator summarizes the important elements and ends the session. Note that the learners in this case were at a point in their education where they should be able to deliver a reasonable amount of quality and safe care. Thus, they are permitted to complete the simulation without interruption.

Simulations can be used for either formative or summative assessment. Either way, simulations must be designed so they can be implemented in a consistent manner. When students are being tested in high-stakes situations, such as assessing their mastery of content or competence, then uniformity is essential. Objective Structured Clinical Examinations (OSCEs), a form of simulation, have been used in the education of physicians to evaluate competence since the 1970s (Turner & Dankoski, 2008; Warner et al., 2020) and are increasingly being used in other professional disciplines. The overarching philosophy for OSCEs is that all students (candidates) are presented with the same clinical tasks to be completed in the same time frame. Examiners score the students using structured marking schemes, being careful not to introduce bias (Gormley, 2011). During the OSCE, candidates are observed and evaluated as they go through a series of stations in which they interview, examine, and treat standardized patients who present with some type of medical problem. The length of the OSCE station is generally 5 to 20 minutes, and candidates are expected to participate in the encounter as they would in an actual clinical setting. In some OSCEs, an examiner (usually a licensed professional in the same profession as the student) is present to assess clinical and communication skills using a standardized checklist. Some OSCEs are video recorded and are later assessed by more than one examiner (OSCEhome, n.d.).

Using high-fidelity simulation for high-stakes testing or evaluation in pre-licensure programs is a growing area of interest. *High-stakes testing* is defined as an evaluation process associated with a simulation activity in which learners must demonstrate a pre-determined level of performance or they will experience a major consequence such as failing a course or being unable to progress in a program (Bensfield, Olech, & Horsley, 2012; NLN & Laerdal Medical, 2010; Rizzolo, Kardong-Edgren, Oermann, & Jeffries, 2015). Issues around developing a valid and reliable evaluation tool and establishing inter- and intra-rater reliability between evaluators are being explored and are just beginning to be found in the literature (Kardong-Edgren, Oermann, Rizzolo, & Odom-Maryon, 2017).

Conclusion

Many educators assume the only way to use simulation in the academic setting is to have a large facility outfitted with a full array of high-technology simulators. Although nice, this setup is not a requirement to successfully integrate simulation into an academic program. What is necessary is having educators familiar with educational theory who can develop clinical scenarios, select appropriate simulation methods and equipment based on defined educational objectives, and understand how to effectively debrief a simulation-based educational session. Simulation as a teaching and learning strategy has greatly expanded educators' toolkit. When they are familiar with the full array of simulation methodologies, educators in an academic setting are limited only by their creativity.

References

Agency for Healthcare Research and Quality. (2013). *Making health care safer II: An updated critical analysis of the evidence for patient safety practices.* Retrieved from https://www.ahrq.gov/sites/default/files/wysiwyg/research/findings/evidence-based-reports/services/quality/patientsftyupdate/ptsafetyII-full.pdf

Agency for Healthcare Research and Quality. (2017). *National healthcare quality and disparities report.* Rockville, MD: Author. Retrieved from https://www.ahrq.gov/research/findings/nhqrdr/nhqdr17/index.html

Aldrich, C. (2005). *Learning by doing: A comprehensive guide to simulations, computer games, and pedagogy in e-learning and other educational experiences.* San Francisco, CA: Pfeiffer & Co.

Artino, A. R., Dong, T., DeZee, K. J., Gilliland, W. R., Waechter, D. M., Cruess, D., & Durning, S. J. (2012). Achievement goal structures and self-regulated learning: Relationships and changes in medical school. *Academic Medicine, 87*(10), 1375-1381.

Baldwin, K. B. (2007). Friday night in the pediatric emergency department: A simulated exercise to promote clinical reasoning in the classroom. *Nurse Educator, 32*(1), 24-29.

Bantz, D., Dancer, M. M., Hodson-Carlton, K., & Van Hove, S. (2007). A daylong clinical laboratory: From gaming to high-fidelity simulators. *Nurse Educator, 32*(6), 274-277. doi:10.1097/01.NNE.0000299476.57185.f3

Basak, T., & Cerit, B. (2019). Comparing two teaching methods on nursing students' ethical decision-making level. *Clinical Simulation in Nursing, 29*, 15-23.

Beaubien, J. M., & Baker, D. P. (2004). The use of simulation for training teamwork skills in health care: How low can you go? *Quality and Safety in Health Care, 13*(Suppl. 1), i51-i56. doi:10.1136/qshc.2004.009845

Bensfield, L.A., Olech, M. J., & Horsley, T. L. (2012). Simulation for high-stakes evaluation in nursing. *Nurse Educator, 37*(2), 71-74. doi:10.1097/NNE.0b013e3182461b8c

Blackburn, L. M., Harkless, S., & Garvey, P. (2014). Using failure-to-rescue simulation to assess the performance of advanced practice professionals. *Clinical Journal of Oncology Nursing, 18*(3), 301-306. doi:10.1188/14.CJON.301-306

Bowman, K. (2017). Use of online unfolding case studies to foster critical thinking. *Journal of Nursing Education. 56*(11), 701-702. doi:10.3928/01484834-20171020-13

Bradley, C. S., Johnson, B. K., Driefuerst, K. T., White, P., Conde, S. K., Meakim, C. H., ... Childress, R. M. (2019). Regulation of simulation use in United States prelicensure nursing programs. *Clinical Simulation in Nursing, 33*, 17-25.

Campbell, D., Trojanowski, S., & Smith, L. M. (2020). An interprofessional end-of-life simulation to improve knowledge and attitudes of end-of-life care among nursing and physical therapy students. *Rehabilitation Oncology, 38*, 45-51.

Chang, H. Y., Poh, D. Y. H., Wong, L. L., Yap, J. Y.G., & Yap, K. Y. (2015). Student preferences on gaming aspects for a serious game in pharmacy practice education: A cross-sectional study. *JMIR Medical Education, 1*(1), e2. doi:10.2196/mededu.3754

Clapper, T. C. (2010). Beyond Knowles: What those conducting simulation need to know about adult learning theory. *Clinical Simulation in Nursing, 6*(1), e7-e14. doi:10.1016/j.ecns.2009.07.003

Clapper, T. C., & Kardong-Edgren, S. (2012). Using deliberate practice and simulation to improve nursing skills. *Clinical Simulation in Nursing, 8*(3), e109-3113. doi:10.1016/j.ecns.2010.12.001

Cloud, J. (2008, February 28). The science of experience. *Time.* Retrieved from http://content.time.com/time/magazine/article/0,9171,1718551,00.html

Coates, M., Pillado, E., Kim, J., Vasak, R., Yule, A., & Kim, D. Y. (2017). Role of preventability in redefining failure to rescue among major trauma patients. *JAMA Surgery, 152*(11),1083-1084. doi:10.1001/jamasurg.2017.2351

Coelho, G., & Defino, H. L. A. (2018). Role of mixed reality simulation for surgical training in spine: Phase 1 validation. *Spine, 43*(22), 1609-1616. doi:10.1097/BRS.0000000000002856

Condino, S., Turini, G., Parchi, P. D., Viglialoro, R. M., Piolanti, N., Gesi, M., ... Ferrari, V. (2018). How to build a patient-specific hybrid simulator for orthopaedic open surgery: Benefits and limits of mixed-reality using the Microsoft HoloLens, *Journal of Healthcare Engineering*, article ID 5435097. doi:10.1155/2018/5435097

Creutzfeldt, J., Hedman, L., & Felländer-Tsai, L. (2016). Cardiopulmonary resuscitation training by avatars: A qualitative study of medical students' experiences using a multiplayer virtual world. *JMIR Serious Games, 4*(2), e22. doi:10.2196/games.6448

Decker, S., Sportsman, S., Puetz, L., & Billings, L. (2008). The evolution of simulation and its contribution to competency. *The Journal of Continuing Education in Nursing, 39*(2), 74-80.

Durham, C. F., & Alden, K. R. (2008). Enhancing patient safety in nursing education through patient simulation. In R. G. Hughes (Ed.), *Patient safety and quality: An evidence-based handbook for nurses* (Chapter 51). Rockville, MD: Agency for Healthcare Research and Quality. Retrieved from https://archive.ahrq.gov/professionals/clinicians-providers/resources/nursing/resources/nurseshdbk/nurseshdbk.pdf

Ericsson, K. A. (2006). The influence of experience and deliberate practice on the development of superior expert performance. In K. A. Ericsson, N. Charness, R. R. Hoffman, & P. J. Feltovich (Eds.), *The Cambridge handbook of expertise and expert performance* (pp. 683-703). New York, NY: Cambridge University Press.

Ericsson, K. A. (2008). Deliberate practice and acquisition of expert performance: A general overview. *Academic Emergency Medicine, 15*(11), 988-994. doi:10.1111/j.1553-2712.2008.00227.x

Ericsson, K. A., & Harwell, K. W. (2019). Deliberate practice and proposed limits on the effects of practice on the acquisition of expert performance: Why the original definition matters and recommendations for future research. *Frontiers in Psychology, 10*, 2396. doi: 10.3389/fpsyg.2019.02396

Fraser, K., Peets, A., Walker, I., Tworek, J., Paget, M., Wright, B., & McLaughlin, K. (2009). The effect of simulator training on clinical skills acquisition, retention and transfer. *Medical Education, 43*(8), 784-789. doi:10.1111/j.1365-2923.2009.03412.x

Galloway, S. J. (2009). Simulation techniques to bridge the gap between novice and competent healthcare professionals. *OJIN: The Online Journal of Issues in Nursing, 14*(2), Manuscript 3. doi:10.3912/OJIN.Vol14No02Man03

Gannon, J. M., Egelund, E. F., Genuardi, F., Simon, L. V., Morrissey, T. K., Gautam, S., ... Motycka, C. A. (2020). Multistation simulations and deliberate practice to reinforce huddle behaviors in interprofessional student teams. *Clinical Simulation in Nursing, 40*, 17–24.

Ghaferi, A. A., & Dimick, J. B. (2015). Understanding failure to rescue and improving safety culture. *Annals of Surgery, 261*(5), 839-840. doi:10.1097/SLA.0000000000001135

Gordon, J. A., Wilkerson, W. M., Shaffer, D. W., & Armstrong, E. G. (2001). "Practicing" medicine without risk: Students' and educators' responses to high-fidelity simulation. *Academic Medicine, 76*(5), 469-472.

Gormley, G. (2011). Summative OSCEs in undergraduate medical education. *Ulster Medical Journal, 80*(3), 127-132.

Graafland, M., Schraagen, J. M. C., & Schijven, M. P. (2012). Systematic review of serious games for medical education and surgical skills training. *British Journal of Surgery, 99*(10), 1322-1330. doi:10.1002/bjs.8819

Harder, N., Stevenson, M., & Turner, S. (2019). Using simulation design characteristics in a non-manikin learning activity to teach prioritization skills to undergraduate nursing students. *Clinical Simulation in Nursing, 36*, 18–21.

Ijaz, A., Khan, M. Y., Ali, S. M., Qadir, J., & Kamel Boulos, M. N. (2019). Serious games for healthcare professional training: A systematic review. *European Journal of Biomedical Informatics, 15*(1) 12–28. doi:10.24105/ejbi.2019.15.1.3

Institute of Medicine. (2011). *The future of nursing: Leading change, advancing health.* Washington, DC: The National Academies Press. Retrieved from http://www.nationalacademies.org/hmd/Reports/2010/The-Future-of-Nursing-Leading-Change-Advancing-Health.aspx

Interprofessional Education Collaborative Expert Panel. (2011). *Core competencies for interprofessional collaborative practice.* Retrieved from https://www.aacom.org/docs/default-source/insideome/ccrpt05-10-11.pdf?sfvrsn=77937f97_2

Kardong-Edgren, S., Oermann, M. H., Rizzolo, M. A., & Odom-Maryon, T. (2017). Establishing inter- and intrarater reliability for high-stakes testing using simulation. *Nursing Education Perspectives, 38*(2), 63-68. doi:10.1097/01.NEP.0000000000000114

Kneebone, R. (2003). Simulation in surgical training: Educational issues and practical implications. *Medical Education, 37*(3), 267-277.

Knowles, M. S. (1996). Adult learning. In R. L. Craig (Ed.), *The ASTD training and development handbook: A guide to human resource development* (4th ed., pp. 253-264). New York, NY: McGraw-Hill.

Kolb, D. A. (1984). *Experiential learning: Experience as the source of learning and development.* Englewood Cliffs, NJ: Prentice-Hall.

Kyaw, B. M., Saxena, N., Posadzki, P., Vseteckova, J., Nikolaou, C. K., George, P. P., ... Car, L. T. (2019). Virtual reality for health professions education: Systematic review and meta-analysis by the Digital Health Education Collaborative. *Journal of Medical Internet Research, 21*(1), e12959. doi:10.2196/12959

Lamé, G., & Dixon-Woods, M. (2018). Using clinical simulation to study how to improve quality and safety in healthcare. *BMJ Simulation and Technology Enhanced Learning.* Published Online First: 29 September 2018. doi:10.1136/bmjstel-2018-000370

Lateef, F. (2010). Simulation-based learning: Just like the real thing. *Journal of Emergencies, Trauma, and Shock, 3*(4), 348-352. doi:10.4103/0974-2700.70743

Levett-Jones, T., Everson, N., & Lapkin, S. (2019). Exploring the impact of a 3D simulation on nursing students' intention to provide culturally competent care. *Clinical Simulation in Nursing, 36*, 22–29.

Lineberry, M., Dev. P., Lane, H. C., & Talbot, T. B. (2018). Learner adaptive educational technology for simulation in healthcare: Foundations and opportunities. *Simulation in Healthcare, 13*(3S Suppl. 1), S21-S27. doi:10.1097/SIH.0000000000000274

Mahoney, B., & Saloum, M. H. (2020) Graduate medical education. In B. Mahoney, R. Minehart, & M. Pian-Smith. (Eds.), *Comprehensive healthcare simulation: Anesthesiology.* (pp. 143–169). Cham, Switzerland: Springer. doi:10.1007/978-3-030-26849-7_14

Marcus, H., Vakharia, V., Kirkman, M. A., Murphy, M., & Nandi, D. (2013). Practice makes perfect? The role of simulation-based deliberate practice and script-based mental rehearsal in acquisition and maintenance of operative neurosurgical skills. *Neurosurgery, 72*(Suppl. 1), 124-130. doi:10.1227/NEU.0b013e318270d010

McGaghie, W. C., & Harris, I. B. (2018). Learning theory foundations of simulation-based mastery learning. *Simulation in Healthcare, 13*(Suppl. 1), S15-S20. doi:10.1097/SIH.0000000000000279

McGaghie, W. C., Issenberg, S. B., Cohen, E. R., Barsuk, J. H., & Wayne, D. B. (2011). Does simulation-based medical education with deliberate practice yield better results than traditional clinical education? A meta-analytic comparative review of the evidence. *Academic Medicine, 86*(6), 706-711. doi:10.1097/ACM.0b013e318217e119

Moro, C., Štromberga, Z., Raikos, A. & Stirling, A. (2017). The effectiveness of virtual and augmented reality in health sciences and medical anatomy. *Anatomical Sciences Education, 10*(6), 549-559. doi:10.1002/ase.1696

National Council of State Boards of Nursing. (2014). The NCSBN national simulation study: A longitudinal, randomized, controlled study replacing clinical hours with simulation in pre-licensure nursing education. *Journal of Nursing Regulation, 5*(2) S1-S64. doi:10.1016/S2155-8256(15)30062-4

National League for Nursing & Laerdal Medical. (2010). *Think tank on simulation for high-stakes evaluation in nursing education.* Retrieved from http://www.nln.org/docs/default-source/professional-development-programs/report-of-think-tank-final.pdf?sfvrsn=2

Nestel, D., Groom, J., Eikeland-Husebø, S., & O'Donnell, J. M. (2011). Simulation for learning and teaching procedural skills: The state of the science. *Simulation in Healthcare, 6*(Suppl.), S10-S13. doi:10.1097/SIH.0b013e318227ce96

OSCEhome. (n.d.). What is objective structured clinical examination, OSCEs? Retrieved from http://www.oscehome.com/What_is_Objective-Structured-Clinical-Examination_OSCE.html

Pfandler, M., Lazarovici, M., Stefan, P., Wucherer, P., & Weigl, M. (2017). Virtual reality-based simulators for spine surgery: A systematic review. *The Spine Journal, 17*(9), 1352-1363. doi:10.1016/j.spinee.2017.05.016

Rizzolo, M. A., Kardong-Edgren, S., Oermann, M. H., & Jeffries, P. R. (2015). The National League for Nursing project to explore the use of simulation for high-stakes assessment: Process, outcomes, and recommendations. *Nursing Education Perspectives, 36*(5), 299–303. doi: 10.5480/15-1639

Roberts, E., Kaak, V., & Rolley, J. (2019). Simulation to replace clinical hours in nursing: A meta-narrative review. *Clinical Simulation in Nursing, 37,* 5–13.

Robertson, B., Kaplan, B., Atallah, H., Higgins, M., Lewitt, M. J., & Ander, D. S. (2010). The use of simulation and a modified TeamSTEPPS curriculum for medical and nursing student team training. *Simulation in Healthcare, 5*(6), 332-337. doi:10.1097/SIH.0b013e3181f008ad

Ross, J. G. (2012). Simulation and psychomotor skill acquisition: A review of the literature. *Clinical Simulation in Nursing, 8*(9), e429-e435. doi:10.1016/j.ecns.2011.04.004

Schubert, C. R. (2012). Effect of simulation on nursing knowledge and critical thinking in failure to rescue events. *Journal of Continuing Education in Nursing, 43*(10), 467-471. doi:10.3928/00220124-20120904-27

Sheetz, K. H., Dimick, J. B., & Ghaferi, A. A. (2016). Impact of hospital characteristics on failure to rescue following major surgery. *Annals of Surgery, 263*(4), 692-697. doi:10.1097/SLA. 0000000000001414

Shemanko, G. A., & Jones, L. (2008). To simulate or not to simulate. That is the question. In R. R. Kyle & W. B. Murray (Eds.), *Clinical simulation: Operations, engineering, and management* (pp. 77-84). Burlington, MA: Elsevier, Inc.

Shinnick, M. A., Woo, M. A., & Mentes, J. C. (2011). Human patient simulation: State of the science in prelicensure nursing education. *The Journal of Nursing Education, 50*(2), 65-72. doi:10.3928/01484834-20101230-01

Skillstat, Inc. (2013). *The 6 second ECG.* Retrieved from http://www.skillstat.com/tools/ecg-simulator#/-home

Smiley, R. A. (2019). Survey of simulation use in prelicensure nursing programs: Changes and advancements, 2010-2017. *Journal of Nursing Regulation. 9*(4), 48–61. doi:10.1016/S2155-8256(19)30016-X

Su, W. M., & Juestel, M. J. (2010). Direct teaching of thinking skills using clinical simulation. *Nurse Educator, 35*(5), 197-204. doi:10.1097/NNE.0b013e3181e33969

Tan, A. J. Q., Lee, C. C. S., Lin, P. Y., Cooper, S., Lau, L. S. T., Chua, W. L., & Liaw, S. Y. (2017). Designing and evaluating the effectiveness of a serious game for safe administration of blood transfusion: A randomized controlled trial. *Nurse Education Today, 55,* 38-44. doi:10.1016/j.nedt.2017.04.027

Thomas, A., Menon, A., Boruff, J., Rodriguez, A. M., & Ahmed, S. (2014). Applications of social constructivist learning theories in knowledge translation for healthcare professionals: A scoping review. *Implementation Science, 9,* 54. doi:10.1186/1748-5908-9-54

Turner, J. L., & Dankoski, M. E. (2008). Objective structured clinical exams: A critical review. *Family Medicine, 40*(8), 574-578.

Warner, D. O., Isaak, R. S., Peterson-Layne, C., Lien, C. A., Sun, H., Menzies, A. O. … Harman, A. E. (2020). Development of an objective structured clinical examination as a component of assessment for initial board certification in anesthesiology. *Anesthesia & Analgesia, 130*(1), 258–264. doi:10.1213/ANE.0000000000004496

Weiss, S., Bongartz, H., Boll, S. C. J., & Heuten, W. (2018). Applications of immersive virtual reality in nursing education: A review. 1 Clusterkonferenz Zukunft der Pflege—Innovative Technologien für die Praxis Oldenburg, Germany.

Wilhaus, J., Palaganas, J., Manos, J., Anderson, J., Cooper, A., Jeffries, P., … Mancini, M. E. (2012). *Interprofessional education and healthcare simulation symposium.* National League for Nursing. Retrieved from http://www.nln.org/docs/default-source/professional-development-programs/white-paper-symposium-ipe-in-healthcare-simulation-2013-(pdf).pdf?sfvrsn=0

Ziv, A., Wolpe, P. R., Small, S. D., & Glick, S. (2003). Simulation-based medical education: An ethical imperative. *Academic Medicine, 78*(8), 783-788.

Zook, S. S., Hulton, L. J., Dudding, C. C., Stewart, A. L., & Graham, A. C. (2018). Scaffolding interprofessional education: Unfolding case studies, virtual world simulations and patient-centered care. *Nurse Educator, 43*(2), 87-91. doi:10.1097/NNE.0000000000000430

"Simulation moves the sharp and dangerous edge of the learning curve away from patient care and services."

–Ian Curran, MD

Using Simulation in Hospitals and Healthcare Systems to Improve Outcomes

11

Thomas E. LeMaster, MSN, MEd, RN, CHSE, FSSH
Jennifer L. Manos, MBA, MSN, RN
Mary D. Patterson, MD, MEd, FSSH

OBJECTIVES

- Discuss the various opportunities for using simulation in a hospital or healthcare system.

- Describe how to identify a champion for the simulation program.

- Describe the initial planning for implementation of a simulation program.

- Identify the types of simulators used with different learners and courses.

- Describe the challenges of implementing a simulation program and potential solutions.

Simulation programs in clinical settings such as hospitals and healthcare systems are both similar to and different from those in academic settings. As with simulation programs in academic settings, those situated in clinical settings typically have a significant educational component focused on individuals. Some uses for simulation in clinical settings include (Agency for Healthcare Research and Quality [AHRQ], 2013; Ulrich, 2013):

- Onboarding new employees

- Assessing the competency of new or newly employed healthcare providers

- Assessing and maintaining individual competency

- Building and sustaining high-performing teams

- Testing new equipment for usability prior to implementation

- Testing new clinical services and patient care units

- Assessing processes for latent errors

- Other quality improvement or risk management activities

Page, Fairbanks, and Gaba (2018) identified priorities for improving healthcare safety through simulation. These include:

- Designing simulation-based activities to promote high reliability and cultural change in healthcare

- Creating and maintaining a strong culture of safety

- Testing for and using optimal processes and procedures

- Providing intensive and continuing training for individuals, teams, and larger units

- Conducting thorough prospective and retrospective organizational learning and safety management

- Building and maintaining resilience in healthcare systems

- Evaluating the impact of adverse events in healthcare and how simulation-based activities can be used to determine and potentially prevent their cause

The location in which simulation activities occur may differentiate clinically based simulation programs from those in academic settings. Simulation programs serving hospitals and healthcare systems may be based in a freestanding educational building, within the walls of the clinical setting, or even in a mobile van that travels from site to site. Within a hospital or healthcare system, simulation programs can also exist outside of an actual physical location. They can involve in-situ simulations occurring in the actual clinical environment—for example, in an operating room, patient care unit, or emergency department.

Simulation programs based in a hospital or healthcare system support efforts toward improving patient safety, enhancing the educational experiences of staff, and creating a new system to assist in improving overall system performance. Chapter 12 offers details on using simulation for these purposes.

Leadership

Engaged and active leadership is critical to the success of a simulation program. Healthcare and educational organizations must identify a high-level champion who embraces the value of simulation—for example, a board member or hospital executive—to support the simulation program. This level of leader can champion the program and help pave the way for the engagement of potential stakeholders, the acquisition of physical space and simulation technology, and the implementation of a new approach to learning within the organization.

The complexity of today's healthcare environment and embedded culture can make it difficult to implement a change no matter how valuable or appropriate it may be. Changing a system, a procedure, or a process requires much planning. Although simulation has become an accepted form of education, not all healthcare providers will embrace its use. Therefore, simulation champions must be kept well-informed and involved with their simulation programs. Armed with a thorough understanding of the evidence for and benefits that simulation can bring to the overall quality of patient care services, the champion will be able to facilitate buy-in from the various departments and individuals who can benefit from the simulation program.

Hospitals and healthcare systems also need to have a simulation planning committee and a simulation steering or advisory committee to guide the work of the simulation program. These committees are discussed in detail in Chapter 16.

When designing the organizational reporting structure for the simulation program, consider the message that the positioning of the program might send. If the focus of the simulation program is on hospital-wide or system-wide activities, the program should be positioned accordingly within the organization. If the program is based in a specialty department such as emergency medicine or anesthesia, potential users of the program are likely to view it narrowly as offering simulation activities specific to that department or discipline. For example, if the simulation program is based in emergency medicine, potential users, such as nursing services, might be interested in simulation but think the program offers only emergency response scenarios or training.

Simulation programs may be more likely to succeed if they are established to serve all departments and disciplines in the organization rather than a single one. If the simulation program is envisioned as serving the hospital or health system, consideration can be given to creating the program as a separate department reporting to a position such as the chief quality officer. Another possibility might be to situate the simulation program within an existing organization-wide department such as risk management.

Initial Needs Assessment

Simulation is being incorporated in hospitals and healthcare systems as a learning and quality-improvement modality for practicing healthcare professionals. With the focus on developing a culture of safety within healthcare, patient safety groups are calling on hospitals and healthcare institutions to explore simulation as a means to provide ongoing education and professional development (AHRQ, 2013; Murray, 2010; Smith, 2017). Simulation provides the opportunity for repeated practice, team performance assessment, and potential clinical improvement (Gaba, 2004; McGahie, Issenberg, Petrusa, & Scalese, 2016). Simulation is ideal as an educational modality for a variety of experiences, including high-

risk patient conditions. It has the potential to improve performance and encourage teamwork by engaging learners through the re-creation of real clinical situations in a safe environment (Dahlberg, Nelson, Dahlgren, & Blomberg, 2018; Gilfoyle et al., 2017; Senger, Stapleton, & Gorski, 2012).

Performing a needs assessment is a critical step in determining many aspects of the simulation program. Every hospital or healthcare system has unique learning needs and demands (Beam, 2011). Identifying what types of users the simulation program will serve is important for development, growth, and the incorporation of simulation into the organization.

A needs assessment is a systematic process for identifying and addressing the needs of the organization, or gaps between current conditions and desired conditions. A needs assessment should be done to focus simulation-based activities and to ensure alignment with the organization's outcomes, methods, and measures (Kern, 2016). The needs assessment should consider the types of learners to be served, objectives to be achieved, and critical elements to be assessed. The needs assessment should include the organizational, departmental, unit, course, and anticipated learner groups. It should also be repeated on a regular basis. A systematic assessment of the capabilities of the simulation program will guide the overall goals of the simulation program as well as curriculum development and establish a projected growth plan for simulation within the organization.

Within a hospital or health system simulation program, the types of learners will vary. Examples of specific learner types include:

- Registered nurses
- Physicians

- Allied healthcare professionals
- Unlicensed hospital personnel
- Students
- New graduates
- Experienced staff

In addition to identifying learners, based on a needs assessment, the program should identify how training will occur. Examples of training options include:

- Multidisciplinary training
- Task training
- Lab-based simulation training
- In-situ simulation training
- The use of hybrid simulations
- Discipline- or specialty-specific training

Ensuring that the simulation program is developed based on an objective measure of organizational needs will allow simulation staff to develop well-designed, effective, and efficient simulation experiences.

Initial Program Development

When the needs assessment is complete, program development can begin. The first step in developing a hospital-wide or healthcare system–based simulation program is to consider the purposes of the program.

The development of a clear and concise mission and vision will identify the purpose of the program and whom it serves. The vision guides the program into the future. An example of a mission statement could be, "The simulation program is to provide simulation training to individuals and teams to promote patient safety." The vision may be to be a leader in simulation in the region.

As you begin to develop the program, the answers to these basic questions will guide your efforts:

- Who are the key stakeholders at each level, and what are their priorities?
- Who will be the learners in the simulation center?
- What will be the focus of the training (teams, individuals, or both)?
- What training is prioritized?
- Based on the needs assessment, what are the most urgent priorities?
- If you need to start with a limited scope due to budget or space limitations, are you prepared to respond to a broad array of needs now, in the short term, or further out?
- If starting with a limited scope, can you create a long-term approach to the integration of simulation in a phased-in approach?

Early engagement of stakeholders is important. Based on the needs assessment, develop a list of services to be provided by the simulation program. Consider who will be providing the services along with other stakeholders of the simulation program and include them in discussing the development of the program. Leadership will need to understand simulation, the process, and potential benefits. Support from stakeholders will pave the way for program development and eventually facilitate the use of the simulation program by learners.

The next step is to determine the initial goals of the program. This will drive the development of the program. For example: Who are the learners? Will the program be used to train new staff members in orientation? Developing a simulation program to onboard new employees such as RNs can be an effective method to evaluate competencies and develop person-specific onboarding plans. Or, will the program be tasked with developing programs to train and maintain high-performing teams, such as the trauma team, code team, or the anesthesia department? Simulation is now being used to verify competencies and to credential physicians and nurses in specific skill sets before they begin doing clinical rotations. Finally, those implementing the simulation program need to determine whether it will focus on technical or nontechnical skills related to a specific educational program.

When considering the initial focus of the simulation program, identify "low-hanging fruit." That is, choose a group of learners or a department that understands and wants to participate in simulation education. This might be a small group such as a trauma team or code team. After those learners experience simulation education, their behaviors might change in the clinical environment, and they can share information about the experience with others. Others who hear of these positive experiences or witness the positive changes that occur as a result of the simulation program may become interested in using the program themselves. Implementing a program across many groups simultaneously, especially if they are being mandated to participate in simulation, will lead to additional challenges and potentially failure of the program. This is why many programs begin by identifying likely early adopters. Securing early wins with frontline professionals facilitates success of the program moving forward.

To generate enthusiasm for the new simulation program, consider implementing simulation experiences in which learners can participate as a group. Offer the experience as part of a course and emphasize that it is a safe learning environment. One possible approach is to implement simulation into nurse orientation or into new graduate RN residencies. When participants enjoy positive experiences with simulation, they are likely to engage their leadership to facilitate a return to the simulation lab.

Developing a Simulation Lab in a Clinical Setting

Obtaining space for a simulation program in a clinical setting can be very challenging. Space for patients and support services are the priority. That said, providing opportunities to make the environment safer and enhance patient outcomes should also be seen as an important organizational priority. Creating a strong argument for the needs and benefits of the simulation program will be critical to obtaining the necessary space for the program. Consider describing the benefits of identifying latent safety threats as a justification for the use of clinical space.

The need to replicate patient care environments might be imperative when developing a lab-based clinical simulation program. Consider visiting established simulation programs to get ideas for your center. You can find a detailed discussion on developing and building simulation centers in Chapter 16.

Initial Simulation Technology Purchases

Justifying the cost of simulators remains a challenge. The decision as to what equipment to buy should be driven by the goals and mission of the program. A wide range of simulator technology is available (see Chapter 1 for a full discussion on simulation options) as well as simulation center management software and hardware.

The most expensive simulator might not be the most appropriate, given restrictions of space or available support. A full-body simulator that would be selected for a lab setting might need to be different from a simulator that can be used for in-situ simulations or task training.

The lab environment might be designed to simulate a critical-care environment, operating rooms, or patient care rooms in the hospital. As such, a simulator that can be placed on a ventilator or programmed to respond to procedures in real time might be the best choice. Several full-body immersive simulators designed for critical-care environments are available. They are, however, expensive.

Equipment should be selected based on assessed need, planned use, and space. In-situ simulations are often conducted using a tetherless simulator that is self-contained and does not need to be attached to an electric or gas source to operate. Most of these mannequins are controlled by a laptop or tablet operating some distance from the simulator. The mannequins adequately simulate

pulses, cardiac rhythms, respiratory movements, breath sounds, and eye opening. In a clinical setting, tetherless simulation devices allow the educator to move the simulator onto patient care units or other locations, which adds realism to the simulation experience and potentially identifies latent (hidden) safety threats to patients, visitors, or staff.

Based on the needs assessment and the targeted learners, other simulation equipment may be needed. For example, there are haptic simulators for learning ultrasonography and surgical techniques. These simulators are also expensive. Consider purchasing equipment that can be used by multiple learners or departments to add value to the purchase. Also consider the use of standardized patients (SPs) as simulators within the program. Using SPs can increase the realism of a simulation and support many learning objectives. SPs are generally paid hourly and supported with meal and parking vouchers. Be sure to include training time for SPs. Additional information on the use of SPs can be found in Chapters 1 and 4.

Extended Warranties

Organizations will need to decide whether to purchase extended warranties (service agreements) for expensive simulators. This is a significant expense added to the purchase of simulators. Some stakeholders or finance departments might not consider the purchase of an extended warranty to be worthwhile, but the technology used in human patient simulators is unique. When repairs are needed and upgrades are required, having the manufacturer complete the work under a warranty can be more efficient and cost-effective than having an organization's simulation staff attempt to complete the work. Questions to consider when reviewing warranties include the turnaround time for service and whether a loaner program for the simulator exists. Consider the impact on learners and the effect on the program if the simulator is out of service for an extended period of time.

Creating Global and Curriculum-Based Objectives

In both academic and clinical settings, developing global and curriculum-specific learning objectives is essential. Clearly defined learning objectives help facilitate planning for all aspects of the simulation (Naylor & Torres, 2019; Phrampus, 2010). Creating defined objectives focuses the goals of the program as well as course curricula and provides a level of consistency in approach and design. Creating objectives will guide the training priorities for both the healthcare organization and the simulation program. For example, an objective that aims to increase the knowledge of general care nurses related to pediatric codes might require a specific pediatric patient simulator. In contrast, development of a difficult airway course for ear, nose, and throat residents might require the purchase of a specific task trainer.

Objectives for a hospital simulation program may differ from objectives related to a simulation program in an academic setting. The hospital-based program may offer experiences primarily to healthcare professionals with a variety of educational and experiential backgrounds. In addition, the objectives will help determine where the simulation activity will occur—in a lab, in situ, or a combination of both.

In addition to a different type of learner, a hospital-based simulation is likely to have a different focus. Often the hospital leadership will be interested in areas related to onboarding new staff (e.g., nursing orientation or residency), competency, and quality and safety concerns (surgical site infections, codes outside of intensive care units, team functions, and evaluation of facilities, systems, and processes). The stakeholders for these areas are different from those in a college or training program. With hospital-based simulation, it is important to engage relevant leaders and help them to understand how simulation can solve their problems. Patient-safety and risk-management leaders are almost always interested in using simulation. It is helpful to do a needs assessment to understand the pain points of a particular institution with regard to safety and quality. The chief nursing officer (CNO) and the chief medical officer (CMO) are additional obvious leaders to engage. The CNO is typically responsible for the largest workforce in a healthcare organization and has needs related to onboarding, retention, competency, and the work that is accomplished on various units. A CMO typically has overall responsibility for patient safety, licensed independent providers, and the hospital's overall function and reputation. The key to engaging these leaders is to help them understand how the use of simulation can solve a problem that they are charged with solving. This requires local simulation experts to be familiar with the evidence for simulation as well as how to present some sort of return or value on investment.

Creating "Real" Simulations in a Lab

Creating a simulation center (or lab) in a clinical setting can be challenging, time-consuming, and expensive, but it can also provide many benefits to the organization. Organizations can provide many simulation activities in a lab setting, including:

- Simulation-based courses

- Training for procedural skills

- Teamwork and communication training

- Multidisciplinary provider training

For example, one initiative to decrease adverse medical events required that a hospital-based simulation lab design specific adverse medical event courses for identified patient care units. The courses were four hours long and included all members of the care team. The simulation experience needed to occur in a safe location that allowed for serious or uncommon scenarios to unfold and for the team to participate in a debriefing designed to identify opportunities for improvement and reflection on practice.

Training in a dedicated simulation space has both advantages and disadvantages. Several advantages have been identified when hospital staff train in a dedicated simulation lab (Deering, Johnston, & Colacchio, 2011):

- **The learning environment is tightly controlled:** This can help to standardize the experience for all participants and allows for assessment activities and educational activities to occur.

- **Audiovisual (AV) components are more easily accessed:** AV components are often essential to the simulation experience. Making these components more easily available enables hospital staff to benefit from video-assisted debriefings that can provide them with unique experiences to assess their own performance and potentially learn from both themselves and colleagues.

- **It can accommodate a large and diverse group of learners:** The group can be predefined and allow for large numbers of care providers to attend specified training at different times to accommodate clinical scheduling issues.

- **Data obtained can be used for research:** Data obtained during simulations within a designated laboratory in a controlled environment can be used for research to further the field of simulation in healthcare.

In addition, there is evidence that team performance is similar in center-based and in-situ resuscitations (Couto, Kerrey, Taylor, FitzGerald, & Geis, 2015; Kaba & Barnes, 2019; Sørensen et al., 2015).

Disadvantages to consider include:

- **Learner frustration:** There is the potential to frustrate the learners when the simulation laboratory does not accurately or entirely reflect the clinical environment. This can lead to disengagement and lack of involvement in the simulation (Deering et al., 2011). Unfamiliar equipment, environments that are different from the ones in which they practice, and unfamiliar team members can cause frustration and have the potential to distract the learners from the experience being provided.

- **Travel time:** If the simulation center (or laboratory) is located at a different site from the hospital, travel time can be a limiting factor.

- **Difficulty identifying and fixing systems issues:** It's difficult for simulation staff to identify and fix systems issues that are inherent to a particular clinical environment. This may include an operating room. For example, the simulation laboratory might not be able to identify latent safety threats that are created by a specific physical space, process, or organizational structure. Such disadvantages can be mitigated with appropriate planning. It is possible to replicate a clinical environment with detailed planning. This is especially true for environments that typically run a high census or may be too expensive to take out of service for training. This could include operating rooms and certain specialty intensive care units.

In-Situ Simulation: Simulation in the "Real" World

In-situ (Latin for "in position") simulation is a blended approach to simulation that commonly involves embedding simulators within an actual clinical environment (Rosen, Hunt, Pronovost, Federowicz, & Weaver, 2012). In-situ simulations are an important aspect of a hospital-based simulation program because they have the potential to drive deep individual, team, unit, and organizational learning (Goldshtein, Krensky, Doshi, & Perelman, 2020; Josey et al., 2018; Paltved, Bjerregaard, Krogh, Pedersen, & Musaeus, 2017). They allow experienced healthcare providers to participate in simulation activities within their own clinical environment, which results in more contextually relevant learning and identification of actual process improvement opportunities. In-situ simulation provides more realistic experiences than lab-based simulations and thus can provide more accurate evaluation of patient care systems and teams (Patterson, Geis, Falcone, LeMaster, & Wears, 2013).

Hospitals and healthcare systems that embrace in-situ simulation find that it provides a means to identify workarounds, knowledge gaps, and latent safety threats that few other methods are capable of matching (Campbell et al., 2016; Mark et al., 2015; Patterson et al., 2013). In-situ simulations

can provide learning opportunities to both individuals and teams of healthcare professionals and can reinforce competencies acquired in more traditional learning environments (Rosen et al., 2012). Beyond the educational benefits, in-situ simulations provide the opportunity to identify latent safety threats that have the potential to affect patient safety within the organization and to stimulate efforts to address them. In a study performed by Geis, Pio, Pendergrass, Moyer, & Patterson (2011), an in-situ program developed in a high-risk emergency department identified a total of 73 latent safety threats—a rate of 1 for every 1.2 in-situ simulations performed. This use of in-situ simulation can close the loop in process improvement by creating an assessment, training, and evaluation system for individual, team, and organizational learning.

The first step in implementing a hospital-based in-situ simulation program is to determine the outcomes the in-situ simulation is designed to target. As discussed, a needs analysis is crucial to uncovering what you want to achieve with an in-situ simulation program. Rosen et al. (2012) identified key questions to ask when developing in-situ simulation:

- What level of the system is targeted for improvement? Do you want to evaluate individual, team, unit, or organizational improvement?

- Who will participate in the simulation, and who will serve as facilitators or instructors?

- What are the specific objectives for the in-situ simulation?

- Where and when will the in-situ simulation occur?

- How will the in-situ simulation be evaluated?

- How will the information gained from the program be used?

Asking these questions will assist in developing an effective in-situ simulation program and producing the ancillary materials needed (facilitator education, simulators, supplies).

Although in-situ simulation is an essential tool in the delivery of education to healthcare providers, it also has limitations. Considering these issues when developing the program allows the simulation educator to prepare for potential issues before they arise. For example, scheduling and time constraints are a major issue when developing in-situ simulations (Deering et al., 2012; Geis et al., 2011). Because the simulation occurs on the unit, the potential for affecting the care of patients on the unit must be considered (Bajaj, Minors, Walker, Meguerdichian, & Patterson, 2018). There might also be anxiety among the caregivers involved. Finally, when in-situ simulation requires educators and simulators to travel to outlying clinical sites, travel time, wear and tear on simulators, and increased workload for the simulation staff must be factored into the effort. Even with the limitations noted, in-situ simulation has been shown to provide a valuable experience for healthcare providers and organizations (Lighthall, Poon, & Harrison, 2010; Patterson, Blike, & Nadkarni, 2008).

Facilitators should develop guidelines for running in-situ simulations. This is important because different patient care areas might have specific times when an in-situ simulation is not optimal, such as during patient rounds, shift changes, and times of high acuity or high census. For example, for one in-situ program developed for a pediatric intensive care unit, the unit and the simulation educator established a policy that provided specific instructions on when in-situ simulations should not occur. This policy, which was communicated to all charge nurses and attending physicians, included the following parameters (Bajaj et al., 2018):

1. In-situ simulations are *not* to be performed on the unit:

   - If there is a resuscitation in progress or high-risk procedure being performed

   - If there is only one bed open for an admission

   - If there is a low staffing level

   - If it is between 0600 and 0800, 1400 and 1600, 1800 and 2000, or 2200 and 2400 hours

2. In-situ simulations are limited to 20 minutes (10 minutes for simulation plus 10 minutes for debriefing).

In-situ simulations have a high probability of cancellation. For in-situ simulations in emergency departments, Patterson et al. (2013) found a cancellation rate of 28%, although they noted that the cancellation rate decreased as the program matured. As a result, they recommend overscheduling the number of in-situ simulations to achieve the desired total number of simulations. Scheduling more in-situ simulations than are needed allows for a backup plan in case of unexpected events and cancellations.

Staffing Simulation Programs in the Clinical Setting

As a simulation program grows in the clinical setting, challenges will occur, such as:

- Inadequate staff to meet demands

- Insufficient workspace and storage space for simulators and supplies

- The need to train new simulation center employees

Simulation educators may need three to 12 months to become comfortable facilitating a simulation scenario. When hiring new staff members, remember that the benefit of additional staff will not be appreciated immediately. As the simulation program continues to grow, additional departments will reach out for simulation education. Developing a system early to set priorities will assist in managing the growing demand.

A staffing model to consider initially is one in which all team members are cross-trained as much as possible in all aspects of simulation. One example is to have the simulation educator trained to set up and run the simulator as well as to debrief. Facilitators may also be crossed-trained in the use of the AV equipment. Another staffing model is one in which content experts from within the hospital or healthcare system are trained to be facilitators. They are supported by simulation technicians or operations specialists. This allows the program to be more responsive to requests and gives the simulation educator time to assist in course development and oversight.

Determining what staffing model to use is a program-specific decision. Healthcare providers and staff in the clinical setting will be accepting of simulation if it is relevant and specific to their work. Thus, involving content experts from the various disciplines or departments will be important for learner acceptance. You can find detailed information on simulation roles and sample position descriptions in Chapter 14.

Conclusion

The implementation of a simulation program in a hospital or healthcare system can offer many benefits to the organization, the staff, and its patients. It is a considerable task to undertake, but one that is made easier and more likely to be successful by committing time, resources, and leadership to the planning and development phases.

When developing a simulation program in a clinical setting, hospitals and healthcare systems must consider the overall outcomes the organization wants to achieve and the needs of learners. Professional organizations offer resources to assist in the planning and development of a high-quality simulation program. The Society for Simulation in Healthcare (SSH, 2016) has developed peer-reviewed standards for accreditation of simulation programs. These standards have been specifically created to provide a resource for developing programs as well as for programs seeking recognition for meeting the established standards. Although a program may not be ready for accreditation, using standards from accrediting organizations such as the SSH will assist in developing the basic infrastructure needed for a successful simulation program. In addition, the International Nursing Association for Clinical Simulation and Learning (2011) has developed standards of best practice in simulation that can be a resource for the development of a simulation program.

Having a successful simulation program in a hospital or healthcare system involves several key steps. Champions at the program and organizational levels should be identified early in the development process. Organizations should also conduct a needs analysis and use it to identify the global direction of the simulation program. Articulating this direction will facilitate the design of the program and strategic prioritization of activities. After the direction is established, those objectives will allow those implementing the simulation program to determine the appropriate equipment, simulation modalities, and simulation educational methodologies to employ. In addition, the program will be able to accurately identify budgetary needs, sustainable funding, and a staffing model.

Implementing a successful strategy for the use of simulation in hospitals and healthcare systems can be a rewarding experience for simulation educators, the organization, its learners, and ultimately its patients. Simulation has been shown to be effective in ensuring safety in other industries that have come to expect ultra-safe performance, such as aviation. In healthcare, simulation programs can result in major improvements in patient care and outcomes.

References

Agency for Healthcare Research and Quality. (2013). *Making health care safer II: An updated critical analysis of the evidence for patient safety practices.* Rockville, MD: Author. Retrieved from https://www.ahrq.gov/sites/default/files/wysiwyg/research/findings/evidence-based-reports/services/quality/patientsftyupdate/ptsafetyII-full.pdf

Bajaj, K., Minors, A., Walker, K., Meguerdichian, M., & Patterson, M. (2018). "No-go considerations" for in-situ simulation safety. *Simulation in Healthcare, 13*(3), 221-224. doi:10.1097/SIH.0000000000000301

Beam, B. (2011). Lessons learned from planning, conducting, and evaluating in-situ healthcare simulations for Nebraska hospitals. *Nebraska Nurse, 44*(3), 7.

Campbell, D. M., Poost-Foroosh, L., Pavenski, K., Contreras, M., Alam, F., Lee, J., & Houston, P. (2016). Simulation as a toolkit—Understanding the perils of blood transfusion in a complex health care environment. *Advances in Simulation, 8*, 32. doi:10.1186/s41077-016-0032-z

Couto, T. B., Kerrey, B. T., Taylor, R. G., FitzGerald, M., & Geis, G. L. (2015). Teamwork skills in actual, in situ, and in-center pediatric emergencies: Performance levels across settings and perceptions of comparative educational impact. *Simulation in Healthcare, 10*(2), 76-84. doi:10.1097/SIH.0000000000000081

Dahlberg, J., Nelson, M., Dahlgren, M. A., & Blomberg, M. (2018). Ten years of simulation-based shoulder dystocia training—Impact on obstetric outcome, clinical management, staff confidence, and the pedagogical practice—A time series study. *BMC Pregnancy and Childbirth, 18*(1), 361. doi:10.1186/s12884-018-2001-0

Deering, S., Johnston, L. C., & Colacchio, K. (2011). Multidisciplinary teamwork and communication training. *Seminars in Perinatology, 35*(2), 89-96. doi:10.1053/j.semperi.2011.01.009

Gaba, D. M. (2004). The future vision of simulation in health care. *Quality and Safety in Health Care, 13*(Suppl. 1), i2-i10. doi:10.1136/qshc.2004.009878

Geis, G. L., Pio, B., Pendergrass, T. L., Moyer, M. R., & Patterson, M. D. (2011). Simulation to assess the safety of new healthcare teams and new facilities. *Simulation in Healthcare, 6*(3), 125-133. doi:10.1097/SIH.0b013e31820dff30

Gilfoyle, E., Koot, D. A., Annear, J. C., Bhanji, F., Cheng, A., Duff, J. P., … Teams4Kids Investigators and the Canadian Critical Care Trials Group. (2017). Improved clinical performance and teamwork of pediatric interprofessional resuscitation teams with a simulation-based educational intervention. *Pediatric Critical Care Medicine, 18*(2), e62–e69. doi:10.1097/PCC.0000000000001025

Goldshtein, D., Krensky, C., Doshi, S., & Perelman, V. S. (2020). In situ simulation and its effects on patient outcomes: A systematic review. *BMJ Simulation and Technology Enhanced Learning, 6*(1), 3–9.

International Nursing Association for Clinical Simulation and Learning Board of Directors. (2011). Standards of best practice: Simulation. Standard I: Terminology. *Clinical Simulation in Nursing, 7*(4S), s3-s7. doi:10.1016/j.ecns.2011.05.005

Josey, K., Smith, M. L., Kayani, A. S., Young, G., Kasperski, M. D., Farrer, P. … Raschke, R. A. (2018). Hospitals with more-active participation in conducting standardized in-situ mock codes have improved survival after in-hospital cardiopulmonary arrest. *Resuscitation, 133*, 47-52. doi:10.1016/j.resuscitation.2018.09.020

Kaba, A., & Barnes, S. (2019). Commissioning simulations to test new healthcare facilities: A proactive and innovative approach to healthcare system safety. *Advances in Simulation, 4*, article 17. doi:10.1186/s41077-019-0107-8

Kern, D. E. (2016). Overview: A six-step approach to curriculum development. In P. A. Thomas, D. E. Kern, M. T. Hughes, & B. Y. Chen (Eds.), *Curriculum development for medical education* (3rd ed., pp. 5-10). Baltimore, MD: John Hopkins University Press.

Lighthall, G. K., Poon, T., & Harrison, T. K. (2010). Using in-situ simulation to improve in-hospital cardiopulmonary resuscitation. *Joint Commission Journal on Quality and Patient Safety, 36*(5), 209-216.

Mark, L. J., Herzer, K. R., Cover, R., Pandian, V., Bhatti, N. I., Berkow, L. C., ... Mirski, M. A. (2015). Difficult airway response team: A novel quality improvement program for managing hospital-wide airway emergencies. *Anesthesia & Analgesia, 121*(1), 127-139. doi:10.1213/ANE.0000000000000691

McGaghie, W. C., Issenberg, S. B., Petrusa, E. R., & Scalese, R. J. (2016). Revisiting 'A critical review of simulation-based medical education research: 2003-2009.' *Medical Education, 50*(10), 986-991. doi:10.1111/medu.12795

Murray, J. S. (2010). Walter Reed National Military Medical Center: Simulation on the cutting edge. *Military Medicine, 175*(9), 659-663.

Naylor, K. A., & Torres, K. C. (2019). Translation of learning objectives in medical education using high- and low-fidelity simulation: Learners' perspectives. *Journal of Taibah University Medical Sciences, 14*(6), 481–487. doi:10.1016/j.jtumed.2019.10.006

Page, J. T., Fairbanks, R. J., & Gaba, D. M. (2018). Priorities related to improving healthcare safety through simulation. *Society for Simulation in Healthcare, 13*(3S Suppl. 1), S41–S50. doi:10.1097/SIH.0000000000000295

Paltved, C., Bjerregaard, A. T., Krogh, K., Pedersen, J. J., & Musaeus, P. (2017). Designing in-situ simulation in the emergency department: Evaluating safety attitudes amongst physicians and nurses. *Advances in Simulation, 8*(2), 4. doi:10.1186/s41077-017-0037-2

Patterson, M. D., Blike, G. T., & Nadkarni, V. M. (2008). In-situ simulation: Challenges and results. In K. Henriksen, J. B. Battles, M. A. Keyes, & M. L. Grady (Eds.), *Advances in patient safety: New directions and alternative approaches (Vol. 3: Performance and tools)*. Rockville, MD: Agency for Healthcare Research and Quality. Retrieved from http://www.ahrq.gov/downloads/pub/advances2/vol3/advances-patterson_48.pdf

Patterson, M. D., Geis, G. L., Falcone, R. A., LeMaster, T., & Wears, R. L. (2013). In-situ simulation: Detection of safety threats and teamwork training in a high risk emergency department. *BMJ Quality and Safety in Health Care, 22*(6), 468-477. doi:10.1136/bmjqs-2012-000942

Phrampus, P. E. (2010). Simulation best practices: Must-haves for successful simulation in prehospital care. *JEMS, 35*(9), Suppl. 4-7.

Rosen, M. A., Hunt, E. A., Pronovost, P. J., Federowicz, M. A., & Weaver, S. J. (2012). In-situ simulation in continuing education for the health care professions: A systematic review. *Journal of Continuing Education in the Health Professions, 32*(4), 243-254. doi:10.1002/chp.21152

Senger, B., Stapleton, L., & Gorski, M. S. (2012). A hospital and university partnership model for simulation education. *Clinical Simulation in Nursing, 8*(9), e477-e482. doi:10.1016/j.ecns.2011.09.002

Smith, C. (2017). *Embedding safety culture training into quality improvement projects and organizational processes.* The Joint Commission. Retrieved from https://www.jointcommission.org/high_reliability_healthcare/embedding_safety_culture_training_into_quality_improvement_projects_and_organizational_processes/

Society for Simulation in Healthcare. (2016). *SSH accreditation of healthcare simulation programs.* Wheaton, IL: Author. Retrieved from https://www.ssih.org/Credentialing/Accreditation

Sørensen, J. L., van der Vleuten, C., Rosthøj, S., Østergaard, D., LeBlanc, V., Johansen, M., . . . Ottesen, B. (2015). Simulation-based multiprofessional obstetric anaesthesia training conducted in-situ versus off-site leads to similar individual and team outcomes: A randomised educational trial. *BMJ Open, 5*(10), e008344. doi:10.1136/bmjopen-2015-008344

Ulrich, B. (2013). Leading an organization to improved outcomes through simulation. *Nurse Leader, 11*(1), 42-45. doi:10.1016/j.mnl.2012.11.011

"Simulation technology and pedagogy have advanced dramatically in recent years and have the potential to improve health professionals' competency and safe practice."

–Amitai Ziv, Stephen D. Small, and Paul Root Wolpe

Using Simulation for Risk Management and Quality Improvement

12

Pamela Andreatta, EdD, PhD, MFA, MA, FSSH
David Marzano, MD
Jody R. Lori, PhD, CNM, FACNM, FAAN

OBJECTIVES

- Discuss how simulation can be used to promote safety in all aspects of healthcare.

- Examine how simulation can be used to inform quality-improvement mechanisms at all levels of the healthcare system.

- Show how simulation can be used to document evidence of performance skills in healthcare practices.

- Demonstrate how simulation can be used to reduce risks associated with healthcare for patients and providers.

A key tenet for healthcare providers is, "First do no harm." Although modern clinicians might consider the earliest healing methods to be a form of sorcery by today's technology and genome-driven clinical techniques, at their root, all healthcare practices still depend on human performance and are, therefore, susceptible to human error. Human imperfection will likely remain in perpetuity; however, it is possible to limit errors and associated adverse effects on patients, their families, and practitioners themselves. Most healthcare professionals learned through apprenticeships under the tutelage of more experienced clinicians. The apprentice method enables students to learn clinical procedures, techniques, reasoning, and decision-making by observing, and subsequently performing, these behaviors while providing patient care. This method has numerous strengths. Its inherent weakness, however, is the lack of adequate opportunities for repetition and deliberate practice, both of which are so essential for developing psychomotor skills. Instead, the learner may receive subjective observations about performance, often in the absence of performance standards and a lack of preceptor training in teaching and performance assessment. The result is wide variability in the quality of training and, therefore, variability in the quality of clinical performance, with the potential to adversely affect patient care.

Safety

Simulation affects safety in a number of different healthcare situations. Most commonly, simulation is seen as an enabler of patient safety. However, there are other domains in which simulation can foster safety, including clinician safety and environmental safety.

Patient Safety

Singular reliance on the apprentice-training model of clinical instruction places patients at greater risk for a potential adverse event. Consider the likelihood that a learner will take more time to assess and treat a patient than a professional provider would. Although this delay might not have an adverse effect in many clinical situations, it inconveniences patients and endangers those with clinical situations that *are* time dependent. For example, a patient presenting with signs and symptoms of a thrombotic stroke requires quick assessment, diagnosis, and administration of potentially lifesaving drugs such as tissue plasminogen activator. However, this patient faces several obstacles to securing optimal care, including timely admission to the emergency department, rapid triage assessment and diagnosis of a potential stroke patient, quick and accurate intravenous (IV) access placement, prompt evaluation by the attending physicians, and accurate treatment protocols implemented by the clinical team (Monks, Pearson, Pitt, Stein, & James, 2015). Experienced clinicians will be able to assess the patient and perform all necessary clinical tasks to restore blood flow to the brain and potentially avert brain damage within three hours of onset of symptoms if the patient presents to their care shortly after symptoms become evident. However, numerous potential delays could directly affect patient care in this situation. For example:

- The nurse triaging the patient could fail to recognize the clinical signs and symptoms of a stroke, which would delay the patient being expedited through the emergency department.

- The admitting nurse might require multiple tries to place an IV, which would delay the initial evaluation by the physician.

- A medical student might see the patient and take a detailed but prolonged history and present the findings to a resident, who subsequently performs another examination and presents the information to the attending physician, who then repeats the essential parts of the examination, further adding to the delays.

- Still more delays can occur as the resident interprets CT scans and lab results and then subsequently reviews and discusses the findings with the attending physician.

- The resident orders the drugs, but the nurse notes that the order includes an incorrect dosage and must request a new order.

- The drug arrives in the correct dose, but the time limit for administering the drug has passed due to delayed care. The patient is no longer a candidate and suffers permanent effects from the stroke.

This example illustrates the frustrations that the current training system imparts on all stakeholders—including practitioners, trainees, patients, families, administrators, etc. Fortunately, advances in clinical teaching methods and technologies offer an alternative approach: simulation.

Simulation-based teaching methods provide an excellent bridge between acquiring clinical skills in a patient-free context and applying clinical skills during patient care. Simulation has been used for clinical training from the earliest days of medical education. Early simulations used animals, human cadavers, fruits and vegetables, and manufactured synthetic models designed to replicate an aspect of clinical performance (such as suturing or venous access) or clinical procedures (such as bowel surgery).

Advances in computer and imaging technologies have led to training solutions in which hardware and software interfaces merge to provide simulators that function like their clinical correlates. These high-technology simulators include human mannequins, surgical trainers, virtual-reality constructs, and augmented reality systems, among other hybrid platforms. They enable learners to practice techniques from IV placement, Foley catheter placement, and identification of abnormal physical examination findings to more complex interactions involving team communication, management of disaster drills, and multidisciplinary teamwork. Additionally, many of these high-technology simulators capture performance data that provide feedback to learners about how well they are performing and where they need to improve to meet expected standards.

Sollid et al. (2019) describe the top five topics that healthcare simulation can address to improve patient safety. These topics, along with examples of patient safety problems for each topic, were identified by an international group of experts:

- **Technical skills:** physician technical competence, introduction of new technologies, high-risk/low-frequency procedures, learning on patients, implementation challenges/resistance to change

- **Nontechnical skills:** fragmentation of care, transitions between routine and nonroutine activities, lack of shared understanding, monitoring error detection and recovery, context complexity, interdependence, dynamics

- **System probing:** unaware of existing patient safety problems, lack of probes to identify processes at individual, team, and system levels, suboptimal link between patient

safety challenges (outcomes) and training interventions, system complexity—lack of appropriate research to deal with dynamic system, suboptimal link between patient/public perception/experience of safety and interventions (educational, system)

- **Assessment:** lack of evidence/paucity of data that demonstrate that simulation is effective and cost-effective

- **Effectiveness:** poor competence leads to patient harm, lack of awareness that mistakes are being made, lack of accountability, punitive patient safety culture

The advantages of mastering specific clinical skills in a simulated context before working with actual patients are obvious. Not only will the patient benefit from timely and accurate care from those beginning their clinical service, but supervising clinicians will be able to focus on more advanced or critical aspects of clinical care, thus further increasing the overall quality of care for patients. Consider the previous example of the stroke patient. At minimum, simulation-based training would facilitate repeated practice for (Garside, Rudd, & Price, 2012; Ross, Reedy, Roots, Jaye, & Birns, 2015):

- Recognizing the signs and symptoms of a stroke

- IV placement

- Expedited history taking

- Assessing lab results

- Evaluating CT scans

- Developing appropriate treatment plans

Simulation-based training also facilitates the opportunity for learners and practitioners to rehearse and hone communication skills between the multiple team members involved in patient care, identify and correct any perceived errors, and ultimately decrease the time from admission to administration of correct treatment (Blum, Raemer, Carroll, Dufresne, & Cooper, 2005; Lateef, 2010).

The use of debriefing during these types of team-based simulation activities facilitates the identification and review of actions and behaviors that could potentially lead to errors or compromise patient safety (Cantrell, 2008). More importantly, the ability to identify these potential problems before they occur during actual patient care makes it possible for remedies and retraining to happen before any harm befalls an actual patient. Ultimately, it serves to minimize patient risks while at the same time improve clinical efficiencies and quality of care (Barsuk, Cohen, McGaghie, & Wayne, 2010; Hunt, Fiedor-Hamilton, & Eppich, 2008; Hunt, Shilkofski, Stavroudis, & Nelson, 2007; Issenberg, McGaghie, Petrusa, Lee Gordon, & Scalese, 2005; Van Sickle, Ritter, & Smith, 2006).

Clinician Safety

The apprenticeship model of traditional healthcare education, in which learning in the context of actual patient care is widely accepted, has clear disadvantages for patient safety. It also has clear disadvantages for clinician safety. The additional stress associated with providing patient care while feeling ill-prepared or incompetent can impose significant negative affective overload that impedes both performance and the learning process (Easterbrook, 1959; Humara, 1999; Mandler, 1979; van Galen & van Huygevoort, 2000; Van Gemmert & van Galen, 1997).

Negative affective elements can influence the performance of both trainees and instructors. Trainees might experience cognitive overload

as a result of one or more stressors in the environment, including being nervous or fearful of performing tasks or making an incorrect clinical decision (Fletcher et al., 2004; Hassan et al., 2006; Langan-Fox & Vranic, 2011; Stucky et al., 2009). Instructors might experience stressors associated with divided attention while concomitantly providing patient care and teaching, as well as managing multiple patients and their families (Firth-Cozens, 2003; Lepnurm, Lockhart, & Keegan, 2009; Rutledge et al., 2009; Song, Tokuda, Nakayama, Sato, & Hattori, 2009).

Negative affect has a direct and adverse impact on cognition and psychomotor skills, both of which decline as the magnitude of stressors and the number of concurrent stressors increase (Andreatta et al., 2010; Dandoy & Goldstein, 1990; Finn et al., 2018; Heatherton & Wagner, 2011; Kirchbaum, Pirke, & Hellhammer, 1993; Schuetz et al., 2008; Wiswede, Münte, & Rüsseler, 2009). This increases the risk of clinicians not only injuring patients but also themselves by performing tasks incorrectly.

In addition to increasing the probability for error, these adverse effects put clinicians at risk for incorrect assimilation of the learning context, making it more difficult to build a strong knowledge framework and resulting in extended training periods for discrete cases and in aggregate (Barsuk et al., 2010; Bond et al., 2004; Desai & Desai, 2018; Hunt et al., 2008). Negative affect builds on itself if unmitigated (Santesso et al., 2012). This is particularly true when stress adversely affects performance in the clinical setting in which a trainee is having difficulty, the patient is uncomfortable or annoyed, and the instructor is increasingly concerned about the patient and the amount of time it is taking to perform the clinical tasks. Communication between these constituents, and potentially the patient's family, can further worsen an already stressful context (DiGiacomo & Adamson, 2001).

Healthcare requires high-quality, reliable, and accurate performance to achieve optimal clinical outcomes. Clinicians are expected to perform to these high standards upon licensure. All too often, however, they are not afforded adequate opportunity to practice their skills with sufficient frequency to achieve those standards during training. For example, placing an IV catheter requires knowledge of the various instruments and supplies and how they work and connect with the others, as well as the manual dexterity to control each instrument or multiple instruments concurrently, all of which must be done in a way that does not harm the patient, the clinician, or other clinicians working with the patient.

To achieve mastery in any given area of expertise requires concerted and repeated practice, supported by constructive feedback and assessment (Chancey, Sampayo, Lemke, & Doughty, 2019; Ericsson, 2004, 2011; McKinley, Boulet, & Hambleton, 2005). This is especially true for psychomotor skills. Clearly, it is unethical to conduct prolonged or multiple attempts at intervention to facilitate learning, or to repeat interventions for the sake of practice in a real clinical setting. Not only would this be uncomfortable for patients, it increases the risk for harm or poor quality care. Simulation provides a contextually accurate environment for practicing techniques without adversely affecting real patients.

Consider the example of an elderly patient, who, after being found feverish and delirious by a family member, is brought to an emergency room in septic shock from an untreated infected toe. The attending physician orders an IV to be placed, and the task is assigned to an intern. The patient is dehydrated, the family is anxious, and the healthcare team is working intensely to avert the life-threatening situation. This context has multiple levels of embedded stress to which more experienced providers might be accustomed. For the intern, however, these stressors, coupled with the unfamiliarity of performing the clinical task, can lead to affective overload. This could in turn directly—and adversely—lead to cognitive dissonance that impedes performance.

If the intern has had an opportunity to practice placing an IV in multiple simulated contexts so that performance became automatic, the impact of the situational stressors will be more easily managed. This will prevent delays in care or a prolonged task-related clinical engagement that could potentially worsen the clinical situation. The likelihood of injury to self or others from using instruments incorrectly or using an incorrect technique will also be significantly reduced. In addition, had the team been able to practice performing lifesaving skills together, they might have had sufficient situational awareness to support the intern during the event by using supportive language, providing guidance throughout the task, or even assigning the task to a more seasoned team member because they understand that the difficulty of placing the IV in the critical situation is beyond the intern's abilities. This example is indicative of situations that are not unusual in healthcare and illustrates how simulation can be used to improve clinician safety.

Environmental Safety

Human performance is instrumental to risk management; however, numerous environmental factors influence safety in healthcare. For example:

- Facilities might be designed to prioritize aesthetics over function

- Equipment might be integrated into clinical practice without sufficient prior training for personnel
- Utility hookups might lead to inefficient or unsafe power connections
- Furnishings and room designs might be inconsistent and confounding
- Storage space might be poorly labeled or inadequately maintained

All these environmental factors require clinicians to divert attention from patient care to ensure safety.

Simulation facilitates the optimization of environmental design and orients clinicians to the environments in which they work (Andreatta, Marzano, & Smith, 2012; Bender, 2011; Dearmon et al., 2013). For example, before selecting and integrating new defibrillators, nurses from the entire hospital may be invited to test multiple models using mannequin simulators as patients in various room contexts. Each patient simulator experienced cardiopulmonary arrest that required use of the defibrillator. After using the equipment in these simulated contexts, the nurses evaluated each model and noted specific issues that were challenging for them to use. These data informed the purchasing decisions and provided the equipment vendors with suggestions for how to improve some of the design features of their models.

In another example, concerns over patient safety and quality of care led us to design an immersive simulation-based orientation in new hospital facilities before transferring the clinical care of actual patients (Andreatta & Marzano, 2013). All clinicians participated in simulated patient care necessitating the use of resources required for patient triage, low- and high-risk antepartum care, normal and urgent intrapartum care, and normal and emergent postpartum care, including surgical interventions. In addition to patient care in the new facilities, participants were paged to consult at each of two institutional emergency departments: pediatric and adult. We asked participants to identify areas of concern, causes for delays, and issues they felt could adversely affect patient care. These data identified several significant quality challenges for which we were able to make specific recommendations for improvement.

Practices and Processes

Hospitals and clinics are busy places, where clinicians, technicians, administrators, and staff—who must manage a wide variety of conditions while facing major time limitations—interact with patients and their families. To provide some measure of control and continuity, institutions establish processes, practices, procedures, and protocols—both formal and informal—that serve as a form of governance over actions and activities within and between institutions. These rules and guidelines might be developed proactively or reactively in response to a near miss or adverse event. They are typically created by risk-management administrators in consultation with representatives from the clinical areas affected by directives. However, institutions rarely have a specific method for reviewing existing processes, practices, procedures, and protocols to determine whether there are conflicting rules, obsolete recommendations, inefficient processes, or directives that are practically impossible to implement. The following section presents examples of how the authors use simulation to analyze processes in one clinical area of our institution and to inform improvement recommendations for those processes.

Process Analyses

Simulation provides a platform for analyzing both formal and informal institutional practices and using those analyses for improving associated quality and safety at a system-wide level. Optimally, these types of simulation activities will be supported at the highest levels by institutional management, conducted on a routine basis, and include all clinical specialties and all clinical, administrative, and support staff. Interdisciplinary teams serve this function better than specialty-specific or clinician-focused activities. The debriefing can be used to identify those practices with potential to adversely impact patient care. Capturing and tracking those areas of concern over time will provide a data set from which to analyze trends and reveal the areas requiring review or clarification. Designing interdisciplinary simulated scenarios that require clinicians to implement frequent, infrequent, casual, and critical policies helps reveal those areas where improvements can be made. Likewise, simulated scenarios designed to further improve safety and efficiencies in areas where a single discipline manages tasks, decision-making, or other patient activities could benefit discipline-specific behaviors.

Process Improvement

Simulation-based methods are invaluable for identifying areas where excess or deficiencies weaken processes within a healthcare system. Conducting simulation-based drills that require multispecialty, interdisciplinary teams to engage in patient-care scenarios is especially useful for identifying weak areas that might otherwise go unnoticed until an adverse or near-miss event occurs. For example, the results of a program involving physicians, nurses, residents, and allied health professionals from emergency medicine, obstetrics, anesthesiology, and neonatology tasked with providing care to pregnant patients presenting to an emergency department (simulated) identified five categories of discrepancies between health system policies and procedures and actual clinical practices by clinicians (Andreatta, Frankel, Smith, Bullough, & Marzano, 2011). Conflicts and inconsistencies included:

- The use of discipline-specific practices such as jargon

- Multiple and differing protocols for the same situation

- Policies that were either unknown or unconsidered

- Situations in which policy was needed but absent

- Policies that were impossible to implement practically

These discrepancies were identified during debriefing sessions that followed the simulated clinical management, and at least one discrepancy was revealed during each session. Importantly, each discrepancy had the potential to lead to errors in patient care or delays in expedited care.

Consider a clinical scenario in which a patient arrives to an emergency department and the resident physician asks the nurse to "draw a rainbow." An experienced nurse from that particular emergency department might understand that the order requests that blood be drawn for every color-coded lab vial. However, if the nurse is new to the department, she might not understand what the resident is ordering. At best, this could lead to a delay in the order being implemented; at worst, assumptions about the order could lead to inaccurate care.

The value of simulation-based activities to facilitate this type of quality improvement is tremendous, if only because it would be practically impossible to discriminate the same information through standard evaluation practices of clinical processes. Current quality monitoring typically involves tracking near-miss and adverse outcomes, such as iatrogenic injury or infection, that are reported and analyzed during morbidity and mortality conferences (which are commonly referred to as M & M). Typically, these discussions include participants from one discipline and specialty, thus limiting the ability to analyze system-level weaknesses. Without the information garnered through the types of inclusive simulation described earlier, system-level discrepancies would likely remain hidden until an error brought them to the forefront. Recently, Lobos et al. (2019) studied the use of simulation-based event analysis to investigate adverse events. They found that—compared to traditional event analysis—the use of simulation allowed for immediate debriefing with participation of the clinicians involved, improved the discovery of unique causes for errors, and generated improved strategies for error prevention.

Process Development

In the same way simulation-based activities can help analyze, review, and improve healthcare practices, they can be used to develop processes that are absent but needed (Andreatta, Perosky, & Johnson, 2012; Schulz, Lee, & Lloyd, 2008). For example, clinical care can rapidly change through the development of a new technology, such as advanced scanning devices or redesigned surgical instruments. In these situations, the processes and procedures that regulate how clinical care is provided might also need to be changed to accommodate the new technology. Rather than guessing how those policies should be changed, clinicians can use the technology in simulated contexts to determine how best to approach the creation of clinical and administrative guidelines that affect its use. They can also have the opportunity to test the newly created guidelines with other constituents in simulated contexts before enacting the new technology and new process recommendations in the course of real patient care.

Referring to the example of using simulation to select new defibrillators for the health system, the consensus opinion of those participating in the evaluation was to implement a policy that removed the doors covering the manual controls to minimize the likelihood of delays due to unclear operating instructions. Further simulation-based activities confirmed that removing the doors eliminated all confusion about how to access the manual controls without minimizing the clarity of how to operate the equipment in automatic mode.

Professional Development

The use of simulation to establish performance standards and facilitate performance assessment can significantly enhance professional development for clinicians at all levels of expertise and in all clinical specialties.

Self-Assessment

Established performance standards and validated assessment mechanisms provide clinicians with a platform for demonstrating their clinical abilities; such a platform is presently difficult to achieve through direct observation of clinical practice, written examination, case logs documenting the numbers and types of clinical activities performed, or examination of the clinical records of treated patients. Simulation levels the playing field by having a common platform (controlled contextual variance), validated assessment instruments (controlled measurement variance), consistent case complexity (controlled clinical variance), and prescheduled performance opportunities (controlled extraneous variance due to fatigue, competing demands, and so on; Andreatta & Gruppen, 2009; Andreatta, Marzano, & Curran, 2011). These levels of control facilitate accurate assessment that informs clinicians whether they need to practice or refresh their skills before they degrade or after they have had a break in continuous practice that might have weakened their skills. These types of assessments do not need to be formal; rather, the ability to self-assess privately could lead clinicians to consistently maintain their skills as part of their routine practice and provide evidence of this practice as part of their continuing education toward professional development. The following section discusses this further.

Maintenance of Competency

All licensed healthcare providers are required to provide evidence that they have maintained their professional competency over time. Currently, specialty boards, state boards, and various other national or international accrediting bodies define the requirements for maintenance of certification (competency; Lewis, Gohagan, & Merenstein, 2007). There might be multiple levels and requirements for the initial granting of licensure, as well as for maintenance of licensure. For example, initial granting of specialty board certification is a multitiered process that includes:

- Graduation from an accredited training program
- A passing score on a written examination

- Completion of a specific number of required clinical cases
- A passing score on an oral examination administered by examiners from the specialty board

The board-certification process primarily assesses cognitive skills, with no measurable performance evidence in either the psychomotor or affective domains. After achieving board certification, practitioners enter into a process called maintenance of certification. Requirements for maintenance of certification vary depending on the discipline and specialty, but typically include successfully reading and answering written questions about a set of predetermined articles and achieving a passing score on a written examination every few years. If successful, the clinician reenters another practice period before repeating the maintenance of certification process. Again, this process assesses cognitive skills only.

The credentialing process examines cognitive skills. For multiple reasons, it assumes that psychomotor and affective performance will positively correlate. The primary reason is that it is difficult to measure psychomotor and affective skills in a way that is predictive. This is because few (if any) performance standards are defined for those domains. This is in large part due to two factors:

- The challenge of assessing performance during real-time clinical care
- The variability of clinical cases that confound direct comparison between standards and performance

Simulation provides a platform for resolving this barrier because it facilitates the use of standardized cases and the concomitant establishment of measurable performance standards. As a result, several credentialing bodies have begun to require performance in a simulated clinical context as part of the certification and maintenance of certification processes. For example, the American College of Surgeons (ACS; 2012) now requires candidates to successfully complete the Fundamentals of Laparoscopy simulation that measures psychomotor skills, and the American Board of Anesthesiology (ABA, n.d.) has mandated simulation-based performance as part of the Maintenance of Certification in Anesthesia (MOCA; Levine, Flynn, Bryson, & Demaria, 2012; Sachdeva et al., 2011).

These examples illustrate the move toward performance-based assessment in the certification and maintenance of certification processes. Still, a substantial amount of work remains to be accomplished before these assessment outcomes can be used as competency evidence. Simulation for high-stakes assessment requires rigorous statistical validation to ensure that performance measured in a simulated context predicts competent performance in actual clinical practice. However, simulation has the potential to bridge the existing gap between the evidence required by the current certification process and the optimal evidence required to demonstrate competence across all performance domains. The use of simulation-based assessment can inform clinical training contexts, certification, maintenance of certification, and re-entry and expansion of practice credentialing (Luchtefeld & Kerwel, 2012). One advantage of using simulation-based performance for credentialing processes is that it facilitates assessment in every performance domain. This adds statistical power to the evaluation process because the triangulation of data will provide a greater degree of assurance that the outcomes predict competence.

Privileging, Reentry, and Expansion of Practice

In addition to licensure and board certification, many institutions require additional evidence before granting privileges for clinical practice. These typically include a clinician who has the desired privileges at the institution observing the performance of one desiring privileges or, in more complex areas, the completion of a subspecialty program and its associated credentialing processes. The development of increasingly complex simulation programs, enhanced contextual fidelity, and precisely validated assessment mechanisms will afford the same level of assurance and standardization to the privileging process as described for the certification process in the previous section.

The perpetual technological and procedural advancements in healthcare require clinicians to not only maintain their skills but also to expand them. Simulation provides the opportunity for clinicians to acquire new skills and techniques, acquaint themselves with new technologies and equipment, and practice infrequently performed procedures or clinical tasks (Andreatta, Chen, Marsh, & Cho, 2011; Andreatta et al., 2010; Bennett, Cailteux-Zevallos, & Kotora, 2011). Ideally, practitioners should be able to acquire, practice, review, and rehearse their skills in a simulation environment before performing them in applied clinical care. In this way, simulation serves as a form of gatekeeping that minimizes risks for clinicians and patients.

Team Development

Individual competence alone is not sufficient. All practitioners work as part of a team, not just as individuals. Team-based factors are known contributors to adverse and sentinel events.

Team-development efforts have accordingly been recommended as part of quality and safety practices in most hospitals and clinics (Leape & Berwick, 2005).

Studies evaluating the extent to which these types of activities will affect actual patient care are ongoing and not yet conclusive. However, using simulation to facilitate these types of activities makes logical sense. Team-based performance requires contextually accurate circumstances that cause the types of challenges typical of quality and safety concerns. It would be unethical to enact these types of team exercises in actual clinical practice, so simulation provides the next best alternative.

Numerous opportunities are possible, but interdisciplinary cases derived from actual cases from the institution's records have the greatest potential for eliciting relevant team-based factors, as well as minimizing the perception that the case scenario is improbable or contrived (which can reduce the engagement of some clinicians). All aspects associated with individual performance can be considered for team performance as well, and especially the uses of routine performance drills have been shown to have direct effect on clinical performance and patient outcomes (Andreatta, Saxton, Thompson, & Annich, 2011).

Medical-Legal Issues

Simulation can be used effectively to address medical and legal issues such as obtaining informed consent and simulating events in preparation for litigation.

Informed Consent

Informed consent is a contract made between a patient and those responsible for the patient's care (Terry, 2007). The contract is made when the patient requires medical care. This puts patients at a disadvantage because they are vulnerable due to a diagnosed medical condition or injury. Patients are asked to sign a form essentially releasing the medical establishment from all responsibility for any and all complications that might occur during the provision of clinical care. Patients are required to choose between signing the contract and not receiving the care required to maintain their health or in some cases to avoid death.

The process of contracting informed consent involves a physician reviewing the indications for the required treatment or procedure(s) that will be performed along with any associated risks of the prescribed care plan, such as bleeding, infection, and up to and including death. The informed consent process typically takes less than 30 minutes, during which time patients must interpret unfamiliar medical terminology to evaluate the potential risks versus outcomes for their particular medical circumstances. Patients have become more proactive about asking questions as a result of information available to them through the internet, including online forums and patient information sites. However, they remain at a disadvantage because of the threat to their health and well-being if they do not agree to the providers' terms, as well as their relative lack of clinical knowledge.

Simulation has the potential to improve this process for patients by providing them with more information presented in a more understandable way, which is also accessible through multiple viewings repeated at will. For example, consider a patient who has been diagnosed with a tumor, which is an indication for surgery. The typical informed consent process involves a surgeon explaining the step-by-step procedure to the patient. However, a videotaped simulation of key portions of the surgery could be used to actually show the patient the step-by-step process. The surgeon would typically review the potential complication risks using terms such as bleeding, infection, damage to bowel, bladder, ureters, and blood vessels, but a simulator could be used to demonstrate what these complications are, as well as how they would be repaired. A videotaped simulated procedure could also help orient the patient to the preoperative, operative, and postoperative contexts in the same way that hotel websites show guests what to expect on arrival. Patients could be given a DVD or provided with web access to this information so that they could review it multiple times as needed. Additional information could include postoperative information such as how to care for wounds, manage side effects, or perform physical therapy exercises.

Providers could also use simulators to demonstrate their skills while orienting patients to their individual care plans and any associated risks. Mannequin simulators, procedural trainers, virtual-reality models, and standardized patient actors can support the informed consent process by demonstrating to patients exactly what will take place during their care. Although resource-intensive, these types of simulations could occur through small group activities to review common aspects of care, with private review of individual details. As simulation technologies continue to improve, the ability for clinicians to demonstrate exactly what they will do using a model derived from patient care data (see "virtual simulations" in Chapter 7) will further improve the integrity of the informed consent process.

The use of simulation as part of the informed consent process could provide five major improvements to the current system:

- It would likely result in more well-informed patients due to the multiple modalities through which the information is presented, including sequential audio, video, text, and illustrations. More informed patients will likely feel more empowered to ask appropriate questions.

- It could allow patients to review the information later so that if new questions arise, they can ask them before the scheduled procedure or treatment.

- It could enhance the security of the medical-legal environment for providers by documenting the information provided to patients during the informed consent process.

- It could provide a more standardized informed consent process, eliminating the variability that currently exists depending on which physician provides the information.

- Access to these types of simulations—especially if they are in a format that facilitates on-demand access—could decrease the amount of time spent during clinic appointments for these consultations, as well prepare patients to participate in their own care.

Litigation

Litigation is an unfortunate reality of healthcare practice in many countries. Currently, several factors work against healthcare providers and institutions when a legal complaint is filed.

Documentation is a key factor in a clinical practice defense. However, most lawsuits don't end up in court until several years after the actual event.

Medical documentation is rarely sufficient to adequately describe the details around clinical events. Moreover, jury members typically do not have medical backgrounds. This disadvantages defendants because lawyers might play on the sympathies of a jury in cases regarding an adverse patient outcome, regardless of whether the outcome was actually a result of a medical error or negligence. This is a situation in which simulation can provide a useful means for reducing costs associated with medical malpractice.

Simulation provides the opportunity for the jury to witness what happened during clinical care, what was typical or atypical about the case, why and how complications could be expected, how they were managed, and why the patient outcome resulted. Rather than listening to verbal interpretations of clinical information that is abstract, the jury would be able to see exactly how things occurred and why decisions were made the way they were (Clifford & Kinloch, 2008). Simulation can allow the jury to see inherent challenges to a procedure or demonstrate that correct medical practice was delivered, despite the patient outcome. In conjunction with using simulation as part of the informed consent process, the jury could assess whether the patient understood the potential complications of his or her care plan.

Consider the following real-life example. A patient was admitted to the hospital in labor, with expressed desires to have a completely natural labor. Her fetus began to show signs of compromise, as demonstrated by a fetal heart rate tracing. The physicians and nurses explained the need for an emergency cesarean delivery to the patient and her partner; however, the patient and her partner refused to consent to the procedure. Note that in most states, performance of a cesarean delivery without patient consent is considered assault. The healthcare team tried to explain the severity of the situation to the patient and her partner for 45 minutes, at which time the patient consented. She was moved to the operating room. The fetal heart tones were no longer present, and the baby was stillborn via cesarean delivery. Despite exhaustive resuscitative efforts, the baby could not be revived and was declared dead.

Despite the accurate clinical management of the case, the documentation did not adequately reflect the tone and obstinacy of the patient's refusal to sign the consent. When the first depositions for the legal case were being taken three years later, the patient recalled that she and her partner were not adequately informed of the urgency of the situation. Several members of the healthcare team who were present at the time of the event had moved and were unavailable. During the deposition, the physician reviewed the fetal heart rate tracing under questioning and noted that the patient refused to sign the consent, which led to the delay in performing the cesarean delivery. The jury was left to decide which accounting of events to believe, while facing a grieving couple whose baby died.

Simulation could demonstrate the staging of the actual events that occurred for the jury so that the defendant's lawyer could walk them through the case, step-by-step, demonstrating the actual events and the timeline where information was provided to the patient and when consent was granted. The jury would then be able to deliberate with a realistic depiction of the occurrence. Along with seeing a grieving patient and her partner, the jury would also see a physician who did everything possible to provide the best care for the patient and her baby within the law. At minimum, the jury would have witnessed the facts and challenges of the case rather than simply heard a description of them in abstraction.

Simulation can also provide a platform for preparing healthcare workers for the courtroom by helping them learn how the legal system examines care records and how to provide testimony during a malpractice trial. A simulated trial enables participants to learn about all stages of a malpractice suit, including a trial, which prepares them to provide accurate and comprehensive information to the jury (Jenkins & Lemak, 2009). This is an important part of medical education that is lacking, especially given its importance in applied clinical practice.

Conclusion

How can you begin using simulation to manage and mitigate risk and improve quality and safety at your institution? Start by working with your quality-improvement and risk-management groups to identify areas in which adverse, sentinel, or near-miss events have occurred in the past five years and in which clinical outcomes from your institution are below the national level. Working with these offices will serve multiple purposes:

- You will identify areas in which improvements will be most visible. This will make it easier to capture evidence about performance effects tied to simulation activities.

- You will gain insight into concerns at the institutional level, as well as gain multilateral partnerships in developing objectives and implementing activities.

- These groups possess expertise that is critical for analyzing the healthcare metrics required to evaluate outcomes.

- You will build a collaborative program that can serve the quality and safety needs of the institution itself in all the ways discussed in this chapter.

Building a culture in which quality and safety are integral components of clinical practice is essential for high-performing healthcare institutions. Simulation resources and methods provide a framework for introducing and maintaining this type of culture. The Society for Simulation in Healthcare (2010) offers guidance for building programs designed to support the acquisition and maintenance of clinician performance factors through processes that have resulted in system-level change at many healthcare institutions.

References

The American Board of Anesthesiology. (n.d.). *About MOCA 2.0.* Raleigh, NC: Author. Retrieved from http://www.theaba.org/MOCA/About-MOCA-2-0

American College of Surgeons. (2012). *Joint statement by the ACS and SAGES on FLS completion for general surgeons who perform laparoscopy.* Chicago, IL: Author. Retrieved from https://www.facs.org/about-acs/statements/fls-completion

Andreatta, P., Chen, Y., Marsh, M., & Cho, K. (2011). Simulation-based training improves applied clinical placement of ultrasound-guided PICCs. *Supportive Care in Cancer, 19*(4), 539–543. doi:10.1007/s00520-010-0849-2

Andreatta, P., Frankel, J., Smith, S. B., Bullough, A., & Marzano, D. (2011). Interdisciplinary team training identifies discrepancies in institutional policies and practices. *American Journal of Obstetrics & Gynecology, 205*(4), 298–301. doi:10.1016/j.ajog.2011.02.022

Andreatta, P., & Marzano, D. (2013). *Comprehensive, simulation-based clinical care orientation informed quality and safety mechanisms prior to moving to new hospital facilities.* In abstracts presented at the 13th Annual International Meeting for Simulation in Healthcare. *Simulation in Healthcare, 8*(1), 66.

Andreatta, P., Marzano, D., & Smith, R. (2012). *Comprehensive clinical care orientation using simulated patients informs quality and safety mechanisms prior to moving to new hospital facilities.* Abstracts from SimHealth 2012, Sydney, AU, September 2012.

Andreatta, P., Perosky, J., & Johnson, T. R. (2012). Two-provider technique is superior for bimanual uterine compression to control postpartum hemorrhage. *Journal of Midwifery & Women's Health, 57*(4), 371–375. doi:10.1111/j.1542-2011.2011.00152.x

Andreatta, P., Saxton, E., Thompson, M., & Annich, G. (2011). Simulation-based mock codes significantly correlate with improved pediatric patient cardiopulmonary arrest survival rates. *Pediatric Critical Care Medicine, 12*(1), 33–38. doi:10.1097/PCC.0b013e3181e89270

Andreatta, P. B., & Gruppen, L. D. (2009). Conceptualising and classifying validity evidence for simulation. *Medical Education, 43*(11), 1028–1035. doi:10.1111/j.1365-2923.2009.03454.x

Andreatta, P. B., Marzano, D. A., & Curran, D. S. (2011). Validity: What does it mean for assessment in obstetrics and gynecology? *American Journal of Obstetrics & Gynecology, 204*(5), e1–e6. doi:10.1016/j.ajog.2011.01.061

Andreatta, P. B., Maslowski, E., Petty, S., Shim, W., Marsh, M., Hall, T., … Frankel, J. (2010). Virtual reality triage training provides a viable solution for disaster preparedness. *Academic Emergency Medicine, 17*(8), 870–876. doi:10.1111/j.1553-2712.2010.00728.x

Barsuk, J. H., Cohen, E. R., McGaghie, W. C., & Wayne, D. B. (2010). Long-term retention of central venous catheter insertion skills after simulation-based mastery learning. *Academic Medicine, 85*(10 Suppl.), S9–S12. doi:10.1097/ACM.0b013e3181ed436c

Bender, G. J. (2011). In situ simulation for systems testing in newly constructed perinatal facilities. *Seminars in Perinatology, 35*(2), 80–83. doi:10.1053/j.semperi.2011.01.007

Bennett, B. L., Cailteux-Zevallos, B., & Kotora, J. (2011). Cricothyroidotomy bottom-up training review: Battlefield lessons learned. *Military Medicine, 176*(11), 1311–1319.

Blum, R. H., Raemer, D. B., Carroll, J. S., Dufresne, R. L., & Cooper, J. B. (2005). A method for measuring the effectiveness of simulation-based team training for improving communication skills. *Anesthesia & Analgesia, 100*(5), 1375–1380.

Bond, W. F., Deitrick, L. M., Arnold, D. C., Kostenbader, M., Barr, G. C., Kimmel, S. R., & Worrilow, C. C. (2004). Using simulation to instruct emergency medicine residents in cognitive forcing strategies. *Academic Medicine, 79*(5), 438–446.

Cantrell, M. A. (2008). The importance of debriefing in clinical simulations. *Clinical Simulation in Nursing, 4*(2), e19–e23. doi:10.1016/j.ecns.2008.06.006

Chancey, R. J., Sampayo, E. M., Lemke, D. S., & C. B. Doughty. (2019). Learners' experiences during rapid cycle deliberate practice simulations: A qualitative analysis. *Simulation in Healthcare, 14*(1), 18–28. doi:10.1097/SIH.0000000000000324

Clifford, M., & Kinloch, K. (2008). The use of computer simulation evidence in court. *Computer Law & Security Review, 24*(2), 169–175. doi:10.1016/j.clsr.2007.11.002

Dandoy, A. C., & Goldstein, A. G. (1990). The use of cognitive appraisal to reduce stress reactions: A replication. *Journal of Social Behavior & Personality, 5*(4), 275–285.

Dearmon, V., Graves, R. J., Hayden, S., Mulekar, M. S., Lawrence, S. M., Jones, L., … Farmer, J. E. (2013). Effectiveness of simulation-based orientation of baccalaureate nursing students preparing for their first clinical experience. *Journal of Nursing Education, 52*(1), 29–38. doi:10.3928/01484834-20121212-02

Desai, B., & Desai, A. (2018). A method of cognitive training of medical students and residents. *Creative Education, 9*(9), 1377–1388. doi:10.4236/ce.2018.99102

DiGiacomo, M., & Adamson, B. (2001). Coping with stress in the workplace: Implications for new health professionals. *Journal of Allied Health, 30*(2), 106–111.

Easterbrook, J. A. (1959). The effect of emotion on cue utilization and the organization of behavior. *Psychological Review, 66*(3), 183–201. doi:10.1037/h0047707

Ericsson, K. A. (2004). Deliberate practice and the acquisition and maintenance of expert performance in medicine and related domains. *Academic Medicine, 79*(10 Suppl.), S70–S81.

Ericsson, K. A. (2011). The surgeon's expertise. In H. Fry & R. Kneebone (Eds.), *Surgical education: Theorising an emerging domain* (pp. 107–122). New York, NY: Springer Science + Business Media.

Finn, K. M., Metlay, J. P., Chang, Y., Nagarur, A., Yang, S., Landrigan, C. P., & Iyasere, C. (2018). Effect of increased inpatient attending physician supervision on medical errors, patient safety, and resident education: A randomized clinical trial. *JAMA Internal Medicine, 178*(7), 952–959. doi:10.1001/jamainternmed.2018.1244

Firth-Cozens, J. (2003). Doctors, their wellbeing, and their stress. *BMJ, 326*(7391), 670–671. doi:10.1136/bmj.326.7391.670

Fletcher, K. E., Davis, S. Q., Underwood, W., Mangrulkar, R. S., McMahon, L. F., Jr., & Saint, S. (2004). Systematic review: Effects of resident work hours on patient safety. *Annals of Internal Medicine, 141*(11), 851–857.

Garside, M. J., Rudd, M. P., & Price, C. I. (2012). Stroke and TIA assessment training: A new simulation-based approach to teaching acute stroke assessment. *Simulation in Healthcare, 7*(2), 117–122. doi:10.1097/SIH.0b013e318233625b

Hassan, I., Weyers, P., Maschuw, K., Dick, B., Gerdes, B., Rothmund, M., & Zielke, A. (2006). Negative stress-coping strategies among novices in surgery correlate with poor virtual laparoscopic performance. *The British Journal of Surgery, 93*(12), 1554–1559.

Heatherton, T. F., & Wagner, D. D. (2011). Cognitive neuroscience of self-regulation failure. *Trends in Cognitive Sciences, 15*(3), 132–139. doi:10.1016/j.tics.2010.12.005

Humara, M. J. (1999). The relationship between anxiety and performance: A cognitive-behavioral perspective. *Athletic Insight, 1*(2), 1-14.

Hunt, E. A., Fiedor-Hamilton, M., & Eppich, W. J. (2008). Resuscitation education: Narrowing the gap between evidence-based resuscitation guidelines and performance using best educational practices. *Pediatric Clinics of North America, 55*(4), 1025-1050. doi:10.1016/j.pcl.2008.04.007

Hunt, E. A., Shilkofski, N. A., Stavroudis, T. A., & Nelson, K. L. (2007). Simulation: Translation to improved team performance. *Anesthesiology Clinics, 25*(2), 301-319. doi:10.1016/j.anclin.2007.03.004

Issenberg, S. B., McGaghie, W. C., Petrusa, E. R., Lee Gordon, D. & Scalese, R. J. (2005). Features and uses of high-fidelity medical simulations that lead to effective learning: A BEME systematic review. *Medical Teacher, 27*(1), 10-28.

Jenkins, R. C., & Lemak, C. H. (2009). A malpractice lawsuit simulation: Critical care providers learn as participants in a mock trial. *Critical Care Nurse, 29*(4), 52-60. doi:10.4037/ccn2009355

Kirschbaum, C., Pirke, K. M., & Hellhammer, D. H. (1993). The 'Trier Social Stress Test'—A tool for investigating psychobiological stress responses in a laboratory setting. *Neuropsychobiology, 28*(1-2), 76-81.

Langan-Fox, J., & Vranic, V. (2011). Surgeon stress in the operating room: Error-free performance and adverse events. In J. Langan-Fox & C. L. Cooper (Eds.), *Handbook of stress in the occupations* (pp. 33-48). Northampton, MA: Edward Elgar Publishing Inc.

Lateef, F. (2010). Simulation-based learning: Just like the real thing. *Journal of Emergencies, Trauma, and Shock, 3*(4), 348-352. doi:10.4103/0974-2700.70743

Leape, L. L., & Berwick, D. M. (2005). Five years after To Err Is Human: What have we learned? *JAMA, 293*(19), 2384-2390. doi:10.1001/jama.293.19.2384

Lepnurm, R., Lockhart, W. S., & Keegan, D. (2009). A measure of daily distress in practising medicine. *Canadian Journal of Psychiatry, 54*(3), 170-180.

Levine, A. I., Flynn, B. C., Bryson, E. O., & Demaria, S., Jr. (2012). Simulation-based Maintenance of Certification in Anesthesiology (MOCA) course optimization: Use of multi-modality educational activities. *Journal of Clinical Anesthesia, 24*(1), 68-74. doi:10.1016/j.jclinane.2011.06.011

Lewis, M. H., Gohagan, J. K., & Merenstein, D. J. (2007). The locality rule and the physician's dilemma: Local medical practices vs the national standard of care. *JAMA, 297*(23), 2633-2637. doi:10.1001/jama.297.23.2633

Lobos, A., Ward, N., Farion, K. J., Creery, D., Fitzgibbons, C., Ramsey, ... Langevin, M. (2019). Simulation-based event analysis improves error discovery and generates improved strategies for error prevention. *Simulation in Healthcare, 14*(4), 209-216.

Luchtefeld, M., & Kerwel, T. G. (2012). Continuing medical education, maintenance of certification, and physician reentry. *Clinics in Colon and Rectal Surg*ery, 25(3), 171-176. doi:10.1055/s-0032-1322546

Mandler, G. (1979). Thought processes, consciousness, and stress. In V. Hamilton & D. M. Washington (Eds.), *Human stress and cognition: An information processing approach* (pp. 179-201). New York, NY: John Wiley & Sons.

McKinley, D. W., Boulet, J. R., & Hambleton, R. K. (2005). A work-centered approach for setting passing scores on performance-based assessments. *Evaluation & the Health Professions, 28*(3), 349-369. doi:10.1177/0163278705278282

Monks, T., Pearson, M., Pitt, M., Stein, K., & James, M. A. (2015). Evaluating the impact of a simulation study in emergency stroke care. *Operations Research for Health Care, 6*, 40-49. doi:10.1016/j.orhc.2015.09.002

Ross, A. J., Reedy, G. B., Roots, A., Jaye, P., & Birns, J. (2015). Evaluating multisite multiprofessional simulation training for a hyperacute stroke service using the Behavior Change Wheel. *BMC Medical Education, 15*, 143. doi:10.1186/s12909-015-0423-1

Rutledge, T., Stucky, E., Dollarhide, A., Shively, M., Jain, S., Wolfson, T., ... Dresselhaus, T. (2009). A real-time assessment of work stress in physicians and nurses. *Health Psychology, 28*(2), 194-200. doi:10.1037/a0013145

Sachdeva, A. K., Buyske, J., Dunnington, G., Sanfey, H. A., Mellinger, J. D., Scott, D. J., ... Burns, K. J. (2011). A new paradigm for surgical procedural training. *Current Problems in Surgery, 48*(12), 854-968. doi:10.1067/j.cpsurg.2011.08.003

Santesso, D. L., Bogdan, R., Birk, J. L., Goetz, E. L., Holmes, A. J., & Pizzagalli, D. A. (2012). Neural responses to negative feedback are related to negative emotionality in healthy adults. *Social Cognitive and Affective Neuroscience, 7*(7), 794-803. doi:10.1093/scan/nsr054

Schuetz, M., Gockel, I., Beardi, J., Hakman, P., Dunschede, F., Moenk, S., ... Junginger, T. (2008). Three different types of surgeon-specific stress reactions identified by laparoscopic simulation in a virtual scenario. *Surgical Endoscopy, 22*(5), 1263-1267. doi:10.1007/s00464-007-9605-1

Schulz, B. W., Lee, W. E. 3rd., & Lloyd, J. D. (2008). Estimation, simulation, and experimentation of a fall from bed. *Journal of Rehabilitation Research and Development, 45*(8), 1227-1236.

Society for Simulation in Healthcare. (2010). *Accreditation FAQ.* Retrieved from https://www.ssih.org/Credentialing/Accreditation/FAQ

Sollid, S. J. M., Dieckman, P., Aase, K., Soreide, E., Ringsted, C., & Ostergaard, D. (2019). Five topics health care simulation can address to improve patient safety: Results from a consensus process. *Journal of Patient Safety, 15*(2), 111–120.

Song, M.-H., Tokuda, Y., Nakayama, T., Sato, M., & Hattori, K. (2009). Intraoperative heart rate variability of a cardiac surgeon himself in coronary artery bypass grafting surgery. *Interactive Cardiovascular and Thoracic Surgery, 8*(6), 639-641. doi:10.1510/icvts.2008.195941

Stucky, E. R., Dresselhaus, T. R., Dollarhide, A., Shively, M., Maynard, G., Jain, S., ... Rutledge, T. (2009). Intern to attending: Assessing stress among physicians. *Academic Medicine, 84*(2), 251-257. doi:10.1097/ACM.0b013e3181938aad

Terry, P. B. (2007). Informed consent in clinical medicine. *Chest, 131*(2), 563-568.

van Galen, G. P., & van Huygevoort, M. (2000). Error, stress and the role of neuromotor noise in space oriented behaviour. *Biological Psychology, 51*(2-3), 151-171.

Van Gemmert, A. W. A., & van Galen, G. P. (1997). Stress, neuromotor noise, and human performance: A theoretical perspective. *Journal of Experimental Psychology, 23*(5), 1299-1313. doi:10.1037/0096-1523.23.5.1299

Van Sickle, K. R., Ritter, E. M., & Smith, C. D. (2006). The pretrained novice: Using simulation-based training to improve learning in the operating room. *Surgical Innovation, 13*(3), 198-204.

Wisewede, D., Münte, T. F., & Rüsseler, J. (2009). Negative affect induced by derogatory verbal feedback modulates the neural signature of error detection. *Social Cognitive and Affective Neuroscience, 4*(3), 227-237. doi:10.1093/scan/nsp015

"What happens if a big asteroid hits Earth? Judging from realistic simulations involving a sledgehammer and a common laboratory frog, we can assume it will be pretty bad."

–Dave Barry

Using Simulation for Research

13

Gary Geis, MD
Stephanie D. Boyd, PhD
Benjamin T. Kerrey, MD, MS

Not all simulation-based interventions produce a straightforward outcome. Despite numerous published studies that indicate the benefit of simulation-based education (SBE), the question "Where is the evidence that simulation makes a difference in learning or patient outcomes?" remains common. Measurements in simulation and dissemination of findings provide pieces of a fuller picture of how SBE affects learning and patient outcomes. This chapter provides a framework for educators who want to explore research and SBE.

Research on Simulation-Based Education

The strength of SBE is its ability to provide learners with opportunities for repetitive practice and timely feedback in settings where actual patients cannot be harmed. Research on SBE activities is needed to justify the implementation of time- and resource-intensive simulation-based curricula. Although practitioners of SBE may have extensive experience with simulation as a teaching tool, experience and knowledge of research are less common. Research provides a structured framework and methodology to measure whether interventions have an actual effect and to identify best practices for integrating simulation into health profession education (Hatala & Cook, 2019).

The published literature for a given subject, including SBE, can be divided into primary and secondary literature. Published studies on a given topic constitute the *primary literature* in the field. These single studies are foundational to the evolution of both research and curriculum development. Any individual study, however, reveals only a limited part of the general effectiveness of SBE. For this reason, experts periodically publish *secondary literature*, or reviews of single studies/primary literature. There are several types of secondary literature reviews, all of which summarize the current state of understanding on a specific topic.

OBJECTIVES

- Discuss the primary areas of study in which simulation-based education has been the focus.

- Discuss the translation of findings from simulation-based research to the bedside.

- Discuss the design and implementation of simulation-based research.

- Understand the nuances of simulation-based training for participants when research is involved.

Key Terms

The following terms are commonly used when describing research.

- **Human subject:** A living person about whom a researcher collects either 1) data through interaction or intervention with the person or 2) identifiable information.

- **Reliability:** The extent to which a measure is reproducible in other settings.

- **Validity:** The extent to which the observed measurement truly measures the outcome or the characteristic it is attempting to measure.

Kane's Validity Framework

Whether you are trying to understand advantages and pitfalls of simulation to create your own SBE or are looking to design your own simulation-based research, a review of existing literature is an essential step to guiding development. A framework may be helpful when interpreting current published research on simulation-based education.

Although it is not the only existing framework, Kane's validity framework can serve as a helpful guide to interpreting and designing simulation-based research. In Kane's framework, an intervention or tool is evaluated in terms of four inferences (Cook, Brydges, Ginsburg, & Hatala, 2015; Kane, 2006):

- **Scoring:** Refers to evidence at the level of the measurement tool. In developing a scoring tool to measure the effectiveness of a given simulation-based program, you would want to assess several aspects of the tool before starting to use it. For example, if multiple people use the tool and similarly score a participant's performance in a simulation, the tool shows excellent *inter-rater reliability*—evidence that the tool can be used reliably.

- **Generalization:** Refers to how the tool works in the educational setting. Generalization in this sense means what happens after the tool is developed and is used to evaluate the simulation-based training. For example, if the tool detects differences between novices and experts during the training, this is an example of validity evidence to support the generalization inference.

- **Extrapolation:** Examines how the tool functions in the real world. For example, demonstrating that those who score well on the tool during training are more likely to perform a task with fewer errors in the clinical setting is evidence to support the extrapolation inference.

- **Implications:** Refers to the consequences of the tool's use for the learner, the healthcare system, or society. For example, a tool that has good validity evidence at the first three levels but requires intensive use of resources may raise many issues when implemented. Could implementing the tool require other educational offerings to be reduced at your institution? Should everyone be assessed with the tool, or is it better directed at a targeted subset of learners? Questions like these should not be overlooked in the assessment of a tool or an intervention's validity.

Systematic reviews employ a rigorous approach to searching the literature—quantitative and experimental research often leads to or supports a meta-analysis, which is a specific form of research that combines results from multiple studies into a new analysis. Meta-analyses are often performed when a large number of rigorous studies show conflicting results or when the available studies were performed with relatively small numbers of subjects. Various types of non-systematic reviews also summarize the existing status of the literature on a topic, but they do not make claims to absolutely systematic selection or analytic processes. In general, these reviews look at the existing body of literature more "selectively, not exhaustively" (McGaghie, Issenberg, Petrusa, & Scalese, 2016, p. 987), with an emphasis on guiding readers to a deeper understanding of the complexities associated with the topic under review (Pawson, Greenhalgh, Harvey, & Walshe, 2005).

This chapter provides an overview of existing SBE research, highlights important questions that remain unanswered, and considers ways in which the literature shows a need for more rigorous reporting standards as the field matures.

Overview of Research on Simulation-Based Education

The published literature, including systematic reviews and meta-analyses, generally suggests that SBE is beneficial and acceptable to learners (Cook et al., 2011, 2012; Issenberg, McGaghie, Petrusa, Gordon, & Scalese, 2005; McGaghie, Issenberg, Cohen, Barsuk, & Wayne, 2011). We also know, however, that some simulation interventions are more effective than others. A review of the existing literature on SBE is helpful as a means of gaining insight into what factors are most associated with success. One large non-systematic review has suggested 12 evidence-based best practices

associated with effective learning (McGaghie, Issenberg, Petrusa, & Scalese, 2010):

- Feedback
- Deliberate practice
- Curriculum integration
- Outcome measurement
- Simulation fidelity
- Skill acquisition and maintenance
- Mastery learning
- Transfer to practice
- Team training
- High-stakes testing
- Instructor training
- Educational and professional context

A full review of the evidence supporting each best practice is beyond the scope of this chapter, but it is worthwhile to explore one example in some detail. Feedback is usually seen as an integral component of simulation education. Indeed, one large systematic review has identified feedback as the most important feature of effective SBE (Issenberg et al., 2005). Moreover, there is evidence that, regardless of approach, feedback contributes to improved learning (Levett-Jones & Lapkin, 2014). Questions remain, however, regarding when feedback should occur, how long *debriefing* (a feedback conversation that typically occurs immediately following a simulation) should last, and whether the use of video playback during debriefing contributes to its effectiveness. Although single studies have shown evidence for a variety of approaches, more recent reviews have concluded that there is not yet enough evidence in the literature to answer any of these questions definitively (Cheng, Auerbach, et al., 2014; Levett-Jones & Lapkin, 2014; Dieckmann et al., 2011).

As the field of SBE has matured, researchers have also begun focusing their efforts on how best to target simulation's use for maximum feasibility. One recent review illustrated that training conducted with low-cost, low-fidelity simulators often produces results that are just as good as those of courses using high-fidelity computerized simulators (Norman, Dore, & Grierson, 2012). This is an important finding for institutions that wish to integrate simulation into the educational process but cannot purchase expensive equipment. Other research has opened questions about the choices institutions must make when deciding for whom and how to distribute SBE. A series of published reviews (Cook, Erwin, & Triola, 2010; Cook et al., 2011, 2012, 2013) concluded that simulation will not be the best choice in every circumstance. We need focused research to understand who benefits most, and in what contexts SBE is the most beneficial use of resources.

Translating Simulation-Based Research to the Bedside

Over the last decade, there has been an increasing emphasis on the need for translational studies that evaluate whether improved learning in the educational environment translates to improved patient care and outcomes (moving from Kane's "generalization" inference to his "extrapolation" inference). This is a newer body of literature, driven in part by identification of patient outcome data as a major literature gap by some of the aforementioned reviews (Cook et al., 2010, 2012; McGaghie, Draycott, Dunn, Lopez, & Stefanidis, 2011). Until recently, there was not a sufficient body of work to support extensive reviews in this area. Consequently, while the preceding section emphasized secondary literature, primary literature will be more prominent as we consider evidence for simulation's impact on patient care and outcomes.

Translational studies have demonstrated that SBE can improve inpatient code team performance (Wayne et al., 2008), patient outcomes following births complicated by shoulder dystocia (Draycott et al., 2008), and the rate of complications and need for overnight stays for surgical patients (Zendejas et al., 2011). More recently, augmented and virtual reality–based interventions have been associated with improved procedural success and better patient outcomes when used to train residents performing both ventricular catheterization (Yudkowsky et al., 2013) and colonoscopies (McIntosh, Gregor, & Khanna 2014; Seymour, 2008).

Perhaps the most prominent example of the translation of SBE to improved patient care is a series of studies on the use of SBE to train residents in central venous catheter (CVC) insertion. The initial study demonstrated resident acquisition of appropriate CVC skills in the educational setting (Barsuk et al., 2009). The second study demonstrated that simulation-trained residents inserted CVCs on actual patients with fewer needle passes and higher success rates than traditionally trained residents (Barsuk et al., 2014). Subsequently, the research team reported an 85% reduction in catheter-related bloodstream infections after simulation-based training compared to the same unit before the intervention and to another intensive care unit in the same hospital (Barsuk et al., 2014). The investigators reported significant cost savings associated with this lower infection rate (Cohen et al., 2010), expanding their validity evidence to the "implications" level under Kane's framework. Finally, after demonstrating the successful translation of SBE to improved care at their own institution, the investigators disseminated the training to another hospital, where they replicated their success in infection reduction (Barsuk et al., 2014). By reproducing their results in a different setting, they strengthened the evidence that the patient-outcome improvements observed were due to the effects of the simulation training and not to another factor specific to the original study site.

SBE has also been shown to improve critical nontechnical skills, such as communication and teamwork, but the need for more translational studies on these outcomes is an acknowledged research priority (Cox, Seymour, & Stefanidis, 2015; McGaghie et al., 2010). Recently, there have been more studies published on SBE's impact on improved patient-to-provider communication and care team communication. The majority of SBE involving patient-to-provider communication uses simulated patients, while team communication has typically been conducted using simulators (Blackmore, Kasfiki, & Purva, 2018). Several recent studies have reported that patients (or their families) give higher ratings for the communication skills of healthcare providers after provision of SBE incorporating simulated patients than those who did not undergo SBE. These studies have involved a variety of patient-provider interactions, including conversations with families in the ICU (Sullivan, Rock, Gadmer, Norwich, & Schwartzstein, 2016), oncologist communication of bad news (Fujimori et al., 2014), and military mental-health screenings for soldiers (Douglas et al., 2016).

Improved communication among healthcare provider teams after simulation-based training has been demonstrated to translate to the clinical care environment in multisite studies of both postoperative teams (Paull et al., 2013) and operating room care teams (Sutherland et al., 2006; Weller et al., 2016). Demonstrating that patient care improves directly as a result of improved communication is more challenging.

One example is a study by Riley et al. (2011) to evaluate both patient outcomes and clinical skills after a simulation-based team communication training. In this study, one hospital received no intervention, one received a didactic (but well-established) team training, and a third received the same didactic training augmented by a series of in-situ simulations. The hospital with the simulation training experienced a significant reduction in perinatal mortality after the training, while the hospitals that received no simulation training experienced no change.

Reports of such post-intervention improvement at the patient level are not common but are increasingly emphasized as a priority. Translational outcomes are now sufficiently reported that literature reviews can begin to identify best practices for achieving changes at this level. There is some emerging evidence that repeated shorter interventions may be more effective than longer single interventions. This has become evident in communication-based simulation training (Blackmore et al., 2018) and is suggested for all learning. The aforementioned ICU study using simulated patients, for example, found no effect until participants had attended multiple sessions (Sullivan et al., 2016). On a related note, there is some evidence that skills gained through simulation-based training may not always persist without continued exposure (Armenia et al., 2018; Blackmore et al., 2018). One illustrative study that reported substantial "real world" improvement in teamwork and communication after a series of in-situ simulations also found a return to baseline scores only five weeks after simulations were ended (Miller, Crandall, Washington, & McLaughlin, 2012).

Simulation as a Research Tool

While the primary focus of this chapter is research *on* simulation—that is, research intended to evaluate simulation's effectiveness as an educational strategy—it is important to be aware that simulation may also be used as a research *tool* to study other topics in healthcare. For example, simulation has been used to:

- Assess new clinical environments for overlooked threats to patient safety (Geis, Pio, Pendergrass, Moyer, & Patterson, 2011)

- Study patient flow through clinical areas (Hung, Whitehouse, O'Neill, Gray, & Kissoon, 2007)

- Prepare an emergency department to participate in a clinical trial of the treatment of status epilepticus (Chan et al., 2019)

This type of research uses simulation's defining attributes to examine a variety of questions in ways that could not be achieved safely, ethically, or feasibly in actual clinical environments (Cheng, Auerbach et al., 2014). Although not the focus of this chapter, studies like these are an important component of the SBE literature.

A Note on Interpreting the Literature

In this overview of the current literature on SBE, we have focused largely on review articles. These sources typically summarize concepts that apply to SBE professionals working in a variety of topical areas. They also help clarify general gaps in the primary literature and focus attention on common flaws in study design and reporting methodologies. For example, many studies fail to provide adequate information about study participants (Lewis, Strachan, & Smith, 2012) or sufficient detail about

debriefing methods (Cheng, Eppich, et al., 2014; Levett-Jones & Lapkin, 2014; Palaganas, Fey, & Simon, 2016) and other elements of interventions (Cheng et al., 2016; Sevdalis, Nestel, Kardong-Edgren, & Gaba, 2016).

The prevalence of these flaws represents one of several important limitations to the utility of review. For example, lack of clear reporting in single studies makes it difficult to analyze findings from multiple studies in aggregate (Sevdalis et al., 2016). Further, even when all these elements are standardized and described in the primary article, other factors may confound results. Researchers in SBE work within varied institutional constraints and are faced with the task of conducting research while also providing education—sometimes in active patient care settings. Methods and practices will inevitably be diverse even with strong efforts at standardization. To an extent, a truly systematic review of the literature may not be possible (Eva, 2008; McGaghie et al., 2010; Pawson et al., 2005). Researchers should be aware of these limitations and should know that non-systematic reviews fill an important role. Similarly, the secondary literature should never be consulted to the exclusion of single studies.

As the field of SBE matures, researchers will continue to summarize current understanding in reviews, which in turn can reveal new areas that are ripe for study. This is part of the process of research. An understanding of this cycle can guide researchers to use best practices for designing rigorous, relevant studies and reporting findings in ways that contribute to SBE's growth as a field.

Resources for the Research Process

When conducting your literature review, consider these resources:

- **Literature databases:** Several online databases make it easier to search references and abstracts in the biomedical literature. This is often the most efficient way to begin your literature review. Medline, Embase, and PubMed are some of the most prominent examples.

- **Your institution's library:** Librarians, particularly at academic institutions, are trained in the science of systematically finding and sorting information. They can provide guidance on search technique and can also help you access full text articles for references you identify.

- **A citation manager:** There are several invaluable software tools for keeping track of references both during your literature review and later, when you are getting ready to publish. These tools will store your references and automatically format your bibliography according to your target journal's guidelines when you publish. However, citation managers are not foolproof, so you will still need to make sure the references are correct.

When you are planning and implementing your study procedures, consider these resources:

- **Your institution's institutional review board (IRB):** Your IRB representative(s) can be an excellent resource as you develop your protocol. They can help you determine what category of review will apply to your research and can often provide institutionally preferred protocol and consent document templates.

- **Published standards for reporting research:** Reporting standards developed by expert consensus define best practices for designing studies and reporting their results. The Standards for Quality Improvement Reporting Excellence (SQUIRE) provides a general framework for publishing healthcare improvement interventions (Ogrinc et al., 2016). Guidelines published by Cheng et al. in 2016 describe additional considerations specific to research in SBE.

- **Standardizing simulations:** In SBE research, it is important to standardize the intervention being studied, so that, to the extent possible, all participants receive the same intervention. The 2016 article by Cheng et al., referenced above, is an excellent resource for understanding the elements of a simulation that should be standardized and for obtaining guidance on how to clearly describe standardization procedures.

- **Your colleagues:** Research is almost always a team endeavor. Your work will be strengthened by collaboration with statisticians and colleagues who have subject matter expertise in areas relevant to your work (Brazil, Purdy, & Bajaj, 2019).

- **SimZones:** The types and variation in SBE activities can make selecting the best simulation-based approach overwhelming. SimZones is an organizational system for SBE. It has four types, or zones, of SBE. These range from solitary learner-directed activities to SBE in the actual care environment (Roussin & Weinstock, 2017). SimZones can help those designing simulation-based activities to understand what type of SBE is appropriate for a given problem and to address issues common to SBE.

Society for Simulation in Healthcare (SSH) Research Resources

SSH has a number of research resources available at https://www.ssih.org/SSH-Resources/Research-Tools:

- Research tools
- Medical literature management
- Planning and conducting research
- Research funding
- Social networking between researchers

Designing Simulation-Based Research

The preceding sections outlined some of the major areas of focus in the literature on simulation-based education and described how recommendations for best practice emerge from the process of research. The rest of this chapter provides a framework to help you begin considering ways of making your own contributions to the collective knowledge of the simulation education community. A comprehensive guide to designing research is well-beyond the scope of this chapter. Rather, we intend to provide a framework for starting research design, tools to develop an initial research plan, an overview of some of the nuances of simulation-based research, and additional resources.

Research studies are classified as either observational or interventional:

- **Observational:** In an observational study, the researcher makes no changes to the study subject or environment. The researcher *observes* only, with the intent of learning something new about the subject.

- **Interventional:** Interventional research requires the investigator to change at least one element of the subject or the environment to specifically measure the effect of that element. Importantly, interventional research also requires observation, so interventional studies use many of the same approaches for design and measurement as observational studies.

Both types of studies may employ the following types of methodologies:

- **Quantitative:** Quantitative methods typically result in findings that can be represented numerically. For example, a researcher may measure the time between patient arrival and initiation of treatment.

- **Qualitative:** Qualitative methods do not rely on numeric representation. Instead, they target a deeper understanding of selected issues. For example, participants might be interviewed or complete open-ended survey questions about factors that they believe cause delays in treatment initiation.

- **Mixed:** Mixed methods studies employ the collection and analysis of both quantitative and qualitative data.

Some observational studies take the form of targeted needs assessments, specifically intended to inform the development of better interventional studies. For example, consider how a needs assessment combining quantitative and qualitative measures could improve intervention design. Completing a needs assessment prior to an intervention is best practice, and not doing so has been cited as a weakness in the published simulation literature (Eppich, Howard, Vozenilek, & Curran, 2011; Weaver et al. 2010).

As suggested by Kane's framework, interventional studies typically progress through multiple phases. For example, an early study assessing the effect of a new course might simply evaluate whether the training is feasible and acceptable to participants, and whether learners demonstrate skill improvement immediately after completion. A second phase might aim to demonstrate sustained skill improvement in the simulated setting several months later.

Ideally, the ultimate goal of simulation-based education research will be to show that improvements in patient outcomes are linked directly to the education you are evaluating. Reaching this level of evidence qualifies the research as translational science (McGaghie, 2010). Starting this process can seem intimidating, but with a clear and well-developed research plan, the process becomes much simpler.

Where to Start: Developing a Research Framework

In daily working life, we often think of questions that could form the basis of important research. We wonder if the educational course we are required to attend really works (our experience tells us no) or why we struggle to remember the material when we need it. We ask ourselves these questions all the time, but they are often vague, unvoiced, and biased by our emotional responses and previous experience.

Conducting good research requires turning general or vague questions into focused questions that are "answerable" and that can guide development of research design (Bragge, 2010). The first step in designing a research project is to develop a specific, structured research question. If a question is vague or poorly developed, then the study results will be, too.

Using a structured framework to develop your question can help you avoid this problem. One of the most widely used frameworks for this purpose is the problem, intervention, comparison, and outcome (PICO) framework (Schardt, Adams, Owens, Keitz, & Fontelo, 2007). PICO is generally a framework for interventional research, but there are a number of PICO variants and similar frameworks, some of which can be used to develop a research question for observational studies. Table 13.1 provides an example of using the PICO framework to design a simulation-based study to improve the recognition of sepsis in medically complicated children.

Using the PICO framework, we now have an answerable question: For nurses who perform the initial evaluation of children in an emergency department (sample setting), does simulation-based training with a new pediatric sepsis simulator result in improved recognition of early-sepsis signs during training (outcome 1) and more rapid treatment of actual patients (outcome 2)?

Table 13.1	PICO Framework	
	Description	**Example**
Problem	What is the problem you are trying to solve?	Improving the care of septic patients requires early recognition and efficient treatment with fluids and antibiotics, especially by front-line providers like nurses. The problem is that sepsis can be especially difficult to recognize in medically complicated children, especially in the early stages.
Intervention	What intervention do you intend to study?	A new (hypothetical) augmented reality simulator has been developed that can mimic many of the signs and symptoms of sepsis, including changes in skin color, pulse, and skin temperature. The intervention is to use this new simulator to train providers to recognize milder physical abnormalities that are present in early sepsis.
Comparison	What is the alternative to the intervention (if relevant)?	Training with a standard human patient simulator.
Outcome	What will you measure to assess change as a result of your intervention?	Outcome 1: Learner performance on the human patient simulator before and after training Outcome 2: Time between patient arrival and completed administration of first intravenous fluids and antibiotics

The next step in designing a good research question is to use your question framework to conduct a comprehensive literature search. This is an additional benefit of using a question framework like PICO: Searching the literature for a refined, specific question is incomparably easier than for a vague, unstructured question. Moreover, an effective literature search almost always helps to refine the study question even more. An effective search also gives insight into the issues that need to be addressed when designing and conducting the study and shows how others have addressed these issues.

As you embark on this search, keep these points in mind:

- Take time to read both primary and secondary literature during your search.

- The references included in a good systematic review are an excellent place to find the highest quality and most relevant studies.

- Consider the strength of the evidence presented in other studies (there are numerous published tools to help with this step, e.g., Joanna Briggs Institute Meta-Analysis of Statistics Assessment and Review Instrument), and review their limitations.

- Previously published articles can suggest pitfalls you can avoid or opportunities to take existing work a step further.

- Consider the setting and study population. If a previous study took place at a large research institution and you are at a small community hospital, determine whether you can implement your work in the same way.

As you continue to plan your study, the existing literature is an invaluable guide and reference.

One pitfall early in the design stage is to let the scope of work get out of hand. You will likely think of many interesting questions and issues related to your main question. Avoid the temptation to chase each one. Instead, write them down and use them for your recommendations for future research—or for your next research study. The question framework can be especially helpful in avoiding this pitfall.

Aims, Hypotheses, and Statistics

After you have refined a specific, structured research question and used this question to comprehensively review the published literature, the next step is to develop the study aims and hypotheses. The *specific aims* of a study are simply the goals of the research, written as brief, focused points. These aims tell a reader what you plan to accomplish and drive the creation of the study design. For each specific aim, there is usually one or more corresponding hypotheses. *Hypotheses* are clear statements of what you believe the truth is with respect to your study aim. Any hypothesis must be finalized before the study starts and should not change until the results are reviewed.

For the sample PICO research question above, an example of the specific aim and hypotheses might look like this:

- **Aim:** To determine whether simulation-based training with a new pediatric sepsis simulator improves pediatric nurse recognition and treatment of sepsis in children.

- **Hypothesis 1a:** Pediatric nurses who participate in simulation-based training with the new pediatric sepsis simulator will more accurately identify physical findings present in early sepsis in children when compared with pediatric nurses who participate in training with a standard simulator, as measured by performance on post-training simulations.

- **Hypothesis 1b:** Patients with early sepsis who are initially evaluated by pediatric nurses who participated in the sepsis-simulator training will have initial intravenous fluids and antibiotics given more quickly when compared with patients initially evaluated by pediatric nurses who participated in standard training, as measured by lower time from patient arrival to completion of first fluids/antibiotic.

With the foundation of a research project in place, you are in an excellent position to take some often-neglected steps that can help maximize the chances for successful study completion. One such step—and perhaps the most important—is to get advice early and often from someone with statistical expertise. A statistical expert will help determine the necessary sample size—that is, the number of participants needed to detect the anticipated difference between groups. Using the previous example, a statistical expert can provide the number of pediatric nurses who need to be included (hypothesis 1a) and the number of patient encounters (hypothesis 1b). A conversation with a statistical expert can also reveal problems with your study design before the study starts, when they can more easily be fixed. Recent review articles have identified problems with sample size and statistical errors as being extremely common in the published research on simulation-based education (Issenberg et al., 2005; Lewis et al., 2012; Zendejas, Brydges, Wang, & Cook, 2013). When these errors are present, they limit the strength of the evidence produced by a study.

Measuring Outcomes

After you have refined your aims and hypotheses and consulted with a statistical expert, you will need to select study outcome measures and develop a data collection plan. You will test your hypotheses by using appropriate tools to measure the outcomes specified in your research question. This is less straightforward in simulation-based research than it is in other fields because the changes you can expect to see are rarely easy to demonstrate with a simple number. For example, if you were studying an investigational cancer drug, you would likely assess effectiveness by comparing the mortality rate among patients who received the drug with those who did not. In contrast, the options for outcomes in SBE research are often indirect (e.g., confidence, social factors, knowledge) and may be more ambiguous if not considered and refined.

SBE outcomes generally fall into four main topical categories:

- **Satisfaction:** Satisfaction outcomes relate to participants' perceptions regarding an intervention and are usually measured via participant surveys. Course evaluations that assess how learners perceive the quality of a training are one example. Other satisfaction measures evaluate confidence in skills or changes in attitude following an intervention. In general, you should not use satisfaction as your only outcome measure. As noted earlier in this chapter, there is already consensus that simulation is perceived as acceptable and useful by learners. However, it can be useful to include a basic satisfaction measure among other outcome measures. You may well learn something that helps you improve the training or better fit it into your institution's general educational landscape.

- **Technical:** Technical outcomes pertain to the participant's ability to perform a skill, such as demonstrating proficiency in central venous catheterization. Competency validation checklists are often used to assess technical outcomes.

- **Nontechnical:** Nontechnical skills are cognitive and interpersonal skills employed during clinical care. Examples include communication behaviors, teamwork, and knowledge (Gordon, Darbyshire, & Baker, 2012). Checklists that observers use to assess team communication and surveys that test knowledge before and after training are examples of measures that assess nontechnical skills.

- **Safety:** Outcomes in this category focus on improving the safety of the care delivered and the prevention of medical errors. These outcomes are the most likely to be translational in nature. The outcome for hypothesis 1b in the preceding example, which relies on the analysis of data from patient charts to demonstrate improved patient care, is one example of a safety-related outcome.

Outcomes can also be categorized by level of impact. In educational research, this is frequently done using Donald Kirkpatrick's (1998) set of descriptors:

- Participation (level 1)

- Attitudes (level 2a)

- Knowledge and/or skills (level 2b)

- Behavior (level 3)

- Organizational practice (level 4a)

- Benefit to patients (level 4b)

Under this system, satisfaction outcomes usually fall at level 1 or 2a. Outcomes related to both technical and nontechnical skills are typically categorized at level 2b if learning is only demonstrated in educational settings, or level 3 if there is a transfer of behavior to the clinical setting. Safety outcomes are most likely to be categorized at level 4a or 4b. As the field of SBE has matured, there has been increased emphasis on prioritizing research at Kirkpatrick levels 3 and 4. While it is not our intent to overwhelm readers with frameworks and hierarchies, it is helpful to have some awareness of the ways in which the outcome measures you select for your own research are likely to be categorized in the context of the broader SBE literature. A basic understanding of both Kane and Kirkpatrick is helpful in this regard.

In the preceding example, the outcome for hypothesis 1a was nurse recognition of specific physical findings on the human patient simulator (a technical skills outcome at Kirkpatrick level 2b). This outcome could be measured as present or not or by time to recognition (verbalization).

There are often a variety of ways to measure a given outcome, each with its own advantages and disadvantages. One benefit of conducting an extensive literature review during research question development is that it can help you identify outcome measures that are already in use. You do not need to develop your own measure to answer your research question; in fact, it is almost always better to use something that already has published evidence for its validity and reliability.

When reviewing a potential measure, look for information about how it was created and validated, and consider the settings in which it

has been used. Keeping Kane's framework in mind as you assess your options will be helpful. You will certainly want to choose a measure with existing evidence at Kane's scoring level. Depending on the nature of your study, you should also consider what evidence exists for the measure's effectiveness in the educational setting or, if applicable to your work, in the clinical setting.

Note that perfect evidence is *not* necessary. If you are doing a clinical investigation and the measure that seems most appropriate to you has so far only been used in the classroom setting, you will still usually be better off than you would be using a new measure—and your work may even help further the validation of this instrument. If you find yourself in that situation, reach out to the corresponding author of the article that initially described the measure. In most cases, they will be delighted to hear from you, answer questions, and possibly even collaborate as you develop this new use for their work.

Although the literature contains many published outcome measures, it is worth mentioning that there are situations in which you might need to develop your own. If you conclude that this is necessary, be sure to consult with experts both in the area you are studying (pediatric sepsis, in our example) and in the science of measure development. Allow ample time for this process. Without thoughtful planning and preparation, you may end up with a measure that is not capable of assessing your outcome.

Other Issues in Designing Simulation-Based Research

After determining the specific outcome (e.g., cool skin temperature) and measure (present or not), all data elements of interest must be identified. Researchers usually collect data for several participant and environmental factors in addition to the study outcome measure. For instance, in the preceding example, you may want to know the prior experience of nurses participating in the training, including how much clinical experience or sepsis training each participant had. This type of information, which is usually displayed in the first table when the study is published, is essential for the scientific community to understand the context for the study results, but it has often been inadequately reported in the SBE literature (Lewis et al., 2012). There was something unique about your participants that made them more (or less) likely to benefit from the training.

A related and important issue is determining whether the study groups were similar to each other aside from the difference in training. (For example, did nurses in both groups have similar levels of experience?) The participant and environmental data are most commonly used to determine whether differences were present. Researchers will specifically look for *confounding* factors—elements other than your intervention that could be responsible for changes observed in the outcome. Taking factors like these into account when you conduct the analysis will strengthen your ability to draw conclusions about the outcome. For example, you might find that nurses with less than three years of experience benefit from your intervention, while more experienced nurses do not. This is a very useful finding that can guide the next steps for curriculum development and research, and even maximize the cost-benefit breakdown at your institution. Recall that recent reviews have identified a lack of evidence on how to best target simulation trainings so they reach the people who can most benefit from them (Cook et al., 2011, 2012, 2013). By making sure you can describe participant backgrounds adequately, you are designing your study in a way that makes it more able to contribute to the broader exploration of this question.

After you have identified an outcome measure and determined the data that need to be collected in relation to that outcome, the participants, and the study environment, you will need to develop a plan for how to collect those data. Again using the preceding example, after determining the specific outcome (e.g., cool skin temperature) and measure (present or not), the most common approach to data collection would be to have an investigator record participant verbalization (i.e., whether participants say, "the hands are cool") or to ask participants to complete a questionnaire after the simulation.

Background data on participants would most commonly be collected by a questionnaire completed by the participants before the training. Consider the various methods of administering such a questionnaire: Will participants complete the questionnaire on paper, online, or in some other way? If you use a standardized checklist, how will you train the raters who use it to assess participants, and how will you make sure all raters use it in the same way?

You will also need to finalize your plans for the intervention itself. Make sure you have a clear plan that standardizes the specific simulation scenarios, simulators, and debriefing methods you will use. These steps are necessary to ensure that participants all receive comparable training, even if courses occur over a long period of time. When factors like these aren't standardized and reported in publication, it becomes hard to assess whether an intervention was successful or to gain insight into what elements of the intervention contributed to its success. You may recall that lack of standardization affects not only the strength of an individual study but also the strength of the general evidence for SBE (Cheng et al., 2016; Sevdalis et al., 2016). Keep this in mind as you finalize plans for your intervention.

Once the research plan is developed, one or more pilot sessions or "dry runs" of the study procedures can be invaluable in refining the plan and avoiding unforeseen errors. In the hypothetical pediatric sepsis study, suppose you wish to integrate video playback of the simulation during debriefings. You pilot this method and learn that the sound quality in the videos is poor. This problem, if not recognized until the study started, could have caused a significant delay and negatively affected the quality of your results.

Human Subjects Research and Informed Consent

By its nature, simulation-based research often involves human subjects and must be reviewed and approved by an institutional review board (IRB) before you can begin recruiting participants or collecting data. The role of the IRB is to protect the rights and welfare of research participants. In the United States, this involves ensuring that studies are conducted in accordance with the Federal Policy for the Protection of Human Subjects (known as the common rule; US Department of Health and Human Services, [DHHS], 2018). In other countries, other regulations will apply.

Depending on your study procedures and the level of risk to participants, the IRB may approve your study in one of several categories. The level of IRB oversight after approval depends largely on this initial approval category. The categories are:

- Full review—risk is high or unknown, and a full review is required

- Expedited—risk is present, relatively low, and requires a short review

- Exempt—risk is found to be minimal

- "Not human subjects"—does not have human subjects in the study

One of the central elements of ethical research is the concept of *informed consent,* which refers to the right of potential participants in your study to have the opportunity to review procedures, learn explicitly about potential risks and benefits of participating, and ask questions about the study. Simulation research is more likely than some other types of research to introduce new complexities to this process. For example, the team-based measures that are common when studying topics like communication can become complicated if you have one person in a team who chooses not to consent. When using team-based measures, you will need a plan to deal with this circumstance.

Simulation-based research is also more likely than some other fields of study to qualify for modifications to the typical consent requirements. The standard for research involving human subjects is to obtain signed documentation of informed consent from every participant. However, in certain circumstances, IRBs may approve either a waiver of documentation of informed consent or a full waiver of informed consent. A waiver of documentation of consent is typically seen when one of the following is true:

- The consent document is the only document linking the participant to the study, and the risk of harm from a breach of confidentiality is a major risk for the research.

- The study is minimal risk and involves no procedures for which written consent is typically required.

When documentation of consent is waived, the participant must still be provided with the information contained in the consent form, but the document will not be signed. In some cases, such as online surveys, this may not happen in person. A potential participant may receive a survey that includes a face or front page presenting information about the research project and the rights of research participants at the beginning. The information includes the statement that choosing to complete the survey constitutes agreement to participate. You should refer to the common rule or your institution's or country's IRB to understand the elements that are required to constitute informed consent, with or without a waiver of documentation.

A full waiver of informed consent is granted when it would not be feasible to obtain consent from participants due to the nature of the research. This is often seen when patient medical records are retrospectively reviewed. For example, in our hypothetical sepsis recognition study, we planned to review patient charts to determine whether time to completion of the first round of intravenous antibiotics and fluids decreased following the intervention. An IRB would likely approve a waiver of informed consent in this case because it would not be feasible to obtain consent from patients months after the hospital encounter, and the waiver would not increase risk to patients.

Vulnerable Populations and Educational Settings

One element of the common rule regulations is a set of requirements for studying vulnerable populations at increased risk of coercion or undue influence. These populations include both students and employees—frequent participants in simulation-based research. This means you must make specific plans with regard to recruitment, consent, and confidentiality. Think about how participants will be recruited. If a senior nurse researcher is approaching junior colleagues to participate, will they feel that it's acceptable to

express concerns or decline? In research protocols involving employee or student populations, it is common to specify that consent will be obtained by someone who does not occupy a position of authority over participants. Additionally, these protocols usually include specific assurances regarding confidentiality. Employee participants may fear that their performance during simulations could result in negative career consequences. Typical protections include written assurance that individual performance will not be reported to leadership.

Another element of simulation-based research that can affect the level of monitoring required by the IRB is the fact that it often blurs the line between research and education, because it so frequently integrates both. In some cases, a simulation study may be research only. For example, the authors of this chapter recently conducted a preliminary observational study to determine whether motion capture technology could identify differences in technique between novices and experts intubating mannequins (Kerrey et al., 2020). In this case, participants were not engaged in education and were present only to participate in research. A full informed consent process is required in studies of this type. Often, though, simulation-based research is integrated into training that is part of participants' standard continuing education. Such research often investigates the impact of the course rather than the performance of the participants. Put more simply, the *course* is the subject of the research, not the participants in the course, and only some learner activities constitute research participation.

A study carried out by Patterson et al. demonstrates how complicated this can become (Patterson, Geis, Falcone, LeMaster, & Wears, 2013). The study had the objective of demonstrating the feasibility of in-situ simulations to identify latent safety threats more effectively than lab-based training. The main outcome measure was number of threats identified, with secondary outcome measures assessing participant perception of the training's value. Emergency department healthcare providers were paged to unannounced simulations during their shifts; afterward, the teams debriefed while a facilitator used a standardized checklist to record safety threats identified by both facilitators and participants. After each event, participants were asked to complete an online survey assessing the value of the training.

What was a research activity and what was not? The answer was complex. Initially, the in-situ simulations were a novel intervention rather than institutionally typical continuing education. They were implemented for research purposes, and informed consent for all procedures was obtained. However, partway through the project, departmental leadership determined that the in-situ simulations were so valuable that they should become mandatory. The simulations themselves were now educational activities, and the IRB waived the requirement to obtain informed consent for new participants. Because learners never filled out the checklist themselves, their consent for its use to assess the course's impact was unnecessary. However, the survey was still a pure research activity. As such, it could not be mandatory, and participants were required to be informed of the nature of the research and their choices regarding participation.

Anonymity, Confidentiality, and Privacy

Simulation-based training is an attractive educational approach because it provides a safe but realistic environment to practice skills and receive timely feedback. To maintain this safe

environment while collecting research data, it is essential that participants feel confident that the data collected will not be used in ways they did not approve. Taking steps to protect privacy and confidentiality can reassure participants that their data will be used only to evaluate the outcomes of the research. This can be done by limiting the amount of identifiable data collected as well as the number of people who have access to these data. Data should be stored securely, and participants should be informed of the precautions you are taking. Where appropriate, team-based measures can increase confidentiality, as can anonymous data collection, which is often possible for survey data. Attention to these details will help participants feel confident that their responses will not have negative consequences.

Conclusion

Publications in simulation-based healthcare education and training have increased over the past decade. The topics discussed in this chapter can help you place your ideas, interests, and potential studies into context with what has been shown, while at the same time providing you with a framework for developing future research studies about simulation and using simulation.

How do you know what you are doing is important, effective, and sustainable? We suggest you apply the principles discussed in this chapter toward your next class as a way not only to assess the training, but also to spur improvements within the training and excitement about research in your facility. Keep the scope of the assessment small and the outcome measures simple. Start by performing a quick needs assessment of your learners, and then search the medical education literature for an outcome measure that fits what your learners feel they need from the class. Apply this outcome measure during or after the simulation followed by or as a part of your debriefing session. Have your educators reflect on the feasibility and validity of the instrument and then discuss reliability between the assessors. This will enable you to practice creating simulation-based research projects by answering a simple research question in a feasible but valid manner. Then take what you learned and apply it to your current curriculum or to develop a new course.

References

Armenia, S., Thangamathesvaran, L., Caine, A. D., King, N., Kunac, A., & Merchant, A. M. (2018). The role of high-fidelity team-based simulation in acute care settings: A systematic review. *The Surgery Journal, 4*(3), e136-e151. doi:10.1055/s-0038-1667315

Barsuk, J. H., McGaghie, W. C., Cohen, E. R., Balachandran, J. S., & Wayne D. B. (2009). Use of simulation-based mastery learning to improve the quality of central venous catheter placement in a medical intensive care unit. *Journal of Hospital Medicine, 4*(7), 397-403. doi:10.1002/jhm.468

Barsuk, J. H., Cohen, E. R., Feinglass, J., McGaghie, W. C., & Wayne, D. B. (2009). Use of simulation-based education to reduce catheter-related bloodstream infections. *Archives of Internal Medicine, 169*(15), 1420-1423. doi:10.1001/archinternmed.2009.215

Barsuk, J. H., Cohen, E. R., Potts, S., Demo, H., Gupta, S., Feinglass, J., ... Wayne, D. B. (2014). Dissemination of a simulation-based mastery learning intervention reduces central line–associated bloodstream infections. *BMJ Quality & Safety, 23*(9), 749-756. doi:10.1136/bmjqs-2013-002665

Blackmore, A., Kasfiki, E. V., & Purva, M. (2018). Simulation-based education to improve communication skills: A systematic review and identification of current best practice. *BMJ Simulation & Technology Enhanced Learning, 4*(4), 159-164. doi:10.1136/bmjstel-2017-000220

Bragge, P. (2010). Asking good clinical research questions and choosing the right study design. *Injury, 41*(Suppl. 1), S3-S6. doi:10.1016/j.injury.2010.04.016

Brazil, V., Purdy, E. I., & Bajaj, K. (2019). Connecting simulation and quality improvement: How can healthcare simulation really improve patient care? *BMJ Quality & Safety, 28*(11), 862–865.

Chan, S., Babcock, L., Geis, G., Frey, M., Robinson, V., & Kerrey, B. (2019). In situ simulation to mitigate threats to participation in a multicenter clinical trial in high-acuity, low-frequency setting. *Simulation in Healthcare, 14*(1), 1-9. doi:10.1097/SIH.0000000000000328

Cheng, A., Auerbach, M., Hunt, E. A., Chang, T. P., Pusic, M., Nadkarni, V., & Kessler, D. (2014). Designing and conducting simulation-based research. *Pediatrics, 133*(6), 1091-1101. doi:10.1542/peds.2013-3267

Cheng, A., Eppich, W., Grant, V., Sherbino, J., Zendejas, B., & Cook, D. A. (2014). Debriefing for technology-enhanced simulation: A systematic review and meta-analysis. *Medical Education, 48*(7), 657–666. doi:10.1111/medu.12432

Cheng, A., Kessler, D., Mackinnon, R., Chang, T. P., Nadkami, V. M., Hunt, E. A., ... Auerbach, M. (2016). Reporting guidelines for health care simulation research: Extensions to the CONSORT and STROBE statements. *Simulation in Healthcare, 11*(4), 238-248. doi:10.1097/SIH.0000000000000150

Cohen, E. R., Feinglass, J., Barsuk, J. H., Barnard, C., O'Donnell, A., McGaghie, W. C., & Wayne, D. B. (2010). Cost savings from reduced catheter-related bloodstream infection after simulation-based education for residents in a medical intensive care unit. *Simulation in Healthcare, 5*(2), 98-102. doi:10.1097/SIH.0b013e3181bc8304

Cook, D. A., Brydges, R., Ginsburg, S., & Hatala, R. (2015). A contemporary approach to validity arguments: A practical guide to Kane's framework. *Medical Education, 49*(6), 560-575. doi:10.1111/medu.12678

Cook, D. A., Brydges, R., Hamstra, S. J., Zendejas, B., Szostek, J. H., Wang, A. T., ... Hatala, R. J. (2012). Comparative effectiveness of technology-enhanced simulation versus other instructional methods: A systematic review and meta-analysis. *Simulation in Healthcare, 7*(5), 308-320. doi:10.1097/SIH.0b013e3182614f95

Cook, D. A., Erwin, P. J., & Triola, M. M. (2010). Computerized virtual patients in health professions education: A systematic review and meta-analysis. *Academic Medicine, 85*(10), 1589-1602. doi:10.1097/ACM.0b013e3181edfe13

Cook, D. A., Hamstra, S. J., Brydges, R., Zendejas, B., Szostek, J. H., Wang, A. T., ... Hatala, R. (2013). Comparative effectiveness of instructional design features in simulation-based education: Systematic review and meta-analysis. *Medical Teacher, 35*(1), e867-e898. doi:10.3109/0142159X.2012.714886

Cook, D. A., Hatala, R., Brydges, R., Zendejas, B., Szostek, J. H., Wang, A. T., ... Hamstra, S. J. (2011). Technology-enhanced simulation for health professions education: A systematic review and meta-analysis. *JAMA, 306*(9), 978-988. doi:10.1001/jama.2011.1234

Cox, T., Seymour, N., & Stefanidis, D. (2015). Moving the needle: Simulation's impact on patient outcomes. *The Surgical Clinics of North America, 95*(4), 827-838. doi:10.1016/j.suc.2015.03.005

Dieckmann, P., Phero, J. C., Issenberg, S. B., Kardong-Edgren, S., Ostergaard, D., & Ringsted, C. (2011). The first Research Consensus Summit of the Society for Simulation in Healthcare: Conduction and a synthesis of the results. *Simulation in Healthcare, 6*(Suppl.), S1-S9. doi:10.1097/SIH.0b013e31822238fc

Douglas, S. R., Vides de Andrade, A. R., Boyd, S., Leslie, M., Webb, L., Davis, L., ... Bickman, L. (2016). Communication training improves patient-centered provider behavior and screening for soldiers' mental health concerns. *Patient Education and Counseling, 99*(7), 1203-1212. doi:10.1016/j.pec.2016.01.018

Draycott, T. J., Crofts, J. F., Ash, J. P., Wilson, L. V., Yard, E., Sibanda, T., & Whitelaw, A. (2008). Improving neonatal outcome through practical shoulder dystocia training. *Obstetrics & Gynecology, 112*(1), 14-20. doi:10.1097/AOG.0b013e31817bbc61

Eppich, W., Howard, V., Vozenilek, J., & Curran, I. (2011). Simulation-based team training in healthcare. *Simulation in Healthcare, 6*(Suppl.), S14-S19. doi:10.1097/SIH.0b013e318229f550

Eva, K. W. (2008). On the limits of systematicity. *Medical Education, 42*(9), 852-853. doi:10.1111/j.1365-2923.2008.03140.x

Fujimori, M., Shirai, Y., Asai, M., Kubota, K., Katsumata, N., & Uchitomi, Y. (2014). Effect of communication skills training program for oncologists based on patient preferences for communication when receiving bad news: A randomized controlled trial. *Journal of Clinical Oncology, 32*(20), 2166-2172. doi:10.1200/JCO.2013.51.2756

Geis, G. L., Pio, B., Pendergrass, T. L., Moyer, M. R., & Patterson, M. D. (2011). Simulation to assess the safety of new healthcare teams and new facilities. *Simulation in Healthcare, 6*(3), 125-133. doi:10.1097/SIH.0b013e31820dff30

Gordon, M., Darbyshire, D., & Baker, P. (2012). Non-technical skills training to enhance patient safety: A systematic review. *Medical Education, 46*(11), 1042-1054. doi:10.1111/j.1365-2923.2012.04343.x

Hatala, R., & Cook, D. A. (2019). Reliability and validity. In D. Nestal, J. Hui, K. Kunkler, M. W. Scerbo, & A. W. Calhoun (Eds.), *Healthcare simulation research: A practical guide* (pp. 191–197). Cham, Switzerland: Springer.

Hung, G. R., Whitehouse, S. R., O'Neill, C., Gray, A. P., & Kissoon, N. (2007). Computer modeling of patient flow in a pediatric emergency department using discrete event simulation. *Pediatric Emergency Care, 23*(1), 5-10.

Issenberg, S. B., McGaghie, W. C., Petrusa, E. R., Gordon, D. L., & Scalese, R. J. (2005). Features and uses of high-fidelity medical simulations that lead to effective learning: A BEME systematic review. *Medical Teacher, 27*(1), 10-28.

Kane, M. T. (2006). Validation. In R. L. Brennan (Ed.), *Educational measurement* (4th ed., pp. 17-64). Lanham, MD: Rowman & Littlefield Publishers.

Kerrey, B. T., Boyd, S. D., Geis, G. L., MacPherson, R. P., Cooper, E., & Kiefer, A. W. (2020, March 11). Developing a profile of procedural expertise: A simulation study of tracheal intubation using 3-dimensional motion capture. *Simulation in Healthcare*, published online ahead of print.

Kirkpatrick, D. L. (1998). *Evaluating training programs: The four levels* (2nd ed.). San Francisco, CA: Berrett-Koehler Publishers.

Levett-Jones, T., & Lapkin, S. (2014). A systematic review of the effectiveness of simulation debriefing in health professional education. *Nurse Education Today, 34*(6), e58-e63. doi:10.1016/j.nedt.2013.09.020

Lewis, R., Strachan, A., & Smith, M. M. (2012). Is high fidelity simulation the most effective method for the development of non-technical skills in nursing? A review of the current evidence. *The Open Nursing Journal, 6*, 82-89. doi:10.2174/1874434601206010082

McGaghie, W. C. (2010). Medical education research as translational science. *Science Translational Medicine, 2*(19), 19cm8. doi:10.1126/scitranslmed.3000679

McGaghie, W. C., Draycott, T. J., Dunn, W. F., Lopez, C. M., & Stefanidis, D. (2011). Evaluating the impact of simulation on translational patient outcomes. *Simulation in Healthcare, 6*(Suppl.), S42-S47. doi:10.1097/SIH.0b013e318222fde9

McGaghie, W. C., Issenberg, S. B., Cohen, E. R., Barsuk, J. H., & Wayne, D. B. (2011). Does simulation-based medical education with deliberate practice yield better results than traditional clinical education? A meta-analytic comparative review of the evidence. *Academic Medicine, 86*(6), 706-711. doi:10.1097/ACM.0b013e318217e119

McGaghie, W. C., Issenberg, S. B., Petrusa, E. R., & Scalese, R. J. (2010). A critical review of simulation-based medical education research: 2003-2009. *Medical Education, 44*(1), 50-63. doi:10.1111/j.1365-2923.2009.03547.x

McGaghie, W. C., Issenberg, S. B., Petrusa, E. R., & Scalese, R. J. (2016). Revisiting 'A critical review of simulation-based medical education research: 2003-2009.' *Medical Education, 50*(10), 986-991. doi:10.1111/medu.12795

McIntosh, K. S., Gregor, J. C., & Khanna, N. V. (2014). Computer-based virtual reality colonoscopy simulation improves patient-based colonoscopy performance. *Canadian Journal of Gastroenterology & Hepatology, 28*(4), 203-206.

Miller, D., Crandall, C., Washington C. 3rd, & McLaughlin, S. (2012). Improving teamwork and communication in trauma care through in situ simulations. *Academic Emergency Medicine, 19*(5), 608-612. doi:10.1111/j.1553-2712.2012.01354.x

Norman, G., Dore, K., & Grierson, L. (2012). The minimal relationship between simulation fidelity and transfer of learning. *Medical Education, 46*(7), 636-647. doi:10.1111/j.1365-2923.2012.04243.x

Ogrinc, G., Davies, L., Goodman, D., Batalden, P., Davidoff, F., & Stevens, D. (2016). SQUIRE 2.0 (Standards for Quality Improvement Reporting Excellence): Revised publication guidelines from a detailed consensus process. *BMJ Quality & Safety, 25*(12), 986–992. doi:10.1136/bmjqs-2015-004411

Palaganas, J. C., Fey, M., & Simon, R. (2016). Structured debriefing in simulation-based education. *AACN Advanced Critical Care, 27*(1), 78–85. doi:10.4037/aacnacc2016328

Patterson, M. D., Geis, G. L., Falcone, R. A., LeMaster, T., & Wears, R. L. (2013). In situ simulation: Detection of safety threats and teamwork training in a high risk emergency department. *BMJ Quality and Safety in Health Care, 22*(6), 468–477. doi:10.1136/bmjqs-2012-000942

Paull, D. E., DeLeeuw, L. D., Wolk, S., Paige, J. T., Neily, J., & Mills, P. D. (2013). The effect of simulation-based crew resource management training on measurable teamwork and communication among interprofessional teams caring for postoperative patients. *Journal of Continuing Education in Nursing, 44*(11), 516–524. doi:10.3928/00220124-20130903-38

Pawson, R., Greenhalgh, T., Harvey, G., & Walshe, K. (2005). Realist review—A new method of systematic review designed for complex policy interventions. *Journal of Health Services Research & Policy, 10*(Suppl. 1), 21–34.

Riley, W., Davis, S., Miller, K., Hansen, H., Sainfort, F., & Sweet, R. (2011). Didactic and simulation nontechnical skills team training to improve perinatal patient outcomes in a community hospital. *The Joint Commission Journal on Quality and Patient Safety, 37*(8), 357–364.

Roussin, C. J., & Weinstock, P. (2017). SimZones: An organizational innovation for simulation programs and centers. *Academic Medicine, 92*(8), 1114–1120. doi:10.1097/ACM.0000000000001746

Schardt, C., Adams, M. B., Owens, T., Keitz, S., & Fontelo, P. (2007). Utilization of the PICO framework to improve searching PubMed for clinical questions. *BMC Medical Informatics and Decision Making, 7*, 16–21. doi:10.1186/1472-6947-7-16

Sevdalis, N., Nestel, D., Kardong-Edgren, S., & Gaba, D. M. (2016). A joint leap into a future of high-quality simulation research—Standardizing the reporting of simulation science. *Simulation in Healthcare, 11*(4), 236–237. doi:10.1097/SIH.0000000000000179

Seymour, N. E. (2008). VR to OR: A review of the evidence that virtual reality simulation improves operating room performance. *World Journal of Surgery, 32*(2), 182–188. doi:10.1007/s00268-007-9307-9

Sullivan, A. M., Rock, L. K., Gadmer, N. M., Norwich, D. E., & Schwartzstein, R. M. (2016). The impact of resident training on communication with families in the intensive care unit. Resident and family outcomes. *Annals of the American Thoracic Society, 13*(4), 512–521. doi:10.1513/AnnalsATS.201508-495OC

Sutherland, L. M., Middleton, P. F., Anthony, A., Hamdorf, J., Cregan, P., Scott, D., & Maddern, G. J. (2006). Surgical simulation: A systematic review. *Annals of Surgery, 243*(3), 291–300.

US Department of Health and Human Services. (2018). *Code of federal regulations title 45, part 46.* Washington, DC: Author. Retrieved from https://www.hhs.gov/ohrp/regulations-and-policy/regulations/45-cfr-46/index.html

Wayne, D. B., Didwania, A., Feinglass, J., Fudala, M. J., Barsuk, J. H., & McGaghie, W. C. (2008). Simulation-based education improves quality of care during cardiac arrest team responses at an academic teaching hospital: A case-control study. *Chest, 133*(1), 56–61.

Weaver, S. J., Salas, E., Lyons, R., Lazzara, E. H., Rosen, M. A., Diazgranados, D., … King, H. (2010). Simulation-based team training at the sharp end: A qualitative study of simulation-based team training design, implementation, and evaluation in healthcare. *Journal of Emergencies, Trauma, and Shock, 3*(4), 369–377. doi:10.4103/0974-2700.70754

Weller, J. M., Cumin, D., Civil, I. D., Torrie, J., Garden, A., MacCormick, A. D., … Merry, A. F. (2016). Improved scores for observed teamwork in the clinical environment following a multidisciplinary operating room simulation intervention. *The New Zealand Medical Journal, 129*(1439), 59–67.

Yudkowsky, R., Luciano, C., Banerjee, P., Schwartz, A., Alaraj, A., Lemole, G. M. Jr., … Frim, D. (2013). Practice on augmented reality/haptic simulator and library of virtual brains improves residents' ability to perform a ventriculostomy. *Simulation in Healthcare, 8*(1), 25–31. doi:10.1097/SIH.0b013e3182662c69

Zendejas, B., Brydges, R., Wang, A. T., & Cook, D. A. (2013). Patient outcomes in simulation-based medical education: A systematic review. *Journal of General Internal Medicine, 28*(8), 1078–1089. doi:10.1007/s11606-012-2264-5

Zendejas, B., Cook, D. A., Bingener, J., Huebner, M., Dunn, W. F., Sarr, M. G., & Farley, D. R. (2011). Simulation-based mastery learning improves patient outcomes in laparoscopic inguinal hernia repair: A randomized controlled trial. *Annals of Surgery, 254*(3), 502–509. doi:10.1097/SLA.0b013e31822c6994

"All the world is a stage, And all the men and women merely players. They have their exits and entrances; Each man in his time plays many parts."

–William Shakespeare

Defining Roles and Building a Career in Simulation

14

Carol Noe Cheney, MS, CCC-SLP
Karen Josey, MEd, BSN, RN, CHSE
Linda Tinker, MSN, RN

Careers in simulation, the roles of individuals involved in simulation, and the variety of simulation program opportunities have rapidly evolved. Healthcare simulation opportunities exist in areas such as academia, fire departments, hospitals, military, and freestanding simulation and education centers.

Simulation in healthcare is a specialty with identified knowledge and competencies. All individuals working in simulation must be well versed in simulation as well as competent in their clinical or technical roles.

This chapter provides an overview of the roles needed in simulation programs. Whether you are on a limited budget with a small center or have a huge multi-hub center and an unlimited budget, there are basic roles that must be filled to be successful. Roles to plan, design, implement, and evaluate simulation-based learning and development outcomes support the achievement of facility and regional strategies and initiatives to meet organizational goals.

In many cases, the designers of the simulation center or simulation proposal serve in the initial roles of administrator, facilitator, debriefer, educator, simulation curricula designer, and delivery expert, as well as in supportive roles such as the scheduler.

Individuals working in simulation can learn on the job or from additional sources such as fellow pioneers, publications, and programs offered by hospital or university-based simulation centers. Conferences and workshops are available, such as the International Medical Simulation in Healthcare Conference, the International Nursing Association for Clinical Simulation and Learning (INACSL), and the Society for Simulation in Healthcare (SSH).

OBJECTIVES

- Describe the basic roles essential to simulation.

- Know the basic skills needed in simulation.

- Identify different position titles and sample position descriptions utilized in simulation centers.

- Understand certifications and resources that might assist in advancing a career in simulation.

- Define the four Society for Simulation in Healthcare simulation educator competencies.

Simulation certification programs are available through a variety of institutions for leadership and for simulation educator and technologist roles.

Simulation Program Roles

As simulation programs continue to grow, so do the number and types of roles in these programs. The result has been increasing specialization of roles and distinctive role descriptions. This chapter section covers some of the common roles needed for the operation of a simulation program or center (see Table 14.1). Each role is unique to required knowledge and competence (e.g., simulation manager should have knowledge in management and administration, technology, and education, while a simulation technologist should have knowledge in audiovisual (AV) and mannequin technology as well as clinical

aspects). Roles are needed to meet organizational goals and requirements by identification of training needs, subject matter experts (SME), simulation curriculum development, and measurement and evaluations leading to learning and clinical outcomes.

Roles, job titles, and job functions vary depending on a variety of reasons, including the budget, scope, staffing, and resources allocated. Although larger programs might have multiple individuals in each of the roles, smaller simulation programs might consolidate several roles into one position. Freestanding simulation and education centers may have organizational roles such as information technologist (IT), engineers, chief financial officers (CFOs), and marketing professionals, whereas, if the simulation center is a part of an organization, the resources may come from other departments.

Table 14.1   Role, Job Title, and Job Function Examples

Roles	Job Titles	Job Function
Leader	Simulation Program Manager Simulation Director Simulation Medical Director Executive Director Education Director Operations Manager Simulation Operations Manager Medical Director Simulation Coordinator	Budgeting Hiring Managing operations Planning, developing, and implementing policies and strategies
Simulation scenario and curricula development	Simulation Specialist Instructional Designer Surgical Training Specialist	Building scenario, writing objectives, and constructing educational checklists Programming mannequins Moulaging simulated patients
Subject matter expert (SME)	Clinical Experts from varying disciplines Clinical Instructors Clinical Educators	Building and facilitating scenarios Providing feedback on simulations

Roles	Job Titles	Job Function
Simulation programmer/ operator	Simulation Technologist Simulation Specialist	Building, programming, and running mannequins Operating task trainers and simulators Moulaging simulated patients
Simulation educator facilitator	Simulation Educator Standardized Patient Educator Simulation Specialist	Building scenarios, writing objectives, and constructing process checklists Debriefing
Debriefer	Simulation Specialist	Guiding and evaluating learners throughout simulation to meet desired outcomes in debriefing
Data analyst	Systems Consult	Analyzing metric reports
Technical support	IT Support Audiovisual	Supporting educational activities through computer, audiovisual, mannequin, and IT systems Maintaining programs and equipment
Scheduler/administrative assistant	Simulation Coordinator Administrative Assistant	Serving as receptionist Scheduling events and staffing
Engineers	Human Factors, System, Mechanical, Logistics, Reliability	Supporting, assessing, evaluating, and creating educational activities through medical equipment, human factors processes, healthcare systems testing, and assessment
Other roles and skill sets	Evaluator Researcher Finance Director Business Director Marketing Fellowships	Varies

It is especially important for organizations to clearly define the roles and responsibilities of each simulation position and for individuals considering positions in simulation programs to understand what is expected by the organization. Two sample position descriptions, the Simulation Director and the RN Simulation Specialist, are provided at the end of this chapter in Tables 14.2 and 14.3. Some centers have specialty specific positions such as surgical educators and technicians. Accreditation and certification guidelines help to define standards in the roles for a quality program.

Regardless of the role, team members need to have a strong core knowledge base and an understanding of how the following are accomplished in relation to the programs they serve:

- What simulation is and how it applies to adult learning

- How simulation can be utilized with existing education or in building new learning opportunities

- Best equipment for the learning objectives

- How simulation scenarios are built

- How effective and measurable goals are developed

- How to conduct an effective debriefing

- How to facilitate group and individual learning

- How to incorporate evaluations and checklists

- How to gain buy-in for a simulation program

- Effectiveness of simulation compared to other learning modalities

Leadership Roles

Leadership roles and responsibilities vary and may include strategic direction, operations, budgeting, performance reviews, staffing, and program development. The leader may also market and communicate capabilities and benefits of simulation utilization. Many simulation accreditation programs require administrative or operational leadership as well as clinical leadership. A dedicated medical, nursing, or clinical director for simulation might be required. There are undergraduate and graduate degree programs, conferences, national organizations such as American College of Healthcare Executives (ACHE), and other extensive resources and opportunities to develop leadership skills. There are simulation leader-specific resources through simulation organizations such as the Society for Simulation in Healthcare (SSH) and National League for Nursing Simulation Innovation Resource Center (NLN SIRC).

Simulation Scenario/Curricula Development Role

As Alinier notes, "The development of appropriate scenarios is critical in high-fidelity simulation training" (2011, p. 9). Individuals in the simulation scenario/curricula development role build the curricula into a simulation scenario. These experts use their comprehensive and applied knowledge of simulation to put the subject matter into an effective simulation scenario. The curricula may be developed by a subject matter expert (SME) or someone in simulation who has that subject matter expertise. This role may include the expertise of the simulation educator, the SME, and the simulation curricula developer. In the Banner Health Simulation System, the Simulation Specialist/Educator might have subject matter expertise in some clinical areas with little to no expertise in other clinical areas; no one can be an expert in all clinical practices. Simulation educators find the exposure and opportunity to work with many different experts rewarding.

This role requires comprehensive knowledge of simulation theory and implementation to ensure positive learning outcomes. Knowing the resources available and the likely educational needs might influence whether a simulation educator is hired with specific clinical knowledge in any one given area. Understanding program needs and current simulation technology is valuable in incorporating the curriculum into simulation.

Knowledge of adult learning theory, hierarchy of learning and goal and objective writing, measures, evaluation, and assessment is foundational for this role. The individuals in this role must understand all of these concepts to successfully design and develop simulations. Instructional designers can be instrumental in helping design not only the objectives within the simulation, but also any other aspects of the curricula that might be needed to promote learner achievement (Brown & Green, 2016).

Evaluation planning, designing, implementing, and evaluating simulation-based learning and development outcomes to support the achievement of learning goals, as categorized by Bloom, Englehart, Furst, Hill, & Krathwohl (1956), are:

- Cognitive-knowledge

- Psychomotor-skills

- Affective-attitude

The National League for Nursing (NLN, 2020) has resources for nurse educators to stay current on simulation and technology. Nurse educators can design curricula or can be the SMEs, facilitators, evaluators, and debriefers.

Subject Matter Expert Role

Having access to SMEs is essential in building a simulation scenario. The SMEs may not be knowledgeable about simulation at all. For example, a physician, nurse, or other practitioner who does not have any educator or simulation experience can be a SME. The simulation educator can assist in developing the curricula into an effective simulation to include evaluation and assessment. Examples of clinical SMEs include direct care nurses, nurse educators, clinical nurse specialists, respiratory therapists, paramedics,

physicians, and other specialties, such as those with surgical expertise, depending on the training needs. Budget dollars may need to be allocated for a contract or payment for expert individuals to assist with the simulation as it would be improbable to employ every type of clinical SME.

Simulation Programmer/Operator Role

Programming and operating the mannequin to deliver the scenario to meet objectives are basic simulation functions. The equipment or "trainers" used for simulation can vary from simple to complex and from low technology to high technology. The training tool might be as simple as a latex or plastic body part that neither acts nor reacts (task trainer), or as complex as a high-technology, full-body mannequin that has heart, lung, and bowel sounds and can breathe, sweat, and blink. Individuals in the programmer/operator role must know how to use these simulators and trainers, when to use them, and which simulator or trainer will work best for the job at hand.

> Remember that the highest technology tool does not always equate to the best scenario for the specific learning objective.

Today's high technology mannequins are much more plug and play than the mannequins of yesterday. Simulation programmers/operators learn to run the mannequin on the fly—adjusting blood pressure, heart rate, or respiratory functions in the moment when change is needed as learning opportunities occur.

More comprehensive programming enables the simulation educator to build a scenario in the software that causes the mannequin's physiological state to progress, react, and respond depending on time or the actions of the learner. Programming can become very complex if there is a need to have multiple patient scenarios running over long periods of time. For example, Banner Health has an onboarding process in which multiple patient scenarios run simultaneously for four to six hours. Determining the trending of each simulated patient's responses must be timed, and in some cases, complex storyboards must be written to manage the complexity of coordinating multiple simulated patients. This is important so the learner who cares for these simulated patients is not tasked with handling too many patient situations at one time, and events transpire more realistically as they do in the real environment. Therefore, having comfort with computers, simulation software, and many Microsoft Windows-based applications and technology, in general, is essential for programming and operating the simulators.

The vendor of the simulator/mannequin can be a great resource, especially for simulation newcomers who need to learn the tools of their trade. Many of the vendors provide courses in basic and advanced programming for their simulators. Also, some universities and educational conferences partner with various vendors to offer programming classes and training. Programming and operating the simulators are foundational for any simulation program and are at the heart of the definition of this key player—the simulation programmer/operator.

Educator/Facilitator Role

The role of educator is critical as this role guides and manages the simulation for the learners. It is crucial that the educator acts as a facilitator, providing a supportive climate and creating trust (Fanning & Gaba, 2007). The educator should use clear learning objectives to optimize the simulation (Sawyer, Walter, Brett-Fleeger, Grant, & Cheng, 2016).

The educator is typically the person who sets the stage for the scenario and the pre-briefing of the scenarios. Educators ask open-ended questions to guide the group to self-reflect and assimilate learning. The educator may need to redirect the learner if the wrong path is taken.

Facilitation is a skill set that educators need to possess to create meaningful learning environments. Facilitation skills include clarification, allowing time for answering questions and solving problems, paraphrasing, and staying on track using the objectives as a guide (Fanning & Gaba, 2007). The facilitator guides and directs, asks open-ended questions, rephrases, uses silence, and employs other techniques during the training session.

Debriefer Role

Debriefing is a vital part of simulation, influencing learning and self-discovery, and is at the heart of many adult learning theories as being the most effective part of learning. The debriefer role is one of the most important and maybe the most difficult role; it requires training and practice to be effective.

Debriefing is a facilitative method that guides the learner(s) to sustain or improve performance through self-reflection and to obtain deeper understanding through self-guided discovery and feedback (Fanning & Gaba, 2007). Debriefing can also be more directive, when needed, to obtain the goals and the objectives in the simulation (Archer, 2010; Molloy et al., 2020). Debriefing can be vital in transfer of learning to real life situations, which is the purpose of learning (Rivière, Jaffrelot, Jouquan, & Chiniara, 2019).

There are many debriefing strategies that a debriefer needs to be knowledgeable about to have the best learner results. The selection of the best debriefing strategy will depend on variables such as level of the learner and goals and objectives of the simulation experience (Cheng et al., 2015). The debriefer should understand the overall goals of the scenario as well as techniques such as using open-ended questions, using guided reflection, and drawing out quiet individuals in a group setting.

The debriefing role may be assumed by any number of individuals. This is a role with which the simulation educator must be knowledgeable and proficient. Typically, the person who "owns" the scenario is the one who does the debriefing; the simulation educator/specialists debrief on the curricula they develop; for example, at Banner Health, the Sim Specialists are responsible for onboarding skills and scenarios so they are responsible for those debriefings.

Resources for developing and maintaining debriefing expertise include conferences, workshops, articles, and courses. Detailed information on debriefing can be found in Chapter 5.

Evaluator Role

Evaluation is an essential part of any educational program that occurs on many levels throughout any learning process. Considering Kirkpatrick's (2006) Four Level Training Model (reaction, learning, behavior, and results), feeling comfortable or even confident performing a task (level 1: reaction) is different from competency in performance (level 3: behavior). The evaluator in a simulation program should understand how to standardize experiences that are being evaluated, evaluate without influencing responses and outcomes, and be familiar with identified metrics to evaluate if learning has occurred. An even higher level of evaluation is to determine if that learning has generalized to other environments or patient outcomes, also known as translational research (Rivière et al., 2019).

Evaluation can be formative or summative, and the evaluator must understand the difference and rationale for both. This is detailed in Chapter 6. Checklists are a common method of evaluation in the science of psychometrics. Assessment tools using checklists require psychometric testing to ensure that the tool is valid and reliable (see Chapter 6). Many evaluation tools already tested for validity and reliability exist in the literature, depending on the task or performance being evaluated. A psychometrician, human factor engineer, or instructional designer would be ideal to evaluate on a cognitive, psychomotor, and affective domain, and individuals with evaluation knowledge and ability can also perform this function. All evaluators, prior to performing evaluations, should undergo training to ensure understanding.

Standardized Patient Educator Role

Standardized patients and simulated persons can be used to increase the fidelity of a simulation. Using simulated providers or embedded actors (also known in many simulation programs as "confederates") or standardized patients are other means to design effective simulations. A *simulated person* is a person who is scripted to bring realism to the simulation by providing extra challenges, such as a family member or an ambulance worker. A *standardized patient* is a trained actor who portrays a patient in a consistent scripted manner. The use of these individuals can greatly add to the realism and complexity of a healthcare scenario; however, it takes time and highly specialized knowledge to train the actors to deliver behaviors needed for the learner to experience the desired learning outcomes (Barrows, 1993).

A standardized patient educator has the specific knowledge and skills needed to develop and oversee simulations using standardized patients including orientation, training, and supervision of standardized patients as well as teaching and assessment of training. Standardized patient educators require an understanding of operations, flow, personnel, and training of individuals hired to be standardized patients.

Researcher Role

Organizations, associations, and societies that lead and promote excellence in simulation speak to professional growth, patient safety, standards of practice, and research. "Research will be a key factor in advancing the field of simulation to the benefit of patients and healthcare professionals" (Issenberg, Ringsted, Ostergaard, & Dieckmann, 2011, p. 155). This role can be a vital one in simulation environments, especially in academic settings where research is expected. This role requires specialized skillsets and high-level education and experience. Research is a standard in simulation in organizations that are leading simulation. SSH and INACSL both promote research in their mission statements.

Data Analyst Role

The purpose of the data analyst role is to assist in the entry, analysis, and creation of databases of different types of research methods and psychometric tools such as checklists, evaluations, assessments, and test scores. The data analyst is an important position to assist in aggregating data and in assessing and evaluating simulation utilization and outcomes. Succinctly capturing data on low-level measures like attendance and/or perceptual feedback as well as measuring learning and patient outcomes serve to validate simulation investments and endeavors (Buzachero, Phillips, J., Phillips, P. P., & Phillips, Z. L., 2013). Attendance data (e.g., how many

nurses, physicians, or students utilize the center), usage data (e.g., why they use it), learning outcomes, and so on, can be valuable information in addressing use and operations of the simulation program. An individual with a comprehensive understanding of Excel, Access, database software, and other statistical tools is an incredible asset. This person does not have to have clinical expertise; in fact, a nonclinical person can add a fresh perspective to the team.

Capturing and reporting learner activity data are integral parts of many simulation programs. A systems consult may produce a variety of valuable ways on what data to collect, how to collect it, and how to statistically analyze it for frequent reports.

Simulation Technical Support Role

Simulation technical support roles can meet a variety of needs—simulator set up, maintenance, and troubleshooting; using moulage to increase fidelity; IT and AV support; etc. There are many technical aspects in simulation given the varied equipment—from task trainers to high fidelity mannequins.

Set up includes wireless (e.g., simulators and software) and wired connections (e.g., lines, tubing, and compressors) as well as the start-up and shut down of computers and simulators. Many simulation centers use a technician to fill this role—someone who might not have formal education as a healthcare provider. The individual in the technician support role may program and run the simulator, but a clinical resource might be needed to assist the technical support person to understand how to adjust the clinical parameters. Other responsibilities include preparing and applying moulage, cleaning up, performing routine maintenance, assuring all equipment is working properly, and running system diagnostics from the mannequin to the computer systems.

Moulage is a specialized area of simulation that is very time consuming. It takes training and practice to learn the many formulas, compounds, and "items" to produce realistic moulage that helps to immerse the learner into the simulation. One also needs to understand which compounds and materials could affect the integrity of the mannequins or equipment, so as not to permanently damage or stain the equipment. See Chapter 3 for more information on moulage.

Maintaining and troubleshooting equipment is another aspect of technical support. This includes, for example, installing software upgrades, problem solving a compressor issue, or intervening when equipment does not function as intended, such as when a lung won't inflate or a pulse is not palpable. Often, the greater the understanding of the technology and equipment one has, the greater the opportunities to modify the equipment and creatively develop or re-create clinical issues without purchasing separate mannequins or trainers. Individuals with an advanced understanding of the equipment and technology can often perform quick repairs if there is an equipment malfunction without waiting for separate technical support to arrive or aborting the scenario altogether. This knowledge can not only be a critical element in operations due to time efficiency and needs, but also benefit the organization financially as most simulators come with contracted vendor technical support.

Learning the ins and outs of the mannequins and other simulation technology can be very rewarding. Simulation workshops that focus on basic and advanced aspects of technical support are available. Novices can also learn these skills on the job as they learn more advanced problem solving with the help from vendor technical support. In many cases, the simulation educator also fills the technical support role. Depending

on the size and complexity of the simulation program, simulation educators might also have an information technology (IT) support person or other support staff to assist in maximizing the use of the available simulation equipment.

This role is gradually becoming specialized. It benefits from information technology and clinical backgrounds. Most often, an individual has more of one than the other and will need development to support growth. Also, it is important to keep in mind the differences in the cultures of both fields: Clinical technicians or support staff typically come from a busy culture of being hands-on (i.e., active role fixing and maintaining equipment), and IT personnel typically come from a culture of being busy sitting in front of a computer screen (i.e., programming, organizing software). The simulation technical support role requires both hands-on and screen-time. Hence, it helps to set the expectations of the role and provide modeling and guidance during orientation.

Another technical support role is AV support. A person who can assist with video recording and teleconferencing capabilities will increase efficiencies in the program. Many high-technology simulators include an audiovisual recorder that allows for recording and immediate playback opportunities. Virtual reality 360 videos provide an immersive simulation that can be very efficient in delivering just-in-time education. The IT support role might assist with AV support if the simulation center has that availability. Some programs have separate AV teams to help with this equipment.

Scheduler/Administrative Assistant Role

The scheduler/administrative assistant roles include many time-consuming functions. Scheduling, inventory management, purchasing, data collection and entry, monitoring supply levels, and receptionist duties can take time away from the simulation team's main function of simulation education. Some type of scheduling or management system is needed to track and assign the needed space and resources for simulations. These systems are often obtained using the same systems of the larger institution that houses the simulation program. Scheduling is not limited to coordinating designated simulation space. The people resources, equipment, and number of participants can become a job of its own to juggle. Sometimes the mannequins have their own "social" calendar and are loaned out of the simulation space. Receptionist responsibilities and coordination of scheduling simulations are huge functions that can be combined and will lead to a smoother functioning center. It is often more cost effective to employ a nonclinical person to perform these functions, which allows the clinical or simulation experts to focus on their areas of expertise.

Other Roles and Skill Sets in Simulation

Other roles in simulation include human factors engineers, clinical educators, simulation program managers, administrators, medical simulation technical specialists, simulation coordinators, simulation specialists, simulation technicians, and more.

Free-standing simulation programs may need to hire or cost out all roles, whereas organizations that have those roles in their organization can cross cover. Simulation specialists often work with other roles that are not dedicated to the simulation program such as clinical education, subject matter experts, risk and quality, and patient safety. Other roles in simulation include skill sets that encompass market research to include current practice and trends in simulation training, public relations, budgeting, marketing,

grant writing, and finding funding sources for both operations and research applications.

Healthcare Simulation Educator Certification

The healthcare simulation educator's position might encompass many of the roles described previously in this chapter, or it might involve only one role. The requirements are often based on the size of the program in which the healthcare simulation educator is employed.

The SSH offers two healthcare simulation educator certifications: Certified Healthcare Simulation Educator (CHSE) and the Certified Healthcare Simulation Educator – Advanced (CHSE-A). The SSH (2019a) defines a CHSE as "1) an individual who is involved in delivering healthcare-related simulation education interventions or 2) an individual who directly oversees or administers healthcare-related simulation educational interventions" (p. 5). The CHSE-A certification is described as "a portfolio-based certification for leaders in healthcare simulation. This certification distinguishes those who have proven themselves to be advanced educators in their practice in healthcare simulation and serve as mentors and examples to others in the field" (SSH, 2019b, p. 1).

Both the CHSE and the CHSE-A certifications evaluate applicants in the following areas (SSH, 2016, p. 6):

- Professional values and capabilities

- Knowledge of educational principles, practice, and methodology in simulation

- Implementing, assessing, and managing simulation-based educational activities

- Scholarship—spirit of inquiry and teaching

Eligibility requirements for the CHSE include (SSH, 2019a, p. 6):

- Participate in healthcare simulation in an educational role

- Demonstrated focused simulation expertise with learners in undergraduate, graduate, allied health, or healthcare practitioners

- Have a bachelor's degree or equivalent combination of education and experience

- Documented two years of continued use of simulation in healthcare education, research, or administration.

To achieve certification, the applicant must pass an examination to demonstrate knowledge, skills, and abilities.

Eligibility requirements for the CHSE-A include (SSH, 2016, p. 10):

- Current certification as a CHSE

- A minimum of five years of experience in a healthcare simulation education setting

- Demonstrated simulation expertise focused on learners in healthcare at any level

- Master's degree or equivalent experience

- Demonstrated continued use of simulation in healthcare education, research, or administration in the last five years.

To achieve CHSE-A certification, the applicant must submit a portfolio that includes the following (SSH, 2016):

- Professional information

- Reflective statements on each domain of the standards

- Healthcare simulation educational activity developed by the applicant

- Media submission to support and demonstrate the educational activity

- Additional information

The portfolio is reviewed by peer reviewers to determine if the applicant meets the requirements to be granted the CHSE-A certification.

INACSL has developed Standards for healthcare simulation educators (INACSL 2016a, 2016b, 2016c). With cross-pollination of INACSL members in the working group, the SSH certification sought to work hand-in-hand with INACSL standards and vice versa. Certification for healthcare simulation educators and for operations specialists are described more fully in Chapter 15.

Resources to Get Started and Advance

Many associations and organizations dedicated to healthcare simulation offer resources for those new to the field and to support those who have experience to help them keep up to date on trends and publications as well as research. These organizations are easily accessed online and offer memberships and opportunities for collaboration.

NLN has an online simulation e-learning site called the Simulation Innovation Resource Center (SIRC), which offers courses such as designing and developing simulations, debriefing, simulation research, and curriculum integration (http://sirc.nln.org/). Universities and annual conferences also cover many of these same items and include operational topics, research, debriefing, and evaluation methods to name only a small number of opportunities available. The Interservice/Industry Training Simulation and Education Conference (I/ITSEC) has social media support and puts on a modeling, simulation, and training annual conference and promotes cooperation among users of simulation (http://www.iitsec.org).

The American College of Surgeons is a resource for medical surgical simulation. SSH, a multidisciplinary organization, INACSL, and the Association for Standardized Patients (ASPE) are organizations that have standards for simulation practice and performance that can be extremely helpful in guiding one who is looking for a job in the simulation field. These organizations provide links on their websites to other simulation societies, including international resources. Three journals—*Simulation in Healthcare, Clinical Simulation in Nursing Journal,* and *Advances in Simulation*—are available to members of their respective societies and can be accessed online.

Other support for simulation educators includes career centers that have job postings specific to simulation as well as links to many simulation centers, such as the Center for Medical Simulation (CMS) and the Winter Institute for Simulation Education and Research (WISER). Many of these groups have social networks that include listservs and use Facebook forums that are specific for healthcare professionals who are interested in simulation. News, blogs, and newsletters are also available. Some state and local organizations to help support those locally are also available in some areas. There are modeling and simulation programs present in many different industries for education and training; however, these programs are typically tracks for various types of engineers and programmers.

Other ways to get started in this field include attending workshops, conferences, and webinars; engaging in vendor education; and visiting simulation centers. Academic offerings of clinical simulation programs include master's-level courses from Mayo Rochester, Drexel University, Harvard, MGH Institute for Health Professions,

and University of Southern Indiana, to name a few. SSH has a comprehensive literature review for the Certified Healthcare Simulation Educator (CHSE) and CHSE-A and Certified Healthcare Operations Specialist (CHOS) that can be accessed by anyone interested in simulation.

Conclusion

Individuals in many different roles are required for a successful simulation program. The basic roles identified in this chapter can be of assistance when compiling a job description for a simulation center or applying for a simulation job position. Roles discussed include leaders, technical set up and support, AV, SME, facilitator, debriefer, programmer/operator, scenario/curricula developer, and evaluator. Other support roles are data analyst, researcher, scheduler and administrative assistant, as well as someone to moulage, play the confederate, and train standardized patients. Job titles and positions can be a combination of the roles discussed in this chapter, depending on the need and budgets of a simulation center. Being certified as a simulation educator or operations specialist can assist you in demonstrating your qualifications and expertise in simulation. Many resources exist that can assist in learning what the current needs and trends are in the roles and positions available in the specialty of simulation. In the words of the Japanese Buddhist philosopher Daisaku Ikeda:

> People always have many different roles to play. The crucial thing is to be determined to make a wholehearted effort in everything and be fully engaged in what we are doing at any given moment. The secret to successfully fulfilling a variety of roles is to concentrate fully on the task at hand and give it our best effort with enthusiasm, maintaining a positive, forward-looking attitude and not worrying.

Table 14.2   Sample Position Description—Simulation Director

Banner Health Position Description

Position Title: Simulation Director

POSITION SUMMARY

This position provides leadership in the operations, planning, development, execution, evaluation, and standardization of simulation education and training to achieve system organizational strategies and initiatives. Responsible for the management and operations of a simulation center(s) under the oversight of the Sr. Director. Accountable for operations, finance, policies, and implementation of simulation and innovation strategy and management of simulation and innovation programs and technologies.

ESSENTIAL FUNCTIONS

1. Provides leadership for simulation and operational efforts and participates in program development and implementation for multidisciplinary and interprofessional teams.

2. Demonstrates an understanding of key organization strategies and initiatives and ensures the simulation resources and programs are aligned accordingly. Assures the integration of system simulation and innovation activities to achieve system strategies and objectives.

3. Responsible for and oversees the department budget in conjunction with corporate goals and objectives. This position is accountable for meeting annual budgetary goals.

4. Directs personnel actions including recruiting, new hire actions, interviewing and selection of new staff, salary determinations, training, and performance evaluations. Develops simulation goals and objectives that align with the department and system strategic initiatives.

5. Develops and implements strategic simulation and innovation services and opportunities to support the achievement of workforce goals, quality initiatives, and clinical practice. Role models innovative solutions to impact patient safety and evidence-based practice in the design and delivery of workforce learning and development outcomes. Demonstrates the use of research and best practices knowledge for participation in evaluating the effectiveness of simulation education/ training programs.

6. Responsible for and evaluates simulation learning effectiveness using standardized outcome measurements. Improves program effectiveness using metrics by identifying learning gaps, strengths and opportunities.

7. Responsible for oversight, development, delivery, and/or assessment of simulation curriculum, developmental programs, and related services, which may include system process for and coordination with clinical education training programs.

Performs all functions according to established policies, procedures, and regulatory and accreditation requirements, as well as applicable professional standards. Provides all customers of Banner Health with an excellent service experience by consistently demonstrating our core and leader behaviors each and every day.

NOTE: The essential functions are intended to describe the general content of and requirements of this position and are not intended to be an exhaustive statement of duties. Specific tasks or responsibilities will be documented as outlined by the incumbent's immediate manager.

continues

Table 14.2   Sample Position Description—Simulation Director   (cont.)

SUPERVISORY RESPONSIBILITIES

DIRECTLY REPORTING
May include simulation managers, simulation coordinators, administrative staff, and educators at all simulation training centers.
MATRIX OR INDIRECT REPORTING
None
TYPE OF SUPERVISORY RESPONSIBILITIES
Assigned full authority for employment actions including selection, training, coaching, and performance reviews.

Banner Health Leadership will strive to uphold the mission, vision, and values of the organization. They will serve as role models for staff and act in a people-centered, service excellence-focused, and results-oriented manner.

SCOPE AND COMPLEXITY

Responsible for the integration and standardization of simulation across the system. Provides leadership to support simulation needs and the effective design and delivery of simulation programs and developmental opportunities. Internal customers include but are not limited to leaders, medical staff and employees across the organization. External customers include but are not limited to practicing physicians and regulatory agencies. When planning continuing education events, follows all the requirements of CME, ANA and ANCC.

PHYSICAL DEMANDS/ENVIRONMENT FACTORS

OE – Typical Office Environment: (Accountant, Administrative Assistant, Consultant, Program Manager)

Requires extensive sitting with periodic standing and walking.

May be required to lift up to 20 pounds.

Requires significant use of personal computer, phone, and general office equipment.

Needs adequate visual acuity and ability to grasp and handle objects.

Needs ability to communicate effectively through reading, writing, and speaking in person or on telephone.

May require off-site travel

MINIMUM QUALIFICATIONS

Must possess a strong knowledge of healthcare as normally obtained through the completion of a master's degree in healthcare or a related field.

Requires a current RN license in state of practice.

Must possess a strong knowledge within designated area(s) as normally demonstrated through a minimum of five years' related experience. Requires current knowledge and experience with strategic development, program development, operations, and learning solutions. Demonstrates understanding of adult learning principles and change management. Excellent presentation, facilitation, and computer technology skills.

required. Strong organization and communication skills required. Ability to take initiative, problem solve, and improve processes required. Extensive reading, verbal communication, writing, presentation, financial/statistical analysis, and experience in integrating information technology.

PREFERRED QUALIFICATIONS
Minimum two years in a position with primary responsibility for design and delivery of learning content preferred.

Additional related education and/or experience preferred.

Used with permission of Banner Health

Table 14.3   Sample Position Description—RN Simulation Specialist

Banner Health Position Description

Position Title: RN Simulation Specialist

POSITION SUMMARY
This position implements education programs for several service line workforce needs to achieve successful simulation education and training. Plans, designs, implements, and evaluates simulation-based learning and development outcomes to support the achievement of workforce goals, facility and regional strategies and initiatives. Provides expert consultation and critique to simulation development.

ESSENTIAL FUNCTIONS
1. Serves as an internal consultant for simulation design. Designs workforce learning and development outcomes that support facility strategies and initiatives. Conducts assessment of current and projected workforce development needs and provides efficient, effective, high quality programs and services in response. Provides guidance on clinical issues for various service line areas. Serves as a resource for policy and procedures, standards of care, and external agency requirements.

2. Coordinates and assists in all development of scenarios and training in conjunction with faculty and staff to integrate simulation usage into clinical curriculum. Researches, plans, implements, and evaluates curriculum content and sequence. Incorporates proficient clinical practice, safety, and patient centered care in all educational scenarios. Programs, tests, and runs scenarios with faculty, assuring that faculty and equipment are prepared for teaching scenarios.

3. Directly responsible for the development and delivery of employee development programs and designated learning programs that attract new recruits, retain current staff, and improve quality of care. Ensures timely delivery and integration between plan objectives and design in order to obtain intended program impact and stakeholder/participant satisfaction while managing required resources effectively.

4. Uses advanced knowledge to execute set-up, programming, maintenance, use, disassembly, and troubleshooting of simulation equipment. Demonstrates and teaches technical and philosophical aspects of operating and programming simulators to staff. Develops a schedule of simulator activities to include periodic review and maintenance of equipment.

continues

Table 14.3   Sample Position Description—RN Simulation Specialist   (cont.)

5. Implements, interprets, and evaluates learning goals and objectives. Implements assessment tools to be integrated as competency measures in all aspects of simulation-based education. Evaluates learning effectiveness using standardized outcome measurements. Uses performance measures and workforce needs to drive education plans and learning strategies.

6. Manages and leads program development of new systems, applications, software conversions and upgrades, and media integration, maintaining partnerships and troubleshooting. Identifies opportunities for technology improvement and integration into healthcare education.

7. Conducts regular evaluations and critiques of programs, soliciting recommendations from both internal and external customers.

8. Provides consultation for research projects; guides and/or directs process. Effectively translates research outcomes into actions, working with others to improve overall quality and cost effectiveness of patient care.

Performs all functions according to established policies, procedures, and regulatory and accreditation requirements, as well as applicable professional standards. Provides all customers of Banner Health with an excellent service experience by consistently demonstrating our core and leader behaviors each and every day.

NOTE: The essential functions are intended to describe the general content of and requirements of this position and are not intended to be an exhaustive statement of duties. Specific tasks or responsibilities will be documented as outlined by the incumbent's immediate manager.

SUPERVISORY RESPONSIBILITIES

DIRECTLY REPORTING
None
MATRIX OR INDIRECT REPORTING
None
TYPE OF SUPERVISORY RESPONSIBILITIES
N/A

Banner Health Leadership will strive to uphold the mission, vision, and values of the organization. They will serve as role models for staff and act in a people-centered, service excellence-focused, and results-oriented manner.

SCOPE AND COMPLEXITY
This position designs simulation-based clinical training programs for all levels of clinical staff and providers for both internal and external facilities. This position is also responsible for research and applicable grant funding.

PHYSICAL DEMANDS/ENVIRONMENT FACTORS
DP – Typical Direct Patient Care environment: (Nutrition Rep, Chaplain, RN)

Able to stand, walk, bend, squat, reach, and stretch frequently.

Possess physical agility and adequate reaction time to respond quickly and appropriately to unexpected patient care needs.

Needs adequate hearing and visual acuity, including adequate color vision.

Requires fine motor skills, adequate eye-hand coordination, and ability to grasp and handle objects.

Able to use proper body mechanics to assist patients in ambulating and transferring in and out of bed, chair, or wheelchair.

May be required to lift up to 75 pounds.

Must use standard precautions due to threat of exposure to blood and bodily fluids.

Needs ability to communicate effectively through reading, writing, and speaking in person or on telephone.

May require periodic use of personal computer.

Note, all patient and exposure encounters are simulated but require exercise of caution as required in actual patient care settings.

MINIMUM QUALIFICATIONS
Must possess a strong knowledge of clinical care, education, and/or technology as normally demonstrated through the completion of a bachelor's degree in nursing, healthcare, education, technology, or related field.

Requires a current RN license.

Must possess a strong knowledge and understanding of clinical care as normally demonstrated through five years of recent experience in an acute care setting. Requires two years of experience using adult learning principles. Requires the ability to facilitate shared understanding and creative team processes. Develops collaborative relationships that foster synergy, creative solutions, and successful results. Must have excellent written and oral communication skills.

Must also have familiarity with programming and troubleshooting software.

PREFERRED QUALIFICATIONS
Master's degree in nursing, healthcare, or adult learning preferred.

Additional related education and/or experience preferred.

Used with permission of Banner Health

References

Alinier, G. (2011). Developing high-fidelity healthcare simulation scenarios: A guide for educators and professionals. *Simulation and Gaming, 42*(1), 9–26. http://dx.doi.org/10.1177/1046878109355683

Archer, J. C. (2010). State of the science in health professional education: Effective feedback. *Medical Education, 44*(1), 101–108.

Barrows, H. S. (1993). An overview of the uses of standardized patients for teaching and evaluating clinical skills. *Academic Medicine, 68*(6), 443–451.

Bloom, B., Englehart, M., Furst, E., Hill, W., & Krathwohl, D. (1956). *Taxonomy of educational objectives: The classification of educational goals.* New York, NY: Longmans, Green & Co.

Brown, A. H., & Green, T. D. (2016). *The essentials of instructional design: Connecting fundamental principles with process and practice* (3rd ed.). New York, NY: Routledge.

Buzachero, V. V., Phillips, J., Phillips, P. P., & Phillips, Z. L. (2013). *Measuring ROI in healthcare: Tools and techniques to measure the impact and ROI in healthcare improvement projects and programs.* New York, NY: McGraw-Hill.

Cheng, A., Grant, V., Dieckmann, P., Arora, S., Robinson, T., & Eppich, W. (2015, August). Faculty development for simulation programs: Five issues for the future of debriefing training. *Simulation in Healthcare, 10*(4), 217–222. doi:10.1097/SIH.0000000000000090

Fanning, R. M., & Gaba, D. M. (2007). The role of debriefing in simulation-based learning. *Simulation in Healthcare, 2*(2), 115–125. doi:10.1097/SIH.0b013e3180315539

International Nursing Association for Clinical Simulation and Learning Standards Committee. (2016a). Standards of best practice: SimulationSM. Debriefing. *Clinical Simulation in Nursing, 12*(S), S21–S25. http://dx.doi.org/10.1016/j.ecns.2016.09.008

International Nursing Association for Clinical Simulation and Learning Standards Committee. (2016b). Standards of best practice: SimulationSM. Facilitation. *Clinical Simulation in Nursing, 12*(S), S16–S20. http://dx.doi.org/10.1016/j.ecns.2016.09.007

International Nursing Association for Clinical Simulation and Learning Standards Committee. (2016c). Standards of best practice: SimulationSM. Simulation design. *Clinical Simulation in Nursing, 12*(S), S5–S12. http://dx.doi.org/10.1016/j.ecns.2016.09.005

Issenberg, S. G., Ringsted, C., Ostergaard, D., & Dieckmann, P. (2011). Setting a research agenda for simulation-based healthcare education: A synthesis of the outcome from an Utstein Style Meeting. *Simulation in Healthcare, 6*(3), 155–167. doi:10.1097/SIH.0b013e3182207c24

Kirkpatrick, D. L. (2006). *Evaluating training programs: The four levels* (3rd ed.). San Francisco, CA: Berrett-Koehler Publishers.

Molloy, E., Ajjawi, R., Bearman, M., Noble, C., Rudland, J., & Ryan, A. (2020). Challenging feedback myths: Values, learner involvement and promoting effects beyond the immediate task. *Medical Education, 54*, 33–39. doi:10.1111/medu.13802

National League for Nursing. (2020). *Simulation Innovation Resource Center.* Retrieved from https://sirc.nln.org/

Rivière, E., Jaffrelot, M., Jouquan, J., & Chiniara, G. (2019). Debriefing for the transfer of learning: The importance of context. *Academic Medicine, 94*(6), 796–803. doi:10.1097/ACM.0000000000002612

Sawyer, T., Walter, E., Brett-Fleeger, M., Grant, V., & Cheng, A. (2016) More than one way to debrief: A critical review of healthcare simulation debriefing methods. *Society for Simulation in Healthcare, 11*(3), 209–217.

Society for Simulation in Healthcare. (2016). *SSH certified healthcare simulation educator-advanced handbook.* Wheaton, IL: Author. Retrieved from https://www.ssih.org/Portals/48/Certification/CHSE-A_Docs/CHSE-A%20Handbook.pdf

Society for Simulation in Healthcare. (2019a). *SSH certified healthcare simulation educator handbook.* Wheaton, IL: Author. Retrieved from https://www.ssih.org/Portals/48/Certification/CHSE_Docs/CHSE%20Handbook.pdf

Society for Simulation in Healthcare. (2019b). *SSH CHSE-A: Certified healthcare simulation educator-advanced.* Wheaton, IL: Author. Retrieved from https://www.ssih.org/Credentialing/Certification/CHSE-A

> *"My meaning simply is, that whatever I have tried to do in life, I have tried with all my heart to do well; that whatever I have devoted myself to, I have devoted myself to completely; that in great aims and in small, I have always been thoroughly in earnest."*
>
> –Charles Dickens

Credentialing and Certification in Simulation

15

Andrew E. Spain, MA, EMT-P
Gerald R. Moses, PhD, FSSH
Joseph O. Lopreiato, MD, MPH, CHSE-A

OBJECTIVES

- Summarize how simulation is being used in the credentialing of healthcare personnel.

- Identify the importance and value of certification in simulation.

- Describe various requirements for using simulation to create a certification process that meets accreditation criteria.

- Discuss the development and value of the Certified Healthcare Simulation Educator (CHSE) certification program.

According to the Institute for Credentialing Excellence (ICE; formerly the National Organization for Competency Assurance), the term *credentialing* should be used as an "umbrella term to include professional certification, certificate programs, accreditation, licensure, and regulation" (ICE, 2010, p. 1). Credentialing is an accepted part of life in academic and healthcare settings. The process of credentialing typically involves a systematic approach to verifying qualifications, including assessment of whether an individual has the knowledge, skills, and abilities required for a specific position. A number of different credentialing methods have been established to meet the needs of various service sectors and professional disciplines, including licensure, accreditation, certificate programs, and certification (ICE, 2019a). In healthcare, simulation often plays an important role in each of these forms of credentialing. In addition, simulation is increasingly being used as a mechanism for assessment of personnel for the purpose of granting or retaining clinical privileges.

Licensure

Licensure, according to ICE (2019a), "tests an individual's competence but is a mandatory process by which the government grants time-limited permission for that licensed individual to practice his or her profession" (p. 1). Many healthcare professions have multiple steps to obtain licensure, some of which involve the use of simulation to verify competencies or skills. For instance, a paramedic candidate is required to demonstrate competence by successfully completing a number of skill stations as part of the National Registry of Emergency Medical Technicians practical examination. Upon successful completion of the skills assessment and a written examination, the candidate becomes a nationally registered paramedic and can submit the registry certificate to the home state as part of the process to become licensed.

The US Medical Licensing Examination (USMLE) also uses simulation as part of the process to obtain a license as a healthcare provider. This multiple-part examination assesses "the ability to apply knowledge, concepts, and principles, and to demonstrate fundamental patient-centered skills" (USMLE, 2019, p. 1). A portion of this examination requires candidates to demonstrate their professional, interpersonal, and technical skills through the use of simulated patient encounters.

Accreditation

According to the Society for Simulation in Healthcare (SSH), *accreditation* is "a process whereby a professional organization grants recognition to a simulation program for demonstrated ability to meet pre-determined criteria for established standards" (SSH, 2013a, p. 27). The role of accreditation in healthcare simulation is to ensure quality through the assessment of simulation programs and centers. This form of credentialing is focused on competency and performance at the program level rather than the individual performance level that is the focus of licensure, certificate programs, and certification.

SSH has developed standards for simulation programs in healthcare and an accreditation process for simulation programs (SSH Council for Certification, 2019). There are standards in the following areas:

- Core standards and criteria
- Assessment standards and measurement

- Research standards and measurement
- Teaching/education standards and measurement
- Systems integration: Facilitating patient safety outcomes

The SSH Accreditation Standards, Accreditation Instructional Guide, Accreditation Self-Study, Accreditation Application, and a current list of accredited simulation programs are available on the SSH website (www.ssih.org/accreditation). Other organizations, such as the American College of Surgeons (ACS), also have accreditation programs for education institutes, including simulation-based education/training centers (ACS, 2019).

Certificate Programs

In healthcare, the terms *certificate* and *certification* are often used interchangeably, but certificate programs and certification programs are distinctly different. Certificates are awarded after successful completion of a specified course or training session, whereas professional or personnel certification is usually a voluntary process involving an external review that assesses an individual's knowledge, skills, or abilities in a specific area.

There are two types of certificate programs:

- *Certificates of attendance or participation* are "provided to individuals (participants) who have attended or participated in classes, courses, or other education/training programs or events. The certificate awarded at the completion of the program or event signifies that the participant was present and, in some cases, that the participant actively participated in the program or event. Demonstration of accomplishment of the intended learning outcomes by participants is NOT a requirement for receiving the certificate; thus, possession of a certificate of attendance or participation does not indicate that the intended learning outcomes have been accomplished by the participant" (ICE, 2019a, p. 2).

- An *assessment-based certification program* is "a non-degree granting program that (a) provides instruction and training to aid participants in acquiring specific knowledge, skills, and/or competencies associated with intended learning outcomes; (b) evaluates participants' achievement of the intended learning outcomes; and (c) awards a certificate only to those participants who meet the performance, proficiency or passing standard for the assessment(s)" (ICE, 2019b, p. 2).

The primary focus of assessment-based certificate programs is to facilitate the accomplishment of intended learning outcomes, whereas the primary focus of certification is to provide an independent assessment of the knowledge, skills, and/or competencies required for competent performance of an occupational role or specific work-related tasks and responsibilities (ICE, 2010). In addition, oversight for certification programs is provided by an autonomous governing body composed of representatives from relevant stakeholders, while this is not required from assessment-based certificate programs (ICE, 2010).

The use of simulation in certificate-granting programs has become much more prevalent in healthcare. In these programs, simulation can be used to teach, assess, remediate, and evaluate. Certificate programs can be nationally recognized or locally developed. An example of a nationally recognized simulation-based program that provides a certificate is TeamSTEPPS, a program offered by the Agency for Healthcare Research and Quality (n.d.). An example of a locally developed program that uses simulation for teaching and evaluation of a specific competency would be a chemotherapy program developed by a hospital for its RN staff.

Many disciplines, specialties, and aspects of healthcare have certificate programs. Some certificate programs exist to teach educators how to use simulation for the purpose of healthcare education or to improve their skills as simulation educators. Having a certificate from a course may demonstrate exposure to content and/or actual demonstration of competency at completion of the program. However, when presented with any certificate, especially one related to simulation, you need to determine the credibility of the issuing organization, the conditions of the course, and the actual requirements to receive the certificate. For example, a certificate might be given to document that the learner attended a course (certificate of attendance), or it might only be given when the learner has demonstrated achievement of the course objectives.

Evaluation

Whether embedded in a certificate-granting program or being used to determine a healthcare professional's fitness to be granted specific privileges to practice in a clinical setting, using simulation for evaluation requires special attention. When simulation is used for the purpose of high-stakes assessment or evaluation of competency, educators and facilitators need to ensure appropriate, consistent, and fair processes are in place. They need to carefully consider elements such as providing an environment conducive to testing, providing a consistent evaluation experience, and using a reliable and valid tool with proven inter-rater reliability when developing and implementing these types of evaluation programs. Simulation-based credentialing and privileging programs require special attention to ensure the developers and evaluators are well versed in the appropriate simulation techniques to achieve these purposes. See Chapter 6 for information on using simulation for evaluation.

Professional Certification

The concept of certification in the education and healthcare sectors is not new, at least in the US. In this context, certification is a process of verifying and recognizing individuals who meet an established set of standards. It is "designed to test the knowledge, skills, and abilities required to perform a particular job, and, upon successfully passing a certification exam, to represent a declaration of a particular individual's professional competence" (ICE, 2019a, p. 1). In many medical, nursing, and allied health fields, specialty certification is now an expected part of professional development. Individuals often must have a minimum set of certifications to be eligible for certain roles or positions. For instance, physicians, nurses, and other healthcare providers working in a trauma center or emergency department are often expected to obtain and retain specific emergency or trauma certifications. Simulation has now been integrated into almost every specialty certification program in healthcare.

Although a number of certification programs exist that have applicability for those actively involved in healthcare simulation (healthcare simulationists), more comprehensive and globally recognized certifications in this specialty have only recently been developed. The rapid rate of growth in simulation-based activities for healthcare students and professionals has created challenges to establishing core knowledge, skills, and competency standards that are fundamental to the creation of a well-constructed certification program.

Principles of Professional Certification

Some knowledge of the principles of certification is valuable in understanding the role of certification for healthcare simulationists. Competence has been defined as "an expected level of performance that integrates knowledge, skills, abilities, and judgment" (American Nurses Association [ANA], 2014, p. 3). The ANA describes these terms as follows (ANA, 2014, p. 3):

- "*Knowledge* encompasses thinking, understanding of science and humanities, professional standards of practice, and insights gained from context, practical experiences, personal capabilities, and leadership performance.

- *Skills* include psychomotor, communication, interpersonal, and diagnostic skills.

- *Ability* is the capacity to act effectively. It requires listening, integrity, knowledge of one's strengths and weaknesses, positive self-regard, emotional intelligence, and openness to feedback.

- *Judgment* includes critical thinking, problem solving, ethical reasoning, and decision-making."

Of the many evaluation methods used for certification, the most common by far is the multiple-choice question examination designed with a rigorous process and using psychometric principles to establish the required level of competency to be demonstrated. This is not to say there are not alternative approaches to evaluation for certification. Individuals can be certified based on their work and professional history, for instance, through a review of a curriculum vitae. However, these forms of evaluation might have subjective problems, such as poor inter-rater reliability or bias based on personal preference. As a result, multiple-choice questions are the most easily supported knowledge assessment method in certification programs.

Standard procedures and processes for certification have been established and published by accrediting organizations—such as the National Commission for Certifying Agencies, the International Organization for Standardization, and the American Board of Nursing Specialties (ABNS)—that focus on discipline-specific certifications or address specialty areas of practice. Organizations that accredit certification programs establish requirements to ensure fair treatment of candidates. Standards typically include effective governance, identification of resources, inclusion of stakeholders in the certification process, use of valid and psychometrically sound assessment instruments, and establishing rules for recertification (ICE, 2019b). Organizations such as ABNS also provide lists of available certifications as well as resource materials for individuals considering certification (ABNS, 2019).

One final principle of certification is the real-world impact of the process. Initially, when certification programs are introduced to a field, the early adopters view it as a verification of their knowledge and work experience and as a means to seek recognition within their community. As certification programs mature, employers and institutions begin to demand certification as a prerequisite to employment or as an early goal for new employees. Higher salaries might be provided as a reward for a certification, or the loss of a certification might result in suspension

from, or even total loss of, a job for which the certification is required. This reinforces the importance of taking an evidence-based approach when integrating the use of simulation into certification-preparation programs. The potential impact of preparation programs increases when certifications are required for employment.

Value of Professional Certification

A question often asked is, "What's the value of certification?" If healthcare simulationists are seeking to become certified, they need to be able to articulate possible benefits of certification. These benefits include the following (Henderson, Biel, Harman, Wickett, & Young, 2012):

- Protection of the public
- Greater confidence in professional competence
- Increased autonomy in the workplace
- Enhanced marketability, employability, and opportunity for advancement
- Improved monetary rewards
- Better compliance with regulations and conditions of third-party payers
- Raised public opinion
- Lowered risk

A Professional Certification Program for Healthcare Simulationists

Recognizing the value of certification, SSH began work on the creation of an international certification program for simulation in 2009. The initial period of work focused on identifying the knowledge, skills, abilities, and attitudes for which all modalities of simulation had common ground and practice. This was not an easy task given the variety of simulation modalities available. These include task trainers, standardized patients, mannequins, virtual-reality devices, computer simulations, and combinations of these elements. The end result was the development of SSH's *Certification Standards and Elements* (hereafter the Standards; SSH, 2012).

The Standards were developed using a consensus approach involving several meetings of healthcare simulation subject matter experts (SMEs) from North and South America, Europe, and the Asia-Pacific region. These SMEs represented a wide variety of professional societies and stakeholders:

- SSH (Society for Simulation in Healthcare)
- Society in Europe for Simulation as Applied to Medicine
- National League for Nursing
- Association of Standardized Patient Educators (ASPE)
- International Nursing Association for Clinical Simulation and Learning (INACSL)
- Australian Society for Simulation in Healthcare
- Brazilian Association for Simulation in Healthcare
- Canadian Network for Simulation in Healthcare
- Dutch Society for Simulation in Healthcare

This multidisciplinary group of international SMEs met and agreed to create clear expectations in a field where little had existed previously. They shared information, such as INACSL's standards for simulation, created foundational documents, and established a unique collaborative approach to be used in the development of the certification program. The group agreed that the Standards would embrace simulation principles and theories essential for practitioners in the field, regardless of the method of simulation employed. The initial standards were summarized into four core categories:

- Professional values and capabilities
- Knowledge of education principles, practice, and methodology in simulation
- Scholarship—spirit of inquiry and teaching, implementing, assessing
- Managing simulation-based educational interventions

Since this initial work, SSH has developed three certifications to serve the healthcare simulation community:

- Certified Healthcare Simulation Educator (CHSE)
- Certified Healthcare Simulation Educator-Advanced (CHSE-A)
- Certified Healthcare Simulation Operations Specialist (CHSOS)

The educator certifications (CHSE and CHSE-A) are for those healthcare simulationists primarily oriented toward and possessing the knowledge, skills, and abilities in the educational design components of simulation activities. This includes needs assessment, goals and objectives development, scenario design, and evaluation and assessment, including debriefing. The CHSE certification is designed for individuals with two years of competency and experience in the educator role, whereas the CHSE-A is a more advanced certification. There is a five-year experience requirement for this certification and an expectation of demonstrated leadership in the field.

The CHSOS certification was developed for operations specialists (OS). An OS is "an inclusive 'umbrella' term that embodies many different roles within healthcare simulation operations, including simulation technician, simulation technology specialist, simulation specialist, simulation coordinator, and simulation AV specialist. While many of these individuals also design simulation activities, this term refers to the functional role related to the implementation of the simulation activities" (Lopreiato et al., 2016, p. 25). This certification is also examination-based, similar to the CHSE in this respect, and also requires two years of experience in the field.

Practice Analysis

To meet recognized standards for creating a certification examination, it is necessary to conduct an analysis of the typical work experiences in the field. A *practice analysis* (also called a *job analysis*) is:

> a detailed description of current practice in a job or profession. Information from the practice analysis is used at all stages of examination development, including the creation of test specifications, item writing, and examination construction. The practice analysis provides the link between test content and real-world practice; it ensures that the examination is job related, and in this way provides the foundation for examination validity. (Professional Exam Services, 2003, p. 4)

Practice analyses were performed in 2011 for the CHSE and 2013 for the CHSOS certifications independently for the initial development of both. For certifications to maintain currency to practice, the practice analysis must be repeated in a timely manner to support the changes in the industry. It was decided to complete the repeat practice analysis for each certification simultaneously, beginning in 2017. In addition, the decision was made to conduct both with deliberate international involvement, thus ensuring the updated practice analyses would be indicative of worldwide practice in healthcare simulation.

To complete the repeat practice analyses, an outside vendor with expertise in the activity was engaged to work with the SMEs to compile a list of expected knowledge, skills, and abilities (KSAs). The sources for this list included job descriptions, existing statements and compilations of best practice as published by other healthcare simulation associations (e.g., INACSL and ASPE), as well as articles and research that reflected upon the function of an educator and an operations specialist in the healthcare simulation community.

The international compilation and review of the KSAs included representatives from many organizations around the world. Meetings took place in Tampa, Florida, USA; Hong Kong; and Amsterdam, Netherlands. The methodology of review of all the KSAs focused on using the following questions to ensure the KSA was performed globally:

- Is any performance or practice indicated by the KSA illegal in your region?

- Is education on this KSA not available in your region?

- Is any performance or practice indicated by the KSA inconsistent with the religions/ norms and social practices in your region?

- Can the language and phrasing of the KSA not be readily understood by practitioners in your region?

- Are any procedures or practices referred to in this KSA not performed in your region?

When the practice analysis was complete, a survey was sent out to individuals believed to be active in simulation (members of simulation, education, and professional organizations). The survey shared the results of the practice analysis and asked the respondents to comment on the following questions in regard to the compiled list of KSAs:

- Is it important?

- Is it written clearly?

- Is it performed by practitioners regularly?

- Is it redundant with other tasks?

- Does it belong where it is in the outline?

- Is it testable?

The demographic results of the 2018 survey are shown in Table 15.1.

The responses of the surveys were reviewed by a final group of SMEs who met in Tampa, Florida, USA. Key findings in the data indicated that the domains and KSAs were considered accurate and statistically reliable (see Table 15.2).

Table 15.1	2018 KSA Survey Results—Demographics	
Item	**CHSE Survey**	**CHSOS Survey**
Usable sample size*	721	275
Gender	75% female, 25% male	41.2% female, 58.8% male
% certified (SSH certifications)	45.6%	42.2%
≤ 10 years in simulation	71.9%	80.7%
US/international split**	74.2%/25.8%	72.7%/27.3%
# of countries	53	28
Master's or PhD	77.6%	39.3%
English is primary language	83.8%	86.2%

*Completed all demographic and survey elements; **15.5% international for CHSE in 2011; 12% international for CHSOS in 2013*

Table 15.2	2018 Survey KSA Results	
Item	**CHSE Survey**	**CHSOS Survey**
KSAs completely or adequately covered the role	98.6%	97.5%
Cronbach's Alpha	99.6%	99.3%

Cronbach's Alpha is a statistical measure of internal consistency and reliability. Values over 70% (0.7) are generally considered to indicate reliable/consistent results.

In addition, the review of the results by the SMEs included:

- Feedback on missing or unclear items

- Review of feedback from the international SMEs about the KSAs

- Weighting of the importance of each category (domain weight)

With this information in hand, the group of SMEs finalized the list of KSAs, clarifying and improving where needed based on the feedback of the survey, and they determined the final weighting of each of the domains in preparation for the development of the examination. Weighting was assigned as follows (SSH, 2019):

CHSE

- Domain I: Professional Values and Capabilities – 18%

- Domain II: Healthcare and Simulation Knowledge/Principles – 28%

- Domain III: Educational Principles Applied to Simulation – 40%

- Domain IV: Simulation Resources and Environments – 14%

CHSOS

- Domain I: Concepts in Healthcare as Applied to Simulation – 14%

- Domain II: Simulation Technology Operations – 33%

- Domain III: Healthcare Simulation Practices/ Principles/Procedures – 27%

- Domain IV: Professional Role: Behavior and Capabilities – 11%

- Domain V: Concepts in Instructional Design as Applied to Simulation – 15%

Examination Development

The final step in the development of the certification program was to develop the examination. This task required the dedicated work of a number of interdisciplinary SMEs to generate questions, review answers, and develop a reference list. The general process for writing the questions was as follows:

1. Generation of question and answers

   - Questions must be tied to each item on the test blueprint

   - Questions need to be supported by a direct reference (e.g., journal article)

   - Questions must also match actual practice in healthcare simulation

2. Review of questions

   - Improvement of question stems and selections (e.g., no negatives, no humorous distractors)

3. Compilation of items into examination forms

   - For security purposes, two forms of the examination are developed

4. Initial review of the forms by a group of SMEs

   - To ensure each form meets the requirements of the test blueprint (weighting)

5. Final review of the forms by a separate group of SMEs

   - Further review of items and approval of items

Future of Certification in Healthcare Simulation

Although it is difficult to predict what the future holds for healthcare simulation certification, many things are known. Certifications for others involved in simulation in healthcare are likely. For example, administrators are integral to the oversight of simulation programs, and they may well be served by having a certification to recognize their functions and roles. Other advanced certifications may also serve the community through providing a professional development pathway. If these certifications are determined to be appropriate and serve the healthcare simulation community, their development will follow.

No matter the level of certification, it is very clear that professional certification programs for the simulation specialty will need to remain flexible and adaptive as the field of healthcare simulation grows. The rapid growth that is being experienced is wonderful news in almost all ways, but it results in a mandate to continually reevaluate the practice of healthcare simulationists. The typical time period before a repeat practice analysis is needed ranges from five to seven years for established certifications in stable industries. It is possible that, with the amount of research and growth that exists in healthcare simulation, the next practice analysis will occur earlier than this time frame.

The development of certification programs in healthcare simulation has helped to create opportunities for those seeking professional development in the field. With the publishing of the Standards and the examination blueprints, existing certificate programs will likely adapt their educational objectives to ensure that individuals who complete these programs will have success when seeking certification as a healthcare simulation educator.

Conclusion

With increasing emphasis on improving patient safety and enhancing patient outcomes by assuring the competence of providers, credentialing and certification are certain to continue to be important areas of interest for all healthcare organizations. Educators who engage in healthcare simulation will be challenged to integrate simulation into various activities associated with credentialing—either by developing educational programs that leverage the use of simulation to address maintenance of competency or by using simulation techniques to assess the competency of providers for the purpose of privileging.

In this setting, the demand for certification of healthcare professionals is likely to increase. Healthcare simulationists now have the opportunity to demonstrate their competence and expertise by seeking certification themselves. By becoming certified, the HSE professional can become a better practitioner of the science and art of simulation and demonstrate that expertise for others to see.

References

Agency for Healthcare Research and Quality. (n.d.). *TeamSTEPPS*. Rockville, MD. Retrieved from https://www.ahrq.gov/teamstepps/index.html

American Board of Nursing Specialties. (2019). *ABNS - About us*. Aurora, OH: Author. Retrieved from http://www.nursingcertification.org/about

American College of Surgeons. (2019). *Accredited education institutes*. Chicago, IL: Author. Retrieved from https://www.facs.org/education/accreditation/aei

American Nurses Association. (2014). *Position statements: Professional role competence*. Silver Spring, MD: Author.

Henderson, J. H., Biel, M., Harman, L., Wickett, J., & Young, P. (2012). *A look at the value of professional certification*. Washington, DC: Institute for Credentialing Excellence.

Institute for Credentialing Excellence. (2010). *Defining features of quality certification and assessment-based certificate programs.* Washington, DC: Author. Retrieved from http://www.credentialingexcellence.org/p/cm/ld/fid=4

Institute for Credentialing Excellence. (2019a). *About ICE.* Washington, DC: Author. Retrieved from www.credentialingexcellence.org/p/cm/ld/fid=32

Institute for Credentialing Excellence. (2019b). *National Commission for Certifying Agencies (NCCA) Accreditation.* Washington, DC: Author. Retrieved from https://www.credentialingexcellence.org/p/cm/ld/fid=66

Lopreiato, J. O. (Ed.), Downing, D., Gammon, W., Lioce, L., Sitter, B., Slot, V., … the Terminology & Concepts Working Group. (2016). *Healthcare simulation dictionary.* Retrieved from https://www.ssih.org/Dictionary

Professional Exam Services. (2003). Practice analysis: The foundation of examination validity. *PES News, 2*(1), 4–6.

Society for Simulation in Healthcare. (2012). *SSH Certification standards and elements.* Wheaton, IL: Author. Retrieved from http://ssih.org/certification

Society for Simulation in Healthcare. (2013a). *SSH accreditation process.* Wheaton, IL: Author. Retrieved from http://ssih.org/accreditation/how-to-apply

Society for Simulation in Healthcare. (2013b). *SSH certified healthcare simulation educator handbook.* Wheaton, IL: Author. Retrieved from http://ssih.org/certification

Society for Simulation in Healthcare. (2019). *SSH Certification examination blueprint.* Washington, DC: Author. Retrieved from http://www.simcertification.com

Society for Simulation in Healthcare Council for Certification. (2019). *SSH certified healthcare simulation educator handbook.* Retrieved from https://www.ssih.org/Portals/48/Certification/CHSE_Docs/CHSE%20Handbook.pdf

United States Medical Licensing Examination. (2019). *2019 USMLE Bulletin of information.* Philadelphia, PA: Federation of State Medical Boards (FSMB) and National Board of Medical Examiners (NBME). Retrieved from https://www.usmle.org/pdfs/bulletin/2019bulletin.pdf

"We shape buildings; thereafter, they shape us."
—Winston Churchill

Designing Simulation Centers for Health Education

16

Jane Crofut, RN, MAOM
Steve Kopp, AIA, ACHA
Cynthia Walston, FAIA

OBJECTIVES

- Describe a planning process to design a simulation center based on an analysis of curriculum and utilization goals.

- Establish planning parameters to generate a program of spaces for the simulation center.

- Understand the process of engaging and working with an architectural design team to develop a simulation center facility.

A foundational goal of health education at all levels is the preparation of health providers to understand, navigate, and bridge gaps between didactic learning and practice using compassionate, science-based research that improves the human condition. Because healthcare is delivered in a wide variety of physical and cultural settings, from dirt floor huts to robotic operating suites, education facilities must accommodate a similarly broad range of learning experiences. Simulation centers are increasingly seen as flexible locations for experiential learning, fully integrated into academic curricula, and central to interprofessional education in the clinical setting.

This chapter explores the planning needed and suggests physical guidelines to create a new simulation center or to renovate an existing one, as well as considerations for working with facility architects. Purpose-built simulation centers differ in their size, configuration, and organizational structure, based on the specific needs, affiliations, and partnerships of each institution. One shape or one size will not fit all. However, there are evidence-based standards for the size and configuration of the different modalities commonly used to simulate patient care. Where simulation replicates realistic clinical settings, architects employ evidence-based standards for the design of specific room types.

Simulation centers are designed to meet the educational needs of a broad range of users, including nursing and medical students, interns and residents, clinical psychology students, first responders, and professionals at all levels who benefit from advanced, interprofessional training (Society for Simulation in Healthcare, 2019). Today's learners must develop important skills beyond traditional knowledge recall, critical thinking, and task proficiency (Association of American Medical Colleges, 2011). Healthcare delivery is rapidly changing, with an expectation that future healthcare providers will understand, participate in, develop, and advocate for the continuous improvement of integrated health systems in which collaborative teams use evidence-based research, technologies, and social determinants of health to provide streamlined, proactive care. As a result, health and medical educators are researching, developing, and implementing innovative curricula to meet this expectation, leading to numerous emerging trends. Future-forward health education space will be affected by the early integration of the following trends in the curriculum:

- Community-based patient care
- Longitudinal patient experiences
- Big data identification, visualization, and use
- Scholarly, clinical, and translational research
- Merged-degree options with engineering, biomedical sciences, social sciences, and informatics
- Global exposure, work, and educational initiatives
- Socioeconomic determinants of health
- Student self-care and life balance

Pedagogical models for knowledge acquisition and transfer into practice are also evolving, such that curricula are becoming more diverse, with increasing requirements for active, collaborative, and interprofessional learning opportunities, including:

- Team-based active learning activities
- Problem-based collaborative learning

- Skills training with opportunities for self-directed learning and evaluation
- Small group "learning academies" with faculty facilitators
- Formative and realistic immersive patient care management simulation (IPCMS)
- Advanced interactive teaching technologies, including virtual and augmented reality
- Integration of interprofessional education

Today's health education spaces must be easily adaptable to prevent current and future curricula from being bound by schedules, space constraints, pedagogical models, and technology adjuncts. Flexible learning spaces are needed both to meet the needs of current learners and to support inevitable changes in pedagogy and technology over the useful life of a facility. Most, if not all, curriculum-delivery and self-directed learning spaces are potentially capable of multiple uses. Health education and simulation space typologies have strategic alignments and may have shared operational capabilities, allowing one to co-locate and flex between different modalities. To achieve this in a balanced, fiscally responsible, future-forward manner, the following health education space-design precepts are evolving as best practices:

- Learning space size expands or contracts based on the type of use and learner group size.
- Didactic, active, and experiential modes are blended to provide same-session continuum of learning.
- Informal learning and collaboration are promoted by integration of learning spaces with social spaces.

Professional curricula are in a state of almost constant change to prepare graduates to provide care in rapidly changing environments. Curriculum delivery has quickly evolved to encompass blended pedagogical models that require clear definitions of "experiential learning" modalities. Each modality has unique operational requirements that impact the need for facility space, equipment, and other building services, such as air conditioning, electrical power, and AV support. The curricula requirements of immersive patient care management simulation (IPCMS), are a key driver in the evolving design of spaces to support knowledge transfer from clinical skills through interprofessional continuum of patient care management.

Planning for a healthcare simulation center requires a thorough understanding of an institution's goals for pedagogy and research as well as the ability to translate these into a program of physical spaces. There are few widely accepted planning parameters for the design of simulation facilities. There is a need for facility planning guidelines that are based on evidence and best practices, which evolve through time. Such guidelines must enable learners to interact with technology in physical spaces that support the learning goals of the simulation pedagogy.

Structure for Success

The opportunity to design and build a new clinical simulation center comes rarely. When it does come, success requires a structured design process with engaged stakeholders, such as the one depicted in Figure 16.1. Creating the right amount of the right types of spaces so that learners, educators, and researchers can continue to strive to provide better outcomes will necessitate a deep dive into the priorities, unique needs, operational logistics, and funding of the institution, coupled with an analysis of curriculum delivery to ensure customization of proven design precepts that align evolving visions with health education trends.

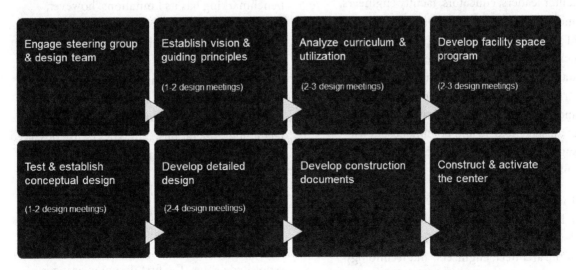

FIGURE 16.1   Recommended design process for a simulation center. In this process, end users are engaged with the architects in multiple meeting sessions for approximately six to 12 months to develop a detailed design plan prior to the start of construction.

A clinical simulation laboratory is a costly venture to build and operate, so decisions need to be based on justified need. Typical construction costs for the build-out of a simulation center can range from $200 to $400 per square foot or more, depending on location. Equipment costs, fees, permits, and inspections can be double or triple this cost depending on the complexity of the project. There is also the continuing cost of operating the facility with staffing, supplies, facility and equipment maintenance, and upgrades of technology.

Steering Group and Design Team

The first step in the design of a simulation center is to onboard and align a steering group with decision-making authority for the project. The inclusion of an organization executive champion is highly beneficial to ensure continued support for the project and to hold members accountable for participation and timely decisions. This group should be kept fairly small and include simulation center leaders, educators, facility engineers, and audiovisual/information technology (AV/IT) specialists. The steering committee should next identify additional internal and external stakeholders and establish a process governance structure to describe their level of inclusion and responsibilities. Relationship mapping of all stakeholders and potential users will suggest opportunities for resource and budget optimization.

The institution's facilities department will engage a design team to assist the steering group in the development of the simulation center, consisting of the architect, engineers, and technology consultants. It is also useful for the institution to engage a construction manager at this time to help establish the allowable cost and create a comprehensive project schedule. At this early stage, preliminary estimates of construction

cost will be based on total area of construction multiplied by a unit cost for a similar type of building escalated to account for inflation in the economy and dependent on geographic location.

If there is an existing simulation center that will be remodeled or expanded, the design team will need to conduct a current-state assessment of the physical facility. This will include a tour of existing campus buildings with end users and maintenance personnel to understand existing conditions and the institution's standards and requirements. The design team will then prepare a facility conditions assessment report, noting opportunities and challenges for the design and construction of the new center.

At this stage, it is useful to conduct benchmark tours of peer institutions to understand comparable simulation programs. This can lead to new ideas that inform the design as well as insight into best practices, lessons learned in earlier projects, and recent innovations. Such benchmarking has its limitations, however, because the use of different spaces, the technology employed, and learner throughput are highly varied across programs. Keep in mind that the curriculum may change so quickly that by the time a new simulation program is funded, designed, and constructed, most of the technology, operations, and types of use observed through benchmarking may be outdated.

Vision and Guiding Principles

Prior to the first meeting with the architect, the steering group should meet independently to establish aspirational goals for the new or renovated center. The first design meeting is typically a visioning session that is facilitated by the architect to identify and validate guiding principles in support of the established goals. These principles should reflect the requirements of leadership, educators, learners, and other partners and thus serve to create a shared mental model for all stakeholders. Measurable success metrics and project priorities are identified at this early stage to aid stakeholders and the design team in making difficult decisions later as the design process evolves.

The role of the architectural team is to translate the project goals and guiding principles into a program of spaces and then bring this forward through the design and construction phases described later in this chapter. Simulation programs rely heavily on AV/IT, so it is important to include technology consultants in initial meetings to prevent redesign at a later stage. Design excellence requires a collaborative team in search of the best ideas. The architect offers leadership to the process and establishes a cooperative effort among the steering group, the end users, and other stakeholders. Architects and designers must be particularly adept at working with multiple—and sometimes conflicting—interests to integrate individual goals and ideas into a unified design. This is achieved through an iterative series of design work sessions with the end users who will ultimately occupy the center. The project will benefit by involving teachers, students, and staff in the planning process during conceptual and design phases. School or hospital leaders should anticipate and commit the time required to be involved in the process.

Curriculum and Utilization Analysis

As discussed in previous chapters, health education includes different modalities of experiential learning: skills and tasks, procedures, standardized patients, immersive simulation, and educator-supervised, hands-on patient care in a hospital or clinic. For each course, the educators must consider learning objectives, evolving best practices, and any existing regulatory and accreditation requirements to determine the number of simulation hours per learner per year in each environment. For example, simulation training hours for undergraduate nursing students will be distributed across skills and tasks, immersive simulation, and standardized patient scenarios. Some programs offer specialized home health or ambulatory care settings as well. A 2014 study by the National Council of State Boards of Nursing comparing the use of simulation and clinical time in undergraduate nursing programs found that up to 50% of clinical time can be substituted with simulation with outcomes equal to or better than the performance of programs using traditional clinical placements (Hayden, Smiley, Alexander, Kardong-Edgren, & Jeffries, 2014). Because available hours and practice opportunities for clinical training with hands-on patient care may be limited by affiliation or geography, programs should consider expanding the number of immersive simulation labs or increasing simulation center hours of operation to serve larger enrollments.

Establishing current and aspirational utilization levels for each experiential learning modality based on, at minimum, a five-year projected enrollment, provides a basis to determine the size and number of each room type, as well as equipment and storage requirements for a new or renovated simulation center.

At this stage, the utilization analysis will reveal:

- Total hours per type of experiential learning space, based on curriculum analysis

- Utilization, based on available hours (per day, week, and year), rather than historical schedules

- Size of each learning space, based on learner group size, station size, equipment, and throughput

- Shared space and operational resources, as well as costs, among different programs

- Transition from dedicated, low-utilization simulation spaces into shared, flexible spaces with improved utilization

- Need for operational support full-time equivalent (FTE) employees

- Technology scope for low voltage systems related to simulation environments.

The designer will identify the key strategic drivers informing the number and size of different simulation spaces and the configuration of room adjacencies in the simulation center. An experienced designer is able to solve challenges in new and unexpected ways by understanding current education processes and the customary learner group size for each type of training session. The designer will document existing workflows to identify patterns, pain points, and opportunities for improvement, resulting in the development of new strategies to optimize the use of simulation in the curriculum and the utilization of individual learning spaces.

Some programs benefit from dedicated-use simulation rooms, such as a mock operating room for training medical students or nurse anesthetists. For most institutions, however, the use of multipurpose "patient flex" rooms with mobile equipment that is adjusted for each scenario provides greater versatility and therefore higher utilization. Utilization of experiential learning spaces should be close to 75%, allowing for downtime to prepare equipment and clean up after each scenario, as well as development time for operational support logistics.

The use of technology is rapidly changing the curriculum. A 2016 survey of nursing schools by the National League for Nursing (NLN) found that larger programs tended to adopt new technology at a faster rate than smaller programs (Wolters Kluwer & NLN, 2016a). In addition, nearly 83% of nursing students believe that using technology enhances their learning experience, and 79% say it will better prepare them for their future careers. According to NLN's survey, 65% of nursing schools use virtual simulation, and 10% leverage virtual reality (Wolters Kluwer & NLN, 2016b).

Facility Space Program

The space program describes the purpose of the center, projected utilization, operational relationships, space requirements, and other basic information relating to the fulfillment of the organization's objectives. The program includes:

- A description of each function

- The operational space required for each function

- The number, type, and area of all spaces; special design features

- Required services and utilities

The size of each space is defined by net square feet (or net square meters), which is the area within the walls of the room. Room size is primarily driven by the purpose of the space and the number of people, the medical equipment, and AV equipment within the space.

During space programming, the design team begins to establish functionality within the space and relationships to adjacent spaces, as well as required equipment and technology that will be employed. Ideally, the space program is based on the learning needs of a standardized curriculum and not the wishes and desires of individuals. The steering group should engage diverse stakeholders to reduce risk in the design process and to increase ownership of the design by the end users. Suggested ranges of areas for the primary rooms in a clinical simulation center are shown in Table 16.1.

Table 16.1	Space Program	
Space Description	**Suggested Area**	**Notes**
Skills and tasks lab – bedside	195–225 ft² per bed position (with classroom seating) 110–160 ft² per bed position (without classroom seating)	Each bed position serves two learners. For example, six positions in the lab would need 660–960 ft² net (without classroom seating).
Skills and tasks lab – partial task	35–50 ft² per learner	Similar to active learning classroom
Immersive simulation room – Large, single position	400–650 ft²	Operating room, trauma room, emergency disaster site (dedicated or flexible)
Immersive simulation room – Small, single position	180–200 ft²	Critical care, emergency care, labor & delivery, procedure (flexible use recommended).
Standardized patient exam room	110–160 ft²	Medical exam and ambulatory care training
Debrief conference	25–30 ft² per learner	Consider movable partitions to combine small rooms into one larger room.
Control room	90–105 ft² per immersive simulation lab	Provide one position with three seats per immersive simulation lab; positions may be centralized or decentralized, with or without observation windows.
Storage/equipment/workroom	400 ft² and larger	Calculate at 35–50% of the simulation space.

The deliverables for the space program will include the following:

- Vision statement and guiding principles, including strategy for and role of simulation in curriculum

- Utilization analysis to translate vision into space types based on curriculum interventions and projected number of learners in each setting

- A tabular listing of the quantity and size of each space type in net square feet

- A written description and/or graphic depiction of the typical configuration and equipment of each space type

- A conceptual plan diagram to show the logical organization of the required spaces to establish programmatic adjacencies and workflow, including the sharing of resources

This is not a comprehensive list of rooms and spaces. The actual space program will also include public and administrative spaces, including a reception area, offices, work rooms, and break areas. Where possible, common building areas, such as the lobby or public toilets, should be shared rather than duplicated. Amenity spaces for learners should also be considered, such as informal collaboration, study, and refreshment areas. Programs often provide dressing and lounge facilities for standardized patient actors as well. After the space program is established, a preliminary construction budget can be developed by using a cost-per-square-foot for each type of space.

Simulation Space Types

Simulation labs for health and medical education include a range of types from multipurpose, flexible classrooms to highly realistic replications of healthcare environments. Technology varies from low tech (low-technology mannequins, partial task trainers) to high tech (advanced teaching and learning task trainers, haptics, AV technology with integrated performance evaluation data capture software). For the simulation center designer, the question is how best to align the modality with the physical space. What size room? What types of equipment? What degree of realism is appropriate for each type of experiential learning? Best practices are evolving toward larger, multipurpose skills and tasks labs that combine bedside or partial task training with traditional classroom furniture and toward flexible immersive labs with mobile equipment.

Skills and Tasks Lab

Skills and tasks labs are multipurpose classrooms for active and experiential learning. Labs include rooms that provide combinations of bedside and task training (see Table 16.1). Low fidelity mannequins in hospital beds and flex-use classroom furniture allow didactic, active, and experiential learning to occur in a single session.

Skills and tasks labs may incorporate AV live feed, record, replay, and data capture typical of an immersive simulation room at one or more bed positions for increased flexibility in instruction. Monitors can be located at each bed position to show live video from a primary teaching station or to present patient case information for a particular lesson (see Figure 16.3).

Bedside skills and tasks labs should have a maximum of two learners per bed per session. This ensures more time on task for each learner and a higher quality engagement with the lesson objective. A mock team communication station with handwashing sink, as well as mobile storage carts, should be provided to support the curriculum delivery.

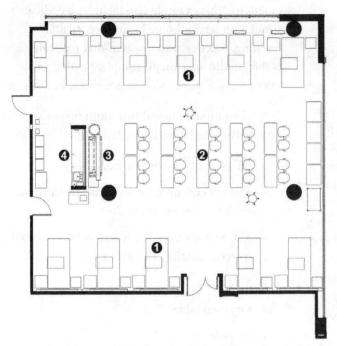

1   BEDSIDE POSITIONS
2   CLASSROOM SEATING
3   TEACHING STATION
4   NURSE STATION / STORAGE

FIGURE 16.2   Plan for a bedside skills and tasks lab. In this example, mobile classroom furniture provides flexibility to combine different learning modes in one session.
Courtesy of CannonDesign.

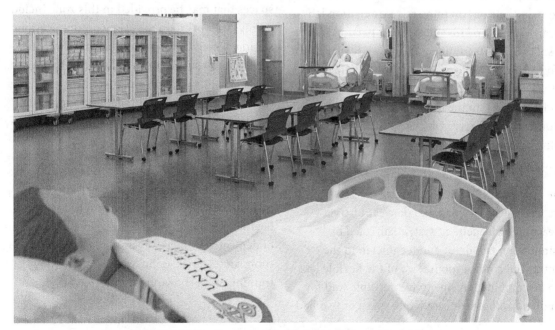

FIGURE 16.3   Example of a bedside skills and task lab.
Image courtesy of GSBS Architects.

Immersive Simulation Labs

Immersive simulation labs support IPCMS learning through realistic, crafted, and facilitated scenarios. Labs replicate various acute care settings, as well as prehospital environments as varied as home healthcare and battlefield triage. Rooms may be dedicated to a single use, such as an operating room, or they may be flexible to support a broad range of experiences. In such "patient flex" rooms, mobile furniture and storage carts are employed to support rapid change among different room types, such as critical care, emergency, obstetrics, and NICU, among others. The physical space includes a patient headwall and a handwashing sink but is otherwise generic. Equipment and furniture are brought in and out of the room as needed to create the scenario.

The floor plan in Figure 16.4 is an example of a "virtual hospital" in a nursing school with six flexible immersive simulation labs and three debriefing conference rooms. Using one debriefing room and one or two immersive simulation labs, a learner group of 10 will alternate participation in six to eight 10-minute patient care scenarios in a four-hour time block. When not participating actively in the exercise in the simulation lab, students return to the debriefing conference room to observe their peers via live AV feed. A session culminates with a post-scenario debriefing to reflect on and evaluate performance.

The pedagogical model is supported by AV live feed, record, replay, and data capture via a learning management system, directed by a simulation facilitator and technician in the centralized control room. Two of the flexible labs can be combined by opening a movable wall for simulations that require a larger space or two bed positions. This example also includes a dedicated simulation lab for home health experiential learning, practice, and research that replicates a 600 ft^2 studio apartment, complete with a small kitchen and a standard, non-accessible bathroom.

Typical equipment found in a multipurpose immersive simulation lab includes:

- 36" W × 80" L hospital bed
- Privacy curtain with 30" clearance around the bed or at the room door
- 8' L wall-mounted headwall with simulated oxygen, medical air, and vacuum
- Side chair
- Overbed table
- IV pole
- 2' W × 4' L × 5' H mobile storage cabinet

Based on program needs, additional simulation spaces that may be provided in this zone include a provider workroom or team communication station, a medication room with handwashing sink, a scrub sink alcove, and a mock bathroom. Informal collaboration and meeting space adjacent to immersive simulation rooms may be provided to support small group learning, as shown in Figure 16.5.

Dedicated immersive simulation labs are appropriate when supported by the curriculum and enrollment levels. In addition to the home health apartment described previously, examples of dedicated immersive labs include an operating room and a mock ambulance for fire/EMS training, both shown in Figure 16.6.

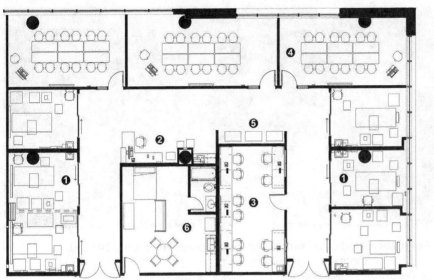

1   IMMERSIVE SIMULATION LABS
2   TEAM COMMUNICATION STATION
3   CONTROL ROOM
4   DEBRIEF CONFERENCE ROOM
5   CASE CART STORAGE
6   HOME HEALTH APARTMENT

FIGURE 16.4   Example of a virtual hospital floor plan in a nursing school.
Image courtesy of CannonDesign.

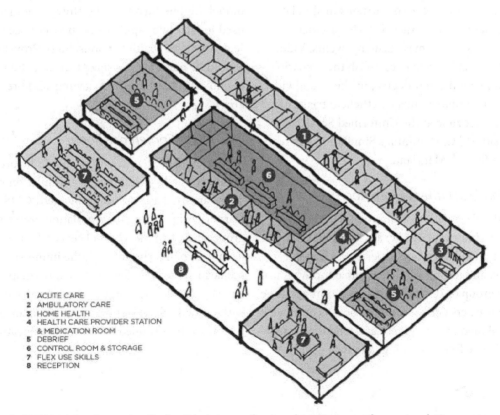

1   ACUTE CARE
2   AMBULATORY CARE
3   HOME HEALTH
4   HEALTH CARE PROVIDER STATION
    & MEDICATION ROOM
5   DEBRIEF
6   CONTROL ROOM & STORAGE
7   FLEX USE SKILLS
8   RECEPTION

FIGURE 16.5   Example of a flexible interprofessional continuum of care simulation center.
Image courtesy of Performance Gap Solutions.

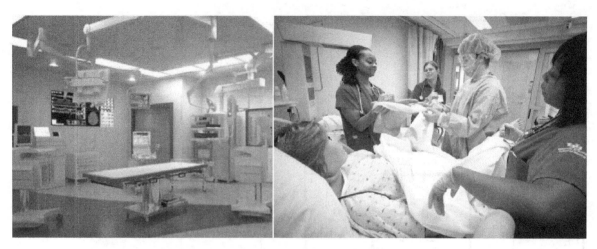

FIGURE 16.6   Examples of dedicated simulation rooms: operating room (left) and mother-baby delivery room.

Images courtesy of CannonDesign and Performance Gap Solution.

Immersive simulation labs may replicate non-hospital spaces, using flexible, multipurpose labs that employ screens or curtains to simulate diverse environments such as traffic accidents, natural disasters, or mass casualty events. Video projection can be used to establish the scenario. An example is the 360-degree, in-the-round video projection used to simulate battlefield triage in an active war zone at the Uniformed Services University Val G. Hemmings Simulation Center in Silver Spring, Maryland.

Standardized Patient Exam Room

A standardized patient exam room (see Figure 16.7) replicates a medical exam room and is used for ambulatory care experiential learning, practice, and testing with a patient actor. A typical learner group of 10 uses five exam rooms at a time (at two learners per room). The room is outfitted with real medical equipment and a handwashing sink. AV live feed, recording, and data capture via the learning management system should be provided in each room to support the pedagogical model. Mobile furniture and storage cabinets are used to facilitate rapid change between scenarios (e.g., women's health to counseling). Provisions should be made for the standardized patients, including access, dressing, staging, and break areas.

Debriefing Conference Room

A debriefing conference room should be provided for every one to two immersive simulation rooms. These are used as classrooms by the IPCMS learner group during the simulation exercises. A group of six to 12 learners observes their peers, usually in pairs, run through the immersive scenario via live AV feed and then participates in a post-scenario experience debriefing discussion with guided self-reflection and performance review led by a trained facilitator or educator.

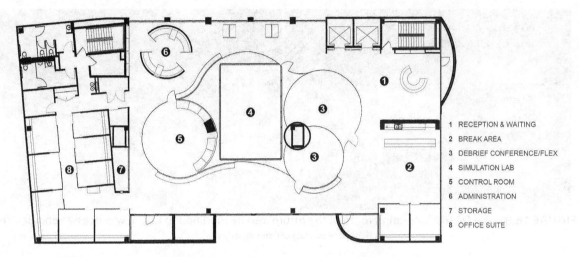

1 RECEPTION & WAITING
2 BREAK AREA
3 DEBRIEF CONFERENCE/FLEX
4 SIMULATION LAB
5 CONTROL ROOM
6 ADMINISTRATION
7 STORAGE
8 OFFICE SUITE

FIGURE 16.7   Example of simulation center designed to flex for specialty experiences.
Image courtesy of CannonDesign.

Debriefing conference rooms require specialized AV systems linked to the simulation control rooms. Remote control of the system should be possible from anywhere in the room. Rooms must have sufficient acoustic privacy to maintain confidentiality. Mobile classroom furniture (flip-top tables, chairs with casters) supports multiple seating configurations, including the ability to sit in a semicircle with a direct view of the simulation monitor. Debriefing rooms are also used for the learning, practice, and testing of small group counseling, patient care conferences, and telehealth.

Control Room

Each immersive simulation lab or cluster of standardized patient rooms requires a dedicated station (see Figure 16.8) for control of communications, the AV system (recording, live feed, playback, and data collection), and the learning management system. Stations may be grouped in one large, central room or distributed at each simulation lab. Each three-seat control position includes one IPCMS technician, one IPCMS facilitator, and one educator content

expert, as needed, to support one learner group at a time. Typical equipment includes AV and learning management system computers, three LCD monitors, a communications microphone, and a telephone.

Storage/Equipment Room

Storage for supplies and equipment is critical to the efficient operation of the simulation center. As a general rule, the storage area should be 35–50% of the area dedicated to immersive simulation. Most centers use part of this space as a work area for equipment repair and maintenance. Bed and stretcher storage is also required. Storage spaces must accommodate various sizes of supplies and equipment from single-use disposables and partial task trainers to adult-sized, computerized mannequins. Both fixed shelving and mobile carts are necessary to support the flexible use of simulation rooms. Mobile carts should be stocked and stored in the storage area and then moved to the simulation room for scenario preparation and staging. This process is similar to the use of "case carts" to prepare the operating room, including the use of preference sheets.

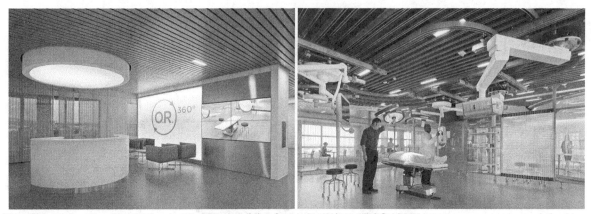

FIGURE 16.8 The OR360 "operating room of the future" can be modified to test new processes and devices.
Image courtesy of CannonDesign.

Innovation Spaces and Trends

Many organizations across the US have created unique, forward-looking simulation spaces for specialty projects and prototype design activities. One example of such a collaborative innovation space is the OR360 simulation lab at Cedars-Sinai Medical Center in Los Angeles (see Figures 16.9 and 16.10). In a partnership with the US Department of Defense, this center focuses on improving outcomes in trauma patients, especially during the critical first hour after a patient is admitted. The center provides a single operating room that's completely flexible with movable walls and a modular ceiling grid. Providers and staff can alter the size of the room and reposition equipment to enact, test, and refine care processes. Workflow is optimized though the use of color-coded trauma bays, collaboration space, and the use of whiteboards to display key patient information.

Among trends in simulation technology, virtual reality and augmented reality are likely to change the status quo in the next decade. It is anticipated that virtual reality will have the greatest increase in adoption (Workman, 2018). Examples include new lesson content conveyed through the use of holograms and 3D visualizations of simulated environments at the iEXCEL Labs at the University of Nebraska. Case Western University has also developed anatomy content for the "mixed reality" HoloLens platform that allows for interaction with instructors and peers while viewing detailed 3D imagery superimposed on the physical environment.

Conceptual Design

After the requirements of the project and the space program are established in the pre-design phase, the building design phases commence. During these phases, the architect gives shape to the institution's vision through drawings and project specifications. Architectural design is traditionally broken into four linear phases:

1. Schematic design

2. Design development

3. Construction documents

4. Construction administration

The level of detail increases with each phase. Stakeholders provide input through design development in multiple rounds of user meetings to ensure that the design stays true to the vision established for the project.

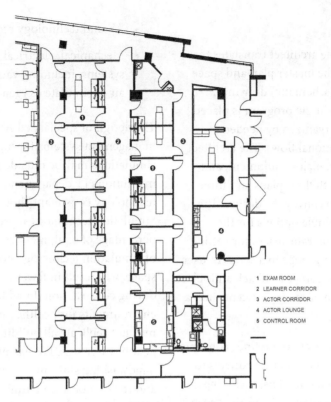

FIGURE 16.9   Example of a plan showing standardized-patient lab realism enhancement with separate hallways and room access for learners and patient actors.
Image courtesy of CannonDesign.

1   EXAM ROOM
2   LEARNER CORRIDOR
3   ACTOR CORRIDOR
4   ACTOR LOUNGE
5   CONTROL ROOM

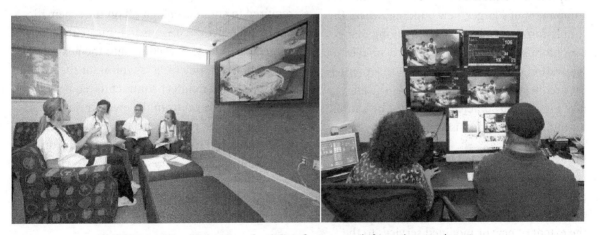

FIGURE 16.10   Examples of a debriefing room (left) and control station.
Images courtesy of GSBS Architects.

Schematic Design

In this initial phase, the architect translates the vision articulated by the master plan and space program into simple (schematic) drawings. Each space developed in the program is placed in the building area, organized by needed adjacencies and operational flows. The architect will show walls, doors, major equipment, and simple cabinetry in both floor plans and three-dimensional images to convey the design. The team may develop multiple options for the configuration of the program spaces for vetting by the stakeholder user groups in a series of user meetings conducted to gather feedback and select a preferred spatial plan or merge concepts into a new plan option.

The architect tests, analyzes, and refines concepts to arrive at an optimal solution that adheres to the established project parameters, including the functionality of the spaces, the project costs (construction, equipment, consultant fees, etc.), and the desired project schedule. Scale affects complexity. A simulation center project that is a component of a larger, new building, where the simulation stakeholders are one among many user groups, is more complex than a smaller renovation of an existing building. In either case, the architect's process is similar, but the effort may take longer, and sufficient time must be allowed for multiple rounds of user meetings.

In the schematic design phase, the architect's consultants for electrical, mechanical/HVAC, plumbing, fire protection, and technology will develop narratives and diagrams to describe the extent of new or modified services to the simulation center. Users will need to provide information required to design these systems, including:

- An equipment list with utility requirements

- AV and technology requirements

- Mechanical, electrical, and plumbing systems, including vacuum and compressed air to simulate oxygen and medical air

The design of specialized AV and learning management systems for high-technology simulations may be outside the scope of the institution's IT department, so a simulation technology consultant should be considered. Simulation technology represents a high percentage of equipment cost. Early incorporation of simulation technology needs, including space, will result in fewer costly changes during construction. In addition, simulation environments for healthcare education may or may not replicate all building services of actual healthcare spaces. For example, functional handwashing sinks may or may not be provided, and the cost of adding functional sinks and other utilities must be evaluated in the context of pedagogical goals for each simulation modality.

At the end of this phase, users are typically required to endorse or sign off on the schematic plans and other documents to indicate their agreement before proceeding into the next phase of design development. It is typical for the owner (organization)/architect contract to require an explicit approval from the owner prior to starting the next phase of design work to ensure agreement on the direction. This set of documents is typically given to cost estimators to verify that the project is on budget.

Design Development

The beginning of the design development phase is a logical extension of the schematic design. In this phase, the architect will develop the design from the approved schematic design to reach a level of completeness that demonstrates the project can be built. The schematic design is overlaid with more detailed information obtained from consultants and team members. The goal of the design development phase is to finalize the design of the rooms and spaces, building materials, and building systems. The design team works out detailed coordination issues while enhancing the project so that major revisions are not needed during construction documentation or, worse, during construction. At this point, the architect will prepare scaled floor plans and elevations for user review and approval.

Three-dimensional drawings or immersive virtual reality walk-throughs of simulation spaces are recommended to give the users a direct spatial understanding of the proposed design (see Figure 16.11). Most users have a difficult time deciphering two-dimensional architectural drawings and visualizing three-dimensional space. Today, the majority of architects use building information modeling software and develop a three-dimensional virtual model of the building that can be inhabited using a virtual reality platform, such as HoloLens. This gives users the visual experience of the space to understand size and spatial relationships with an uncanny sense of veracity. Virtual models can vary from crude gray spaces with block-like elements to highly detailed models with accurate colors and materials. Such detailed computer models are usually an additional design service, not part of an architect's basic services, because they are labor-intensive and time-consuming to produce. However, they may benefit an institution in its marketing and fundraising, and in the context of a large project with a significant capital campaign, it may be a reasonable investment as a marketing tool.

At this point, the design development documents are not yet detailed enough for construction, but they provide sufficient detail to describe construction phasing, integration of simulation technology, communication systems, security, and interior design character and quality for the project. This level of design is typically sufficient for a building contractor to estimate the cost of construction with a high degree of certainty.

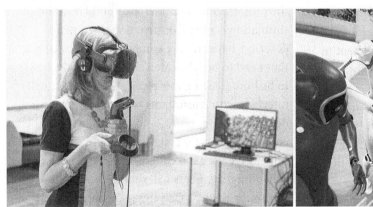
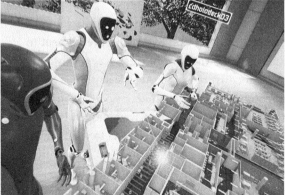

FIGURE 16.11 Architects can provide virtual reality technology that allows users to view, navigate through, and experience the proposed design (in avatar form) prior to finalization of the design.
Image courtesy of CannonDesign.

The deliverables for this phase include product and systems specifications as well as architectural and systems drawings of all building components. These include floor plans with final room locations, doors, and windows; door hardware; room finishes; identification of fixed and movable equipment; and reflected ceiling plans showing lighting fixtures, fire sprinklers, and other devices.

Time spent reviewing and contemplating the design now, during the earlier stages of the process, will save time and potentially expensive changes later. As a note of caution, significant changes made after approval of the design development documents, during the construction drawing phase, may warrant additional fees. Once construction has begun, changes made to the design, especially those involving structural components of the building, can be quite costly; users are encouraged to voice their concerns during this phase of the design process. Stakeholder users are asked again at the end of the design development phase to approve or sign off on these more detailed design documents. User input typically ends with the end of design development.

The project cost estimate and schedule should be updated at the end of design development to manage the owner's resources successfully and prevent costly redesign. At this stage, it is not uncommon for the contractor's cost estimate to exceed the owner's approved budget. In this case, the architect and/or contractor will initiate a process of value engineering (VE) to identify strategies to reduce the cost of the project without reducing quality to an unacceptable level. The VE process allows the owner, architect, or contractor to propose cost reductions that are evaluated relative to the project's vision and guiding principles. Construction costs may be lowered by reducing the area of construction after

revisiting the assumptions of the space program and identifying new ways to serve the same number of learners in a smaller area. This may be achieved by increasing class sizes or extending class hours, although not without an operational cost to the simulation program. Additional opportunities to reduce cost may come from reducing quality of building systems, deferring infrastructure improvements, or eliminating excess capacity for anticipated growth. These are often difficult choices to evaluate, prioritize, and make. The owner may accept some or all of the VE proposals or may halt the design process until the project scope and budget can be reconciled. Where possible, the owner should consider the life-cycle cost of capital investments so that less-costly selections do not wind up costing more in the long run.

Construction Documents

Continuing the design process, the architect prepares drawings and specifications suitable for permit submittal and construction that are referred to as *construction documents*. These drawings are an instrument of communicating the project to the contractor or builder of the simulation center. Construction documents describe, in detail, the components of the project that need to be fabricated and assembled for it to be built. During this phase, the architect will interface with consultants (engineering, interior design, lighting, HVAC, etc.) to ensure a complete coordinated set for construction and will typically not engage user stakeholders. The architect and consulting engineers will submit progress review sets to the owner's facilities team and conduct page-turning sessions with the owner prior to submission of the project for permitting by the local municipality or other authority having jurisdiction.

Construction Administration

In the construction administration phase, as the contractor is physically building the simulation center, the architect supports the owner and contractor by observing construction and notifying both parties of non-compliance where items are not constructed in accordance with the construction documents. The architect reviews the contractor's submittal of product and system information and sub-contractor fabrication drawings, again to affirm or deny that they comply with project requirements. Changes to the design at this stage can be costly to the owner, both in dollars and time lost, so they should be minimized.

It is now time for move-in. Users may be involved in preparing for the move by tagging existing equipment and supplies to be relocated. Once in the new center, users should allow ample time to test equipment and systems and to operationalize new work processes. This may require several weeks, prior to the first official day of operations.

Post-occupancy Evaluation

A post-occupancy evaluation is an examination of the performance of the project after it has been built and occupied. The post-occupancy evaluation answers questions about whether the design goals were met and whether the project satisfies the needs of the users. The design team will evaluate success metrics and make recommendations for changes or remediation if these goals were not satisfied. It is recommended that this process take place 12–18 months after move-in. It typically involves a series of interviews and surveys. Learning from these experiences can impact future design, coordination, and detailing of future simulation projects.

Conclusion

The demand for healthcare providers is growing. To meet this need, we must educate and train highly competent providers using new techniques and processes to achieve effective outcomes at lower costs. Academic and hospital-based simulation centers are used to develop high-performance teams, enhance professionalism, and provide learning experiences to improve communication and coordination skills. Simulation centers in the future will embrace new technologies and evolving research on learning to support these goals (International Nursing Association for Clinical Simulation and Learning Standards Committee, 2016).

Hospitals are creating multiuse simulation rooms near the point of service to support just-in-time simulation to improve patient safety. These centers focus increasingly on interprofessional education to improve the whole team. At most universities, skills and tasks labs and immersive simulation will continue to be the norm for some time. Schools and hospitals should be prepared for new and innovative technologies. Experiential learning in virtual and augmented reality environments is likely to alter the educational and clinical landscape in ways we have yet to predict.

In designing simulation centers, we highlighted several points made in this chapter:

- Development of a shared vision at outset of project
- Evidence-based space programming based on curriculum goals
- Clear decision-making authority
- Expanded stakeholder outreach and inclusion

- Early inclusion of technology experts

- Flexibility of design for future unknown needs

The design process is a creative problem-solving endeavor that transforms ideas and visions into the three-dimensional reality of your simulation center. This chapter was designed to help you better understand what one can expect during the design process. Open communication and collaboration between you and your design team will help ensure a successful project.

References

Association of American Medical Colleges. (2011). *Medical simulation in medical education: Results of an AAMC survey.* Washington, DC: Author. Retrieved from https://www.aamc.org/download/259760/data/medicalsimulationinmedicaleducationanaamcsurvey.pdf

Hayden, J. K., Smiley, R. A., Alexander, M., Kardong-Edgren, S., & Jeffries, P. R. (2014). The NCSBN national simulation study: A longitudinal, randomized, controlled study replacing clinical hours with simulation in prelicensure nursing education. *Journal of Nursing Regulation.* Retrieved from https://www.ncsbn.org/JNR_Simulation_Supplement.pdf

International Nursing Association for Clinical Simulation and Learning Standards Committee. (2016). INACSL standards of best practice: Simulation – Simulation design. *Clinical Simulation in Nursing, 12*(S), S5–S12. http://dx.doi.org/10.1016/j.ecns.2016.09.005

Society for Simulation in Healthcare. (2019). *SSH accreditation self-study guide: Accreditation standards and measurement criteria.* Wheaton, IL: Author. Retrieved from https://www.ssih.org/Credentialing/Accreditation

Wolters Kluwer & National League for Nursing. (2016a). *How nursing education programs are currently using educational technology.* Retrieved from: http://www.nln.org/images/default-source/wolters-kluwer-infographics-2017/wk-infographic1nursingedtech_first-01-(1)-(002).gif?Status=Temp&sfvrsn=2

Wolters Kluwer & National League for Nursing. (2016b). *The what and why of technology use by today's nursing students.* Retrieved from http://nursingeducation.lww.com/content/dam/wk-nes/documents/Student-Technology-Infographic.pdf

Workman, S. (2018, July 30). Mixed reality: A revolutionary breakthrough in teaching and learning. EduCauseReview. Retrieved from https://er.educause.edu/articles/2018/7/mixed-reality-a-revolutionary-breakthrough-in-teaching-and-learning

"The future belongs to those who believe in the beauty of their dreams."

–Eleanor Roosevelt

The Future of Simulation in Healthcare

17

Pamela R. Jeffries, PhD, RN, FAAN, ANEF, FSSH
Eric B. Bauman, PhD, RN, FSSH
Crystel L. Farina, MSN, RN, CNE, CHSE
Pamela W. Slaven-Lee, DNP, RN, FNP-BC, CHSE

The future is bright for simulation, providing numerous possibilities to enhance clinical education for healthcare providers, improve patient safety, and create safer, more efficient systems of care through process improvement and risk management. Simulation is being used today to teach clinical judgment, problem solving, and decision-making skills. In academic settings, clinical simulations are increasingly substituting for actual clinical hours and creating the opportunity for all learners to experience a set of standardized clinical scenarios that prepare them for complex clinical situations. Educators, leaders, and researchers are identifying best practices when designing and implementing simulations and developing the research that will provide the evidence of value in the future. The technical advances and health policy decisions that are emerging today will help dictate the future of simulation in healthcare.

This chapter discusses how simulation, simulation-based education, and gaming will be used in future courses and curricula; the programmatic changes that may occur within the health professions as simulation-based education continues to escalate; the emerging technologies and how these will be integrated within the simulation environment; the issues, challenges, and new opportunities, such as required certification and accreditation of simulation centers, that are evolving around clinical simulations; and the integration of simulation as a process improvement methodology.

OBJECTIVES

- Describe the issues, challenges, and new opportunities that are evolving around the use of simulation in healthcare.

- Discuss programmatic changes that may occur in health professions education as the use of simulation pedagogy escalates.

- Explore how the emerging technologies will be integrated and used in the clinical simulation experiences.

The Use of Simulation, Simulation-Based Education, and Gaming in the Future

While simulation in health professions education is now considered a standard and best practice within the healthcare education paradigm, the technology and variety of simulation offerings continue to expand at a rapid pace. High-fidelity simulators have become synonymous with simulated clinical learning. In recent years, there has been a barrage of sophisticated, multimedia, and virtual educational platforms that allow students to participate in a simulation outside of the traditional education setting. A national study of nursing schools in the US conducted by the National League for Nursing (NLN) and Wolters Kluwer (2016) found that from 2016–2021, virtual reality is expected to have the greatest increase in adoption as a type of simulation. This proliferation of new virtual reality/virtual simulation options is creating its own challenges. For example, given the myriad definitions being used for virtual reality, there is a need for the development of precise definitions of virtual reality and for the adoption of a standardized classification of the levels of virtual reality (Cant, Cooper, Sussex, & Bogassian, 2019; Kardong-Edgren, Farra, Alinier, & Young, 2019).

In screen-based simulation platforms, the learner uses a mouse and keyboard to interact with a computer. These are typically interactive clinical cases in which the user can navigate and make decisions where prompted. The simulation may represent patients, healthcare departments, systems, or other healthcare encounters. Screen-based simulation experiences are changing, providing learners with the opportunity to have a presence within the simulation.

Gaming and virtual-reality platforms are teaching and evaluating clinical skills and decision-making. As this technology expands and improves, faculty struggle to stay current and adapt these innovations into curricula (Bauman, 2016).

Today's learners are not only technologically savvy but also accustomed to learning—often exclusively—through technologies that require learners to try multiple strategies to reach their goals by quickly searching and manipulating the virtual environment throughout the process (Chicca & Shellenbarger, 2018; Ugidos Lozano, Blaya Haro, Ruggiero, Manzoor, & Juanes Mendez, 2019). New gaming platforms are developing quickly that require learners to immerse themselves in the virtual environment. As the technology changes, the terminology changes with it. The rapid increase of digital offerings on the market has created a change in terminology and a recognition that not all digital platforms are the same. *Screen-based simulations* (interactions between learner and computer that require the learner to interact with the mouse and keyboard) are very different from *virtual reality*, interactions in which learners see objects that have a spatial presence (Bauman, 2016; Cant et al., 2019). Learners, wearing an immersive or mixed (immersive and/or augmented) reality headset, experience simulations as if they were present, even when viewing the simulation remotely (Bauman, 2016; Cant et al., 2019; Dang, Palicte, Valdez, & O'Leary-Kelley, 2018).

Gaming is an active learning strategy that requires the learner to use skills and knowledge to reach a specific goal (Gentry et al., 2019; Peddle, 2011). Providing an authentic clinical environment in which either individuals or a group of learners can experiment without risk to the patient is the goal of gaming. When used in the education of health professionals, gaming can help to reinforce knowledge and skills. Kopp and Hanson (2012) used gaming to effectively teach baccalaureate nursing students how to provide end-of-life care. Andersen et al. (2018) found that learners need to have a humanized experience beyond what mannequins and simulators are able to deliver. Virtual reality technology has the ability to provide that human interaction. Learners, wearing virtual reality headsets, can have a virtual presence in the simulation and interact with avatars as if they were having a face-to-face interaction. Motivation and enjoyment may depend on individual learner styles, so not every learner responds to this learning strategy (Blakely, Skirton, Cooper, Allum, & Nelmes, 2008).

Games and applications, particularly those that can be accessed, engaged, or played on mobile devices, offer an interesting paradigm shift in the way a participant or learner can access information. Massive Open Online Courses (MOOCs) are providing access to academic content to millions of people who until just a few years ago had little or no access to college-level or professional training. Very prestigious academic institutions are engaging educational technology like MOOCs as a way to provide a distributed educational experience that transcends the challenges of time, place, and socioeconomic status. Virtual reality simulation software developers are in the process of developing synchronous live multiplayer and distance programs that allow students access and the ability to connect virtually in the same simulation with multiple other learners. Games and simulations are not the only technology available. Learners are accustomed to mobile applications that provide quick and efficient access to references, information, games, and procedures that are efficient tools for all healthcare professionals and are an expectation of society.

Game type formats are evolving to include haptic devices that provide sensory feedback. Butt, Kardong-Edgren, and Ellertson (2018) used virtual reality with haptic devices to enhance skill acquisition. The researchers found that the learners using the virtual reality and haptic devices recalled specific events in the simulation more readily than students who learned skills with a simulator. The learners in the study rated the virtual reality system favorably and were able to demonstrate skill level at two weeks post virtual reality exercise the same as those who practiced with a simulator or task trainer (Butt et al., 2018).

Virtual worlds used in simulation are unique environments constructed so that learners can accomplish specific learning objectives. They allow for interaction and feedback among avatars in the environment so that the learner may modify or change behaviors to adapt to the specific demands of the clinical scenario (Hansen, 2008; Saxena et al., 2018). Because virtual reality platforms are accessible online, they are available around the clock and provide a means for learners to interact without being physically present. This is particularly useful when dealing with distance education (Bauman, 2010) and provides an opportunity for learners to complete virtual simulations on their own time schedule.

Augmented reality—the use of a digital image or artifact superimposed into the actual environment, in some cases onto a physical simulator visible through special lenses or a mobile device—provides the ability to add variables like anatomy and physiology to the simulation experience. Development of the Microsoft HoloLens provides a mixture of augmented and virtual reality environments for enhanced learning.

There are certainly drawbacks to using these new simulation formats. Serious gaming, virtual, and augmented reality simulations require quite a bit of time, as well as financial and technological resources, to create the desired environment (Hansen, 2008). Ultimately, the desire for higher degrees of sophistication and realism will affect the costs to create simulations in the future; however, as the technology evolves, the cost is decreasing as the realism increases.

Virtual simulations have been used in healthcare for skills training, knowledge acquisition, and clinical decision-making (Foronda, Godsall, & Trybulski, 2013). In a prospective cohort study, Burden et al. (2012) used an ultrasound virtual reality simulator to measure competency in obstetrical ultrasonography between trainees and experts. Although the trainees had significantly more deviation from the target measurements on the initial assessment and took significantly longer to conduct the ultrasonography than the expert cohort, there were no significant differences between the trainees and the experts in target ultrasonography measurements after the third repetition (Burden et al., 2012). Virtual reality has also been shown to enhance education and safety training for home healthcare professionals. Darragh et al. (2016) used virtual reality to increase the awareness and safety training of home healthcare professionals. The study was used to develop a virtual reality event that would assist learners to become situationally aware to hazards in the home care setting. Research is ongoing to determine if the program increases situational awareness. LeFlore et al. (2012) used a virtual pediatric hospital unit with virtual patients to determine if this environment was effective in teaching pediatric content. In this study, baccalaureate nursing students who were randomized to receive an experience with a virtual patient trainer had significantly higher knowledge acquisition and better knowledge application compared to those students who received a traditional lecture (LeFlore et al., 2012). Virtual patients have also been used to measure clinical decision-making. Wendling et al. (2011) found that junior anesthesiology residents were more likely to suspect obstructive sleep apnea after interviewing a virtual patient when compared with those residents who interviewed a standardized patient. One can reasonably expect, therefore, to see more virtual patients being used in the future.

Virtual reality has been found to be effective in skill and knowledge acquisition and the retention of knowledge. Associate degree nursing students who received virtually simulated disaster experience in addition to a web-based module were significantly more likely to retain the knowledge two months after the training when compared with those students who only received the web-based module (Farra, Miller, Timms, & Schafer, 2013).

As alternative simulation applications emerge, faculty face challenges of how to incorporate the technology into the curriculum, how to debrief these learning applications, and how to provide student evaluation. Many of the virtual software programs provide data analytics for faculty to determine time in the immersion, decision-making (correct and incorrect actions), and tracking of progression. Verkuyl et al. (2018) explored debriefing of virtual gaming simulations by comparing self-debriefing, virtual debriefing, and in-person debriefing outcomes. Those findings indicate that all three types of debriefing methods for virtual simulations provide positive experiences to learners; however, in this research, virtual and in-person debriefing provided better outcomes. Furthermore, faculty face the need to develop goals of curriculum integration, implementation, and standards of best practice for innovative technology.

Further research is needed to compare the effectiveness of these simulation methods to more traditional methods, determine whether these methods are cost-effective for educating healthcare personnel, and, most importantly, determine whether there is ultimate improvement in patient safety and outcomes because of this simulation (Agency for Healthcare Research and Quality, 2013). Additional research efforts need to determine the most cost-effective methods of creating and delivering education using gaming and virtual reality platforms. Gaming and other virtual reality platforms will surely be powerful tools for healthcare education in the future.

Potential Curriculum and Programmatic Changes

The evolving landscape of healthcare, emphasis on patient safety, and demand for quality clinical education calls for alternative and effective ways to prepare learners. Rapid advances in technology and accessibility have made simulation-based learning an integral part of nursing education.

As programs integrate simulation into the curriculum, it is essential that educators consider best practices for curricular integration and design as well as the International Nursing Association for Clinical Simulation in Nursing (INACSL) Standards of Best Practice in Simulation (INACSL, 2016). As with the adoption of any teaching modality, simulation must be clearly aligned with learning outcomes and requires thoughtful strategic planning, evaluation, assessment, and curricular mapping (Tagliareni & Forneris, 2016).

Robust evidence in support of student learning outcomes has proven to be a driving force in the widespread acceptance of simulation-based learning in nursing education. The National Council of State Boards of Nursing (NCSBN)

National Simulation Study demonstrated that high-quality simulation experiences are a feasible and effective way to reduce the number of traditional clinical hours for pre-licensure nursing students without negatively affecting learning outcomes. The landmark, large-scale, multisite, randomized controlled study demonstrated that up to 50% of clinical hours could be substituted with simulation hours without a statistically significant difference in outcomes measuring knowledge, clinical competency, and NCLEX pass rates. In addition, in a six-month follow-up, there was no difference in clinical competency and practice readiness between study participants that had substituted simulation hours for clinical hours and those who had not. These findings have resulted in regulatory changes permitting the substitution of simulation hours for clinical hours in pre-licensure nursing programs in several states (Hayden, Smiley, Alexander, Kardong-Edgren, & Jeffries, 2014; NCSBN, 2014).

Although significant headway has been made in demonstrating learning outcomes in the pre-licensure nursing programs, evidence to support learning outcomes in graduate nursing education is lacking (Rutherford-Hemming, Nye, & Coran, 2016). Due to this lack of evidence, the National Task Force (NTF) on Quality Nurse Practitioner (NP) Education currently maintains that simulation hours may not substitute the 500 required direct patient care hours required in NP education (NTF on Quality NP Education, 2016). However, as most NP programs require more than the minimum 500 direct patient care hours, high-quality simulation-based learning may be used to augment clinical learning. A recent descriptive study of 133 advanced practice nursing programs in North America found that 98% have currently integrated simulation into the curriculum, using a variety of methodologies (Nye, Campbell, Hebert, Short, & Thomas, 2019). Despite this widespread integration, the expansion and acceptance of simulation in graduate nursing education are dependent, in part, on strong and favorable evidence in support of learning outcomes from rigorous research and faculty development in simulation pedagogy.

With regulatory pressure to ensure healthcare providers are competent to provide care, the question remains as to whether nursing will require students to demonstrate competency by participating in high-stakes simulation testing similar to the Objective Structured Clinical Examination (OSCE). The OSCE first appeared in the 1970s and, over the next 40 years, has become the gold standard in the assessment of clinical skill in medical education. With regulatory pressure to ensure healthcare providers are competent to provide care, the question remains as to whether nursing will require students to demonstrate competency by participating in high-stakes simulation testing similar to the OSCE. A 2014 survey conducted by INASCL demonstrated that 43% of the 605 respondents were currently conducting high-stakes evaluations in nursing (Rutherford-Hemming et al., 2016), with appropriate evaluator training identified as a concern for those considering the use of simulation for this purpose. In a scoping review of literature, 204 studies, published between 1982 and 2018 in 33 countries, revealed that nursing OSCEs were extensively used across various nursing specialties. The authors confirmed validity, reliability, and acceptability of the OSCE in nursing education, noting that nursing OSCEs differ from those used in medical education, owing to the different nature of the discipline and competencies (Goh, Zhang, Lee, Wu, & Wang, 2018). Further investigation is needed into the use of simulation for summative evaluation in nursing education. Moreover, in an effort to achieve a fair testing environment, the NLN urges a thoughtful

and comprehensive review of factors contributing to the potential integration of high-stakes testing (Jeffries, 2012).

When implementing pedagogy of simulation across a program—whether in academia or in a clinical setting—developing facilitator competence and acceptance are critical to appropriate and effective implementation. The INACSL standards call for those involved in the facilitation of simulation to have the education and skill necessary to guide participants toward achieving predetermined learning outcomes. This requires dedication to faculty development in areas relevant to all INACSL standards, including (INASCL, 2016):

- Simulation design
- Outcomes and objectives
- Facilitation
- Debriefing
- Participant evaluation
- Professional integrity
- Simulation-enhanced interprofessional education

As additional evidence is gathered in support of simulation to meet learning outcomes, more faculty must be prepared to use simulation pedagogy. Careful consideration must be given as to how and why simulation is integrated into educational programs. Just as evidence in support of simulation continues to evolve, best practices in the use of this powerful pedagogy have also evolved to support optimal student learning. Growing demand for high-quality clinical education, the establishment of best practices, and a growing body of evidence in support of simulation as a valid and reliable way to achieve learning outcomes will continue to impact the use of simulation in nursing and other healthcare education.

Integrating Emerging Technologies Into Simulation Experiences

Another aspect to consider for the future of simulation includes the integration of additional technologies, such as handheld devices, within the various simulation platforms. Clinical simulations and video games, particularly those that are accessible via mobile devices (for example, tablets and smartphones), represent not only opportunities for interactive knowledge acquisition traditionally obtained through static didactic teaching modalities but also cognitive aids that can be accessed in other learning environments. In other words, the content embedded within these games and applications comes to represent more than just-in-time information. It also models the context of the content being accessed (Bauman, 2010, 2016; Bauman & Games, 2011; Games & Bauman, 2011). In this way, games and mobile applications can also be used in traditional simulation laboratories to support learning objectives, during supervised clinical encounters, and in independent practice.

Game-based and mobile application-based learning are being embraced as pedagogical modalities available for clinical education of healthcare providers as well as a mechanism for patient education. Increasingly, game-based learning is being embraced as a complementary tool available to meet specific learning objectives. Examining fit prior to deploying game-based learning helps to ensure that both educators and learners are ready for this methodology. Without a carefully planned infrastructure, the introduction, integration, and evaluation of game-based learning will leave both learners and educators frustrated (Bauman, 2012). Determining how these modalities best fit alongside other teaching and learning techniques is still to be determined and an area ripe for research.

Despite the challenges associated with reexamining the curricula and determining where new methods, such as game-based learning, can be best leveraged, organizations and educators need to meet this challenge quickly and efficiently. Today's learners are often much more comfortable with digital technology, particularly emerging technology, than their educators. Traditional students are digital natives, whereas their educators are often digital immigrants:

- The term *digital native* refers to those people who have always been part of the digital generation (Prensky, 2001). Smartphones and the internet have always been part of digital natives' day-to-day experience, and journal articles have always been available online. Digital natives have an innate sense of media literacy (Bauman, 2012; Prensky, 2001).

- The term *digital immigrants* refers to individuals who adopted digital technology later in life (Prensky, 2001). For the digital immigrant, digital literacy is a second language.

The number of digital natives in academia and hospital settings will continue to increase, as will the number of patients and healthcare consumers who are digital natives. Educators and other healthcare leaders need to adapt to create effective learning environments that will certainly involve a full array of simulation methodologies (Gilbert & Bauman, 2020).

Certification, Accreditation, and Value Recognition of Simulation

As the use of simulation becomes a best practice in academic and clinical settings in healthcare, there are ample opportunities for professional growth. There are now multiple organizations that are dedicated to advancing the use of simulation (see sidebar that follows). These organizations assist both individuals and professional groups in employing best practices in the use of simulation in healthcare, including how to develop a simulation center, create a simulation scenario, or select valid and reliable tools for evaluation. Many of these organizations publish journals and offer annual conferences to help simulation novices and experts network, collaborate, and disseminate their experiences in simulation.

Certification and Accreditation

As a means for improving patient safety, simulation technology, educational methods, and practitioner assessment, the Society for Simulation in Healthcare (SSH) has launched two programs to set standards and recognize expertise in simulation. Additional information on these programs is provided in Chapter 15.

One program was established to certify individuals with expertise in simulation education in healthcare. A detailed overview of the process is available online in the SSH Certified Healthcare Simulation Educator Handbook (SSH, 2019).

SSH also has developed another program that is designed to provide accreditation for programs dedicated to using simulation technologies and methodologies to improve patient safety and outcomes (SSH, 2013). This accreditation has been designed for simulation programs that use any of the various modalities (mannequins, standardized patients, virtual reality), teach to any type of learner, and are located anywhere in the world. SSH currently offers two types of program accreditation: full accreditation and provisional accreditation.

- *Full accreditation* means that a healthcare simulation program has met core operational standards as well as specific criteria in at least one of four areas: assessment, research, teaching/education, and systems integration. Full accreditation applications will also be required to participate in an onsite survey. Full accreditation is granted for a five-year period with required submission of an annual program report.

Examples of Simulation Organizations

- **Association of Standardized Patient Educators:** http://www.aspeducators.org/
- **International Nursing Association for Clinical Simulation and Learning:** https://inacsl.org/
- **National Center for Simulation:** http://www.simulationinformation.com/
- **NLN Simulation Innovation Resource Center:** http://sirc.nln.org/
- **Society for Simulation in Healthcare:** http://ssih.org

- *Provisional accreditation* allows programs with established structure and processes that have not yet achieved outcomes to apply for provisional accreditation. Interested simulation programs submit a self-study application demonstrating compliance with the standards. Provisional accreditation is granted for a two-year period with required submission of an annual program report.

To date, 138 healthcare simulation programs in 15 countries have been accredited by SSH, making it the largest accrediting body in the field.

Educators who are enthusiastic about the use of simulation technology in their courses and curriculum should consider the best method for their professional growth in the pedagogy of simulation. Initial steps may be to join a simulation organization, become immersed in the simulation literature, and participate in an annual simulation conference. Those who have developed expertise should consider becoming certified. Educators who practice in settings that have actualized their mission to improve patient outcomes and safety through the use of simulation technology should consider seeking program accreditation.

In the future, will certification be required for educators who are engaged in healthcare-related simulations? Will simulation programs be required to be accredited? With an emphasis on documenting competency, this could be a next step in the integration of simulation into the healthcare industry.

Value

The value of simulation, especially as it relates to improving quality and patient safety, must be articulated and disseminated to stakeholders and decision-makers. Through the use of simulation pedagogy, health professionals can be part of a continuous improvement of healthcare teams within the organization. In addition, healthcare organizations can use clinical simulations to drive continuous improvement of healthcare systems and patient outcomes. In academic communities, the value of simulation as a teaching strategy must be measured and the results shared.

With the constant change in the landscape of healthcare, the question is how will simulation-based strategies be positioned as part of the solution to the economic pressures and training challenges? To be relevant in the future, those who embrace and advocate simulation in healthcare will have to ensure that the message to decision-makers is clear. Simulation saves lives and improves efficiency. If this message is not transmitted, the question becomes, "What will happen to simulation programs?" Will they be viewed as an expensive luxury or part of the value equation of affordable, safe patient care with the necessary expansion of a well-trained nursing and physician workforce? Successful simulation programs need to demonstrate that the value of simulation-based strategies is significantly greater than the cost.

The value of simulation must be communicated to stakeholders through translational and economic-based research. To survive, simulation programs may need to diversify their revenue streams as well as work with industry to decrease costs while increasing the ability to report value.

Integration of Simulation as a Process Improvement Methodology

More and more focus is being placed on improving healthcare systems, and the use of simulation for that purpose is becoming increasingly popular. In earlier chapters, in-situ simulations have been discussed as efficient and effective ways to not only improve performance but also identify opportunities for improvements in patient flow, unit design, equipment use, and the development of procedures (Gaba, 2004). Industrial approaches to system analysis and improvement such as Lean and Six Sigma are being adopted in healthcare organizations to help manage complex processes (for example, scheduling) and develop flow for time-sensitive processes (such as stroke or trauma team response; Henriksen et al., 2008). Simulation provides a unique way to assess an existing system or evaluate a proposed new one (Dunn et al., 2013). In the future, simulation-based assessment of in-place and proposed systems has the potential to become an accepted part of all performance improvement programs in healthcare.

Conclusion

Simulation continues to evolve and redefine itself. Gaba (2004) discussed the power of immersive fidelity by comparing the authenticity of future simulation laboratories to the *Star Trek* Holodeck. In the fictional Holodeck, participants are unable to distinguish the difference between a simulation occurring in a created environment (Bauman, 2007) and reality. Created environments are those spaces existing in either a real-time, fixed physical space, such as a simulation laboratory, or within a digital environment (Bauman, 2007, 2010, 2012).

As technology continues to rapidly evolve, so will simulation. Simulation-based technology is already becoming more mobile. The evolution of modern clinical simulation began with mannequin-based simulation laboratories. As simulators became increasingly more portable, educators began to leverage in-situ simulation to increase the authenticity and fidelity of the

learners' experiences. Game-based learning is the natural evolution of screen-based simulation. Early screen-based simulators were often based on decision trees that resembled active multiple-choice scenarios that evolved to some fixed endpoint based on the participants' selection of provided menu choices. Modern game-based learning environments strive to provide immersive experiences. These experiences are often based on situated and unfolding narratives in which players or learners are encouraged to explore their environments and to leave no stone unturned (Bauman, 2010; Gee, 1991, 2003). In the future, as new simulation platforms are developed, gaming and other technology-mediated technologies will increasingly be used to educate health professionals in skills and concepts as well as measure performance.

Academic and clinical expectations are rapidly evolving. Learners have a whole host of expectations about how content will be delivered and accessed and how clinical competence will be acquired and maintained. If educators fail to acknowledge these expectations, the best and brightest students and providers will simply embrace those institutions that are able to meet their expectations (Bauman, 2010). Furthermore, clinical practice is increasingly steeped in digital technology. Embracing teaching methods that include designed experiences that authentically mirror practice settings provides meaningful, situated learning experiences that prepare students for future practice (Squire, 2006).

Evolving technologies, simulators, and platforms have many implications in clinical practice. Healthcare professionals must learn to use the technology associated with contemporary patient care, from patient monitoring systems to electronic medical records. Just as higher education is revolutionizing through the use of

MOOCs, clinical practice is also transforming through the use of a variety of technologies, platforms, and types of simulations. The value of simulation will need to continue to be addressed as educators and practitioners adopt these new technologies for education, training, skill competency, and translating the outcomes of clinical simulations into clinical practice.

References

Agency for Healthcare Research and Quality. (2013). *Making health care safer II: An updated critical analysis of the evidence for patient safety practices.* Comparative Effectiveness Review No. 211. (Prepared by the Southern California-RAND Evidence-based Practice Center under Contract No. 290-2007-10062-I.) AHRQ Publication No. 13-E001-EF. Rockville, MD: Author. Retrieved from www.ahrq.gov/research/findings/evidence-based-reports/ptsafetyuptp.html

Andersen, P., Baron, S., Bassett, J., Govind, N., Hayes, C., Lapkin, S., ... Simes, T. (2018). Snapshots of simulation: Innovative strategies used by international educators to enhance simulation learning experiences for health care students. *Clinical Simulation in Nursing 16,* 8–14. doi:10.1016/j.ecns.2017.10.001

Bauman, E. B. (2007). *High fidelity simulation in healthcare* [Doctoral dissertation, The University of Wisconsin–Madison, United States]. Dissertations & Theses @ CIC Institutions database. (Publication no. AAT 3294196 ISBN: 9780549383109 ProQuest document ID: 1453230861)

Bauman, E. B. (2010). Virtual reality and game-based clinical education. In K. B. Gaberson & M. H. Oermann (Eds.), *Clinical teaching strategies in nursing education* (3rd ed., pp. 183–212). New York, NY: Springer Publishing Company.

Bauman, E. B. (2012). *Game-based teaching and simulation in nursing and healthcare.* New York, NY: Springer Publishing Company.

Bauman, E. B. (2016). Games, virtual environments, mobile applications and a futurist's crystal ball. [editorial]. *Clinical Simulation in Nursing, 12,* 109–114. doi:10.1016/j.ecns.2016.02.002

Bauman, E. B., & Games, I. A. (2011). Contemporary theory for immersive worlds: Addressing engagement, culture, and diversity. In A. Cheney & R. Sanders (Eds.), *Teaching and learning in 3D immersive worlds: Pedagogical models and constructivist approaches* (pp. 248–270). Hershey, PA: IGI Global.

Blakely, G., Skirton, H., Cooper, S., Allum, P., & Nelmes, P. (2008). Educational gaming in the health sciences: Systematic review. *Journal of Advanced Nursing, 65*(2), 259–269.

Burden, C., Preshaw, J., White, P., Draycott, T., Grant, S., & Fox, R. (2012). Validation of virtual reality simulation for obstetric ultrasonography: A prospective cross-sectional study. *Simulation in Healthcare: Journal of the Society for Simulation in Healthcare, 7*(5), 269–273.

Butt, A., L., Kardong-Edgren, S., & Ellertson, A. (2018). Using game-based virtual reality with haptics for skill acquisition. *Clinical Simulation in Nursing, 16,* 25–32. doi:https://doi.org/10.1016/j.ecns.2017.09.010

Cant, R., Cooper, S., Sussex, R., & Bogossian, F. (2019). What's in a name? Clarifying the nomenclature of virtual simulation. *Clinical Simulation in Nursing, 27,* 26–30.

Chicca, J., & Shellenbarger, T. (2018). Connecting with Generation Z: Approaches in nursing education. *Teaching and Learning in Nursing, 13*(3), 180–184. doi.org/10.1016/j.teln.2018.03.008

Dang, B., Palicte, J., Valdez, A., & O'Leary-Kelley, C., (2018). Assessing simulation, virtual reality, and television modalities in clinical training. *Clinical Simultion in Nursing, 19,* 30–37. https://doi.org/10.1016/j.ecns.2018.03.001

Darragh, A., Lavender, S., Polivka, B., Sommerich, C., Wills, C., Hittle, B. ... Stredney, D. (2016). Gaming simulation as health and safety training for home health care workers. *Clinical Simulation in Nursing, 12,* (8), 328–335

Dunn, W., Deutsch, E., Maxworthy, J., Gallo, K., Dong, Y., Manos, J., ... Brazil, V. (2013). Systems integration: Engineering the future of healthcare delivery via simulation. In A. I. Levine, S. DeMaria, A. D. Schwartz, & A. Sim (Eds.), *The comprehensive textbook of healthcare simulation.* London: Springer Publishing.

Farra, S., Miller, E., Timms, N., & Schafer, J. (2013). Improved training for disaster using 3-D virtual reality simulation. *Western Journal of Nursing Research, 35*(5), pp. 655–671.

Foronda, C., Godsall, L., & Trybulski, J. (2013). Virtual clinical simulation: The state of the science. *Clinical Simulation in Nursing, 9*(8), e279–e286. doi:10.1016/j.ecns.2012.05.005

Gaba, D. M. (2004). The future vision of simulation in health care. *Quality and Safety in Health Care, 13*(Suppl. 1), i2–i10. doi:10.1136/qshc.2004.009878

Games, A. I., & Bauman, E. B. (2011). Virtual worlds: An environment for cultural sensitivity education in the health sciences. *International Journal of Web Based Communities, 7*(2), 189–205. doi:10.1504/IJWBC.2011.039510

Gee, J. P. (1991). Memory and myth: A perspective on narrative. In A. McCabe & C. Peterson (Eds.), *Developing narrative structure* (pp. 1–26). Hillsdale, NJ: Lawrence Erlbaum Associates Inc.

Gee, J. P. (2003). *What videogames have to teach us about learning and literacy* (1st ed.). New York, NY: Palgrave Macmillan.

Gentry, S. V., Gauthier, A., L'Estrade Ehrstrom, B., Wortley, D., Lilienthal, A., Tudor Car, L., ... Car, J. (2019). Serious gaming and gamification education in health professions: Systematic review. *Journal of Medical Internet Research, 21*(3), e12994. doi:10.2196/12994

Gilbert, G., & Bauman, E. (2020). New terms for the educator's digital lexicon. EdArXiv Preprints. Retrieved from https://edarxiv.org/fdtym/

Goh, H. S., Zhang, H., Lee, C. N., Wu, X. V., & Wang, W. (2018). Value of nursing objective structured clinical examinations: A scoping review. *Nurse Educator.* doi:10.1097/NNE.0000000000000620

Hansen, M. M. (2008). Versatile, immersive, creative and dynamic virtual 3-D healthcare learning environments: A review of the literature. *Journal of Medical Internet Research, 10*(3), e26. doi:10.2196/jmir.1051

Hayden, J. K., Smiley, R. A., Alexander, M., Kardong-Edgren, S., & Jeffries, P. R. (2014). The NCSBN national simulation study: A longitudinal, randomized controlled study replacing clinical hours with simulation in prelicensure nursing education. *Journal of Nursing Regulation, 5*(2), S1–S64.

Henriksen, K., Battles, J. B., Keyes, M. A., & Grady, M. L. (Eds.). (2008). *Advances in patient safety: New directions and alternative approaches* (Vol. 3: Performance and Tools). Rockville, MD: Agency for Healthcare Research and Quality. Retrieved from http://www.ncbi.nlm.nih.gov/books/NBK43665/

International Nursing Association for Clinical Simulation and Learning Standards Committee. (2016). INACSL standards of best practice: Simulation. Participant evaluation. *Clinical Simulation in Nursing, 12*(S), S26-S29. doi:10.1016/j.ecns.2016.09.009

Jeffries, P. R. (Ed.). (2012). *Simulation in nursing education, from conceptualization to evaluation* (2nd ed.). New York, NY: National League for Nursing.

Kardong-Edgren, S., Farra, S. L., Alinier, G., & Young, H. M. (2019). A call to unify definitions of virtual reality. *Clinical Simulation in Nursing, 31*, 28–34.

Kopp, W., & Hanson, M. A. (2012). High-fidelity and gaming simulations enhance nursing education in end-of-life care. *Clinical Simulation in Nursing, 8*(3), e97–e102. doi:10.1016/j.ecns.2010.07.005

LeFlore, J. L., Anderson, M., Zielke, M. A., Nelson, K. A., Thomas, P. E., Hardee, G., & John, L. D. (2012). Can a virtual patient trainer teach student nurses how to save lives—Teaching nursing students about pediatric respiratory diseases. *Simulation in Healthcare, 7*(1), 10–17. doi:10.1097/SIH.0b013e31823652de

National Council of State Boards of Nursing. (2014). *The NCSBN national simulation study.* Retrieved from https://www.ncsbn.org/jnr_simulation_supplement.pdf

National League for Nursing & Wolters Kluwer. (2016). *Educator forecast for tech usage and growth in nursing education programs.* Retrieved from http://nursingeducation.lww.com/content/dam/wk-nes/documents/Educator-Forecast-Tech-Usage.pdf

The National Task Force on Quality Nurse Practitioner Education. (2016). *Criteria for evaluation of nurse practitioner programs* (5th ed.). Retrieved from https://www.nonpf.org/page/15

Nye, C., Campbell, S. H., Hebert, S. H., Short, C., & Thomas, M. (2019). Simulation in advanced practice nursing programs: A North-American survey. *Clinical Simulation in Nursing, 26*, 3-10. doi:10.1016/j.ecns.2018.09.005

Peddle, M. (2011). Simulation gaming in nurse education: Entertainment or learning? *Nurse Education Today, 31*(7), 647-649. doi:10.1016/j.nedt.2010.12.009

Prensky, M. (2001). Digital natives, digital immigrants part 1. *On the Horizon, 9*(5), 1–6. doi:10.1108/10748120110424816

Rutherford-Hemming, T., Nye, C., & Coran, C. (2016). Using simulation for clinical practice hours in nurse practitioner education in the United States: A systematic review. *Nurse Education Today, 37*, 128–135. doi:10.1016/j.nedt.2015.11.006

Saxena, N., Kyaw, B. M., Vseteckova, J., Dev, P., Paul, P., Lim, K., ... Car, J. (2018). Virtual reality environments for health professional education. *The Cochrane Database of Systematic Reviews, 2018*(10), CD012090. doi:10.1002/14651858.CD012090.pub2

Society for Simulation in Healthcare. (2013). *Accreditation.* Wheaton, IL: Author. Retrieved from ssih.org/accreditation

Society for Simulation in Healthcare. (2019). *SSH certified healthcare simulation educator handbook.* Wheaton, IL: Author.

Squire, K. D. (2006). From content to context: Videogames as designed experience. *Educational Researcher, 35*(8), 19–29.

Tagliareni, E., & Forneris. S. (2016). Sim beyond the sim lab. Lippincott Nursing Education. Retrieved from http://nursingeducation.lww.com/free-resources/resources/white-papers/sim-beyond-the-sim-lab.html

Ugidos Lozano, M. T., Blaya Haro, F., Ruggiero, A., Manzoor, S., & Juanes Mendez, J. A. (2019). Evaluation of the applicability of 3D modes as perceived by the students of health science. *Journal of Medical Systems, 43*(5), 1–6. doi:10.1007/s10916-019-1238-0

Verkuyl, M., Lapnum, J., Hughes, M., McCulloch, P., Romaniuk, D., & Betts, L. (2018). Virtual gaming simulation: Exploring self-debriefing, virtual debriefing, and in-person debriefing. *Clinical Simulation in Nursing, 20*, 7–14.

Wendling, A., Halan, S., Tighe, P., Le, L., Euliano, T., & Lok, B. (2011). Virtual humans versus standardized patients: Which leads residents to more correct diagnosis? *Academic Medicine, 86*(3), 384–388.

Index

A

D